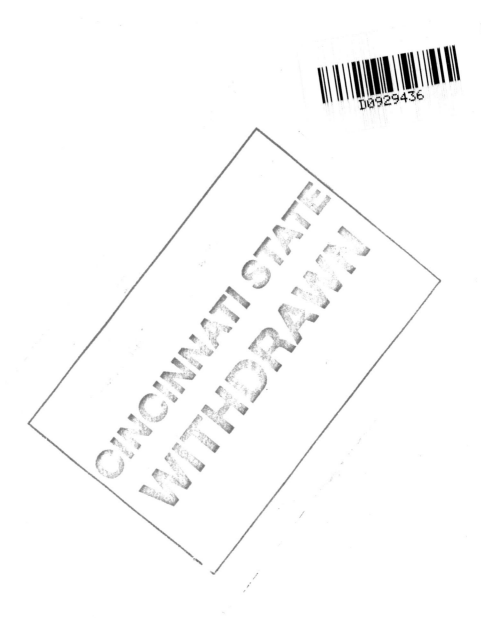

Clinical Anatomy
of the Visual System

Clinical Anatomy
of the Visual System

Lee Ann Remington, O.D., M.S.
Associate Professor of Optometry, Pacific University College of
Optometry, Forest Grove, Oregon

With a contribution by

Eileen C. McGill, B.A., O.D., F.A.A.O.
Senior Optometrist, Department of Veterans Affairs, Ralph H. Johnson
Medical Center, Charleston, South Carolina

Butterworth–Heinemann
Boston   Oxford   Johannesburg   Melbourne   New Delhi   Singapore

Every effort has been made to ensure that the drug dosage schedules within this text are accurate and conform to standards accepted at time of publication. However, as treatment recommendations vary in the light of continuing research and clinical experience, the reader is advised to verify drug dosage schedules herein with information found on product information sheets. This is especially true in cases of new or infrequently used drugs.

 Recognizing the importance of preserving what has been written, Butterworth–Heinemann prints its books on acid-free paper whenever possible.

 Butterworth–Heinemann supports the efforts of American Forests and the Global ReLeaf program in its campaign for the betterment of trees, forests, and our environment.

Library of Congress Cataloging-in-Publication Data

Remington, Lee Ann.
    Clinical anatomy of the visual system / Lee Ann Remington ; with a contribution by Eileen C. McGill.
        p.   cm.
    Includes bibliographical references and index.
    ISBN 0-7506-9558-7 (alk. paper)
    1. Eye--Anatomy. 2. Eye--Histology. 3. Adnexa oculi--Anatomy.
4. Adnexa oculi--Histology. I. McGill, Eileen C.   II. Title.
    [DNLM: 1. Eye--anatomy & histology.   WW 101 R388c 1997]
QM511.R45   1997
611'.84--dc21
DNLM/DLC
for Library of Congress   97-16054
                                                                CIP

British Library Cataloguing-in-Publication Data
A catalogue record for this book is available from the British Library.

The publisher offers discounts on bulk orders of this book.
For information, please contact:

Manager of Special Sales
Butterworth–Heinemann
313 Washington Street
Newton, MA 02158-1626
Tel: 617-928-2500
Fax: 617-928-2620

For information on all B–H publications available, contact our World Wide Web home page at http://www.bh.com

10 9 8 7 6 5 4 3 2 1

Printed in the United States of America

To Dan for his encouragement, understanding, and love

Contents

Preface

Clinical Anatomy of the Visual System was written to provide the optometry and ophthalmology student and clinician a single text that describes the embryology, anatomy, histology, blood supply, and innervation of the globe and ocular adnexa. The pupillary and visual pathways are covered as well.

In the format used in the text, terms and names of structures are noted in bold print when they are first described or explained. The name for a structure that is more commonly used will be presented first, followed by other terms by which that structure is also known. Current nomenclature is moving away from using proper nouns to identify structures and toward a more descriptive name, but that is not always the case.

Clinical comments are included to emphasize that the knowledge of structure is a foundation for recognizing and understanding clinical situations, conditions, diseases, and treatments.

The basis of this text grew from lecture and class notes prepared for students in the Ocular Anatomy and Visual Anatomy classes that I have taught for the last 10 years at Pacific University College of Optometry. I express my gratitude to those students who questioned and corrected and suggested, adding to the usefulness of those notes and eventually this text. Information gathered from historic and current literature is well documented.

My professional colleague Eileen McGill, O.D., contributed her expertise by writing the chapter on the lens; her efforts are greatly appreciated.

My colleague, advisor, and friend Jack Roggenkamp, O.D., gave many hours of his time to edit my work. He read drafts that were at times difficult to wade through and gave valuable advice on the proper usage of vocabulary and punctuation. It would have taken me considerably longer to complete the manuscript without his assistance and encouragement, and I express my wholehearted thanks to him.

The illustrator of most of the original line drawings is a former student, Tracey Asmus-Janetsky, O.D. She spent many hours working with me to ensure that the drawings were accurate. I thank her for her talented contributions.

My thanks also to two of my former students and friends, Michele Bither, O.D., and Kathy Milano, O.D. They read many of the chapters and gave useful insight from the standpoint of the student, reminding me to stay relevant and be very clear in what I was saying.

I thank my children, Tracy and Ryan, for their encouragement and my husband, Dan, for his patience, encouragement, and loving support during the seemingly endless preparation of this manuscript.

I am grateful to Barbara Murphy and Karen Oberheim of Butterworth–Heinemann and Jane Bangley McQueen of Silverchair Science + Communications, Inc., for their guidance throughout this process.

Lee Ann Remington

Clinical Anatomy
of the Visual System

The Visual System

The visual system takes in information from the environment in the form of light and analyzes and interprets it. This process of sight and visual perception involves a complex system of structures, each of which is designed for a specific purpose. The organization of each structure enables it to perform its intended function. The eye houses the elements that take in light rays and change them to a neural signal; it is protected by its location within the bone and connective-tissue framework of the orbit. The eyelids cover and protect the anterior surface of the eye and contain glands that produce the lubricating tear film. Muscles, attached to the outer coat of the eye, control and direct the globe's movement, and the muscles of both eyes are coordinated to provide binocular vision. A network of blood vessels supplies nutrients, and a complex system of nerves provides sensory and motor innervation to the eye and surrounding tissues and structures. The neural signal that carries visual information passes through a complex and intricately designed pathway within the central nervous system, enabling an accurate view of the surrounding environment. This information, evaluated by a process called **visual perception,** influences myriad decisions and activities. This book examines the macroscopic and microscopic anatomy of the components in this complex system and the structures that support it.

THE EYE
Anatomic Features

The eye is a special sense organ made up of three coats or tunics: (1) The outer fibrous layer of connective tissue forms the cornea and sclera; (2) the middle vascular layer is composed of the iris, ciliary body, and choroid; and (3) the inner neural layer is the retina. Within this globe are three spaces: the anterior chamber, the posterior chamber, and the vitreous chamber. The crystalline lens is located in the region of the posterior chamber (Figure 1-1).

The outer dense connective tissue of the eye provides protection for the structures within and maintains the globe's shape, providing resistance to the pressure of the fluids inside. The sclera is the opaque white of the eye. The transparent cornea allows light rays to enter the globe and, by refraction, helps bring these light rays into focus on the retina.

The vascular layer of the eye is the uvea, which is made up of three structures, each having a separate function, though all are connected to one another. Some of the histologic layers are continuous throughout all three structures and are derived from the same embryonic germ-cell layer. The iris is the most anterior structure, and it acts as a diaphragm to regulate the amount of light entering the pupil. The two iris muscles control the shape and diameter of the pupil and are supplied by the autonomic nervous system.

Continuous with the iris at its root is the ciliary body, which produces the components of the aqueous humor and contains the muscle that controls the shape of the lens. The posterior part of the uvea, the choroid, is an anastomosing network of blood vessels with a dense capillary network; it surrounds the retina and supplies nutrients to the outer retinal layers.

The retinal neural tissue, by very complex biochemical processes, changes light energy into a signal that can be transmitted along a neural pathway. The signal passes through the retina, exits the eye via the optic nerve, and is transmitted to various parts of the brain for processing.

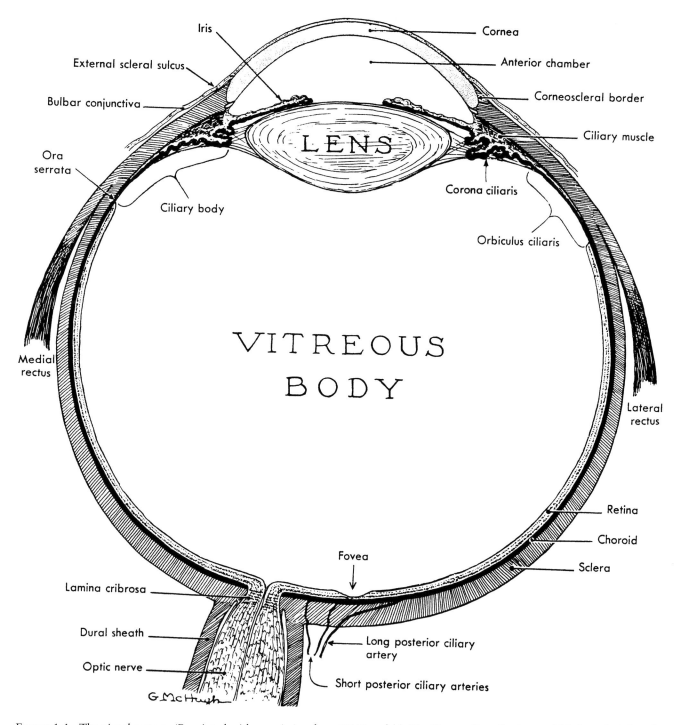

FIGURE 1-1. The visual system. (Reprinted with permission from PC Kronfeld. The Human Eye. Rochester, NY: Bausch & Lomb Press, 1943;5. Copyright Bausch & Lomb.)

The interior of the eye is made up of three chambers. The anterior chamber is bounded in front by the cornea and posteriorly by the iris and anterior surface of the lens. The posterior chamber lies behind the iris and surrounds the equator of the lens, separating it from the ciliary body. The anterior and posterior chambers are continuous with one another through the pupil, and both contain aqueous humor produced by the ciliary body. The aqueous humor provides nourishment for the surrounding structures, particularly the cornea and lens. The vitreous chamber, which is the largest space, lies adjacent to the inner retinal layer and is bounded in front by the lens. This chamber contains a gel-like substance, the vitreous humor.

The crystalline lens is located in the area of the posterior chamber and provides additional refractive power for accurately focusing images onto the retina. The lens must change shape to view an object that is close to the eye; it does this via the mechanism called **accommodation**.

Anatomic Directions and Planes

Anatomy is a very exacting science and specific terminology is basic to its discussion. The following anatomic directions should be familiar (Figure 1-2):

- anterior or ventral: toward the front
- posterior or dorsal: toward the back
- superior or cranial: toward the head
- inferior or caudal: away from the head
- medial: toward the midline
- lateral: away from the midline
- proximal: near the point of origin
- distal: away from the point of origin

The following planes are used in describing anatomic structures (Figure 1-3):

- sagittal: vertical plane running from anterior to posterior locations, dividing the structure into right and left sides
- midsagittal plane: sagittal plane through the midline, dividing the structure into right and left halves
- coronal or frontal: vertical plane running from side to side, dividing the structure into anterior and posterior parts
- transverse: horizontal plane dividing the structure into superior and inferior parts

Because the globe is a spherical structure, references to locations can sometimes be confusing. The following should be kept in mind: In references to anterior and posterior locations of the globe, the anterior pole (i.e., the center of the cornea) is the reference point. For example, the pupil is anterior to the ciliary body (see Figure 1-1). When layers or structures are referred to as **inner** or **outer**, the reference is to the entire globe unless specified otherwise. The point of reference is the center of the globe, which would lie within the vitreous. For example, the retina is inner to the sclera (see Figure 1-1). In addition, the term **sclerad** is used to mean "toward the sclera" and **vitread** is used to mean "toward the vitreous."

Refractive Conditions

If the refractive power of the optical components of the eye (primarily the cornea and lens) correlate with the distances between the cornea, lens, and retina so that incoming parallel light rays come into focus on the retina, a clear image will be seen. This condition is called **emmetropia**. No correction is necessary for clear distance

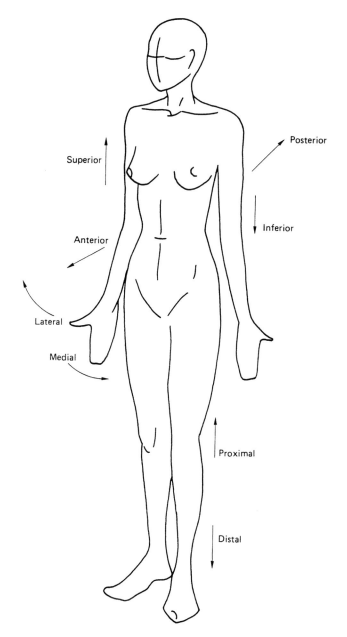

FIGURE 1-2. Anatomic directions. (Reprinted with permission from N Palastanga, D Field, R Soames. Anatomy and Human Movement. Oxford, England: Butterworth–Heinemann, 1989;3.)

vision. In **myopia (near-sightedness)**, because the lens and cornea are too strong or, more likely, the eyeball is too long, parallel light rays are brought into focus in front of the retina. Myopia can be corrected by placing a concave lens in front of the eye, causing the incoming light rays to diverge. In **hyperopia (far-sightedness)**, the distance from the cornea to the retina is too short for the refractive power of the cornea and lens, thereby causing images to come into focus behind the retina. Hyperopia can be corrected by placing a convex lens in front of the eye to

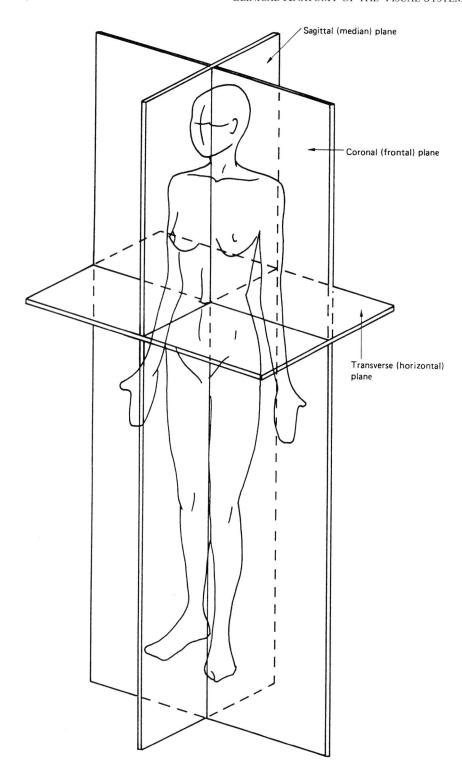

Sagittal (median) plane

Coronal (frontal) plane

Transverse (horizontal) plane

FIGURE 1-3. Anatomic planes. (Reprinted with permission from N Palastanga, D Field, R Soames. Anatomy and Human Movement. Oxford, England: Butterworth–Heinemann, 1989;5.)

increase the convergence of the incoming light rays. Figure 1.4 illustrates these conditions.

OPHTHALMIC INSTRUMENTATION

Various instruments are used to assess the health and function of elements of the visual pathway and its supporting structures. The following is a very brief descrip-

tion of some of these instruments and the structures that can be examined with them.

The curvature of the cornea is one of the factors that determines the cornea's refractive power. A keratometer measures the curvature of the central 3–4 mm of the anterior corneal surface and provides information on the power and toricity at that location. The smoothness of the corneal surface can also be assessed by the pattern reflected from the cornea during the measuring process.

The inside of the eye, called the **fundus**, is examined using an ophthalmoscope, which illuminates the interior with a bright light. The retina, optic nerve head, and blood vessels can be assessed, and information about ocular and systemic health can be obtained. Only here in the body can blood vessels be viewed directly and noninvasively. Various systemic diseases, such as diabetes, hypertension, and arteriosclerosis, can alter ocular vessels. To obtain a more complete view of the inside of the eye, the doctor can instill drugs that will influence the iris muscles, causing the pupil to become enlarged or mydriatic.

The outside of the globe and the eyelids can be assessed with a biomicroscope. This combination of an illumination system and a binocular microscope allows stereoscopic views of various parts of the eye. Particularly beneficial is the view that can be obtained of the transparent structures, such as the cornea and lens. A number of auxiliary instruments can be used with the biomicroscope to measure intraocular pressure and to view the interior of the eye.

The doctor can determine the optical power of the eye with a set of lenses and a retinoscope. This instrument is beneficial also for assessing the accommodative function of the lens.

The visual field is the area that a person sees as he or she looks straight ahead, including those areas seen "out of the corner of the eye." A perimeter is used to test the extent, sensitivity, and completeness of this visual field. Computerized perimeters give very detailed maps of the visual field.

BASIC HISTOLOGIC FEATURES

Because many of the anatomic structures are discussed in this book at the histologic level, included here is a brief review of basic human histology. Other details of tissues are addressed in Chapters 2–7, 9, and 10.

All body structures are made up of one or more of the four basic tissues: epithelial, connective, muscle, and nervous tissue. A tissue is defined as a collection of similar cells that are specialized to perform a common function.

Epithelial Tissue

Epithelial tissue often takes the form of sheets of epithelial cells that either cover the external surface of a structure or line a cavity. The epithelial cells lie on a basement membrane that attaches them to underlying connective tissue. The basement membrane can be divided into two parts: the **basal lamina**, secreted by the epithelial cell; and the **reticular lamina**, a product of the connective-tissue layer.[1] The free surface of the epithelial cell is the apical surface, whereas the surface that

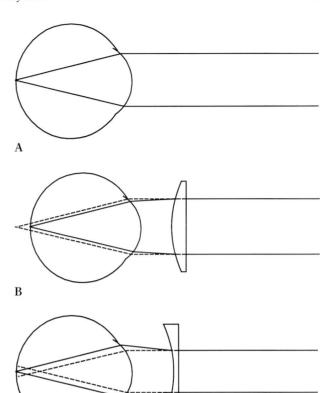

FIGURE 1-4. Refractive conditions. (A) Emmetropia, in which parallel light comes to a focus on the retina. (B) Hyperopia, in which parallel light comes to a focus behind the retina (shown by dotted lines). A convex lens is used to correct the condition and bring the light rays into focus on the retina. (C) Myopia, in which parallel light comes to a focus in front of retina (shown by dotted lines). A concave lens is used to correct the condition and bring the light rays into focus on the retina. (Courtesy of Dr. Karl Citek, Pacific University, Forest Grove, OR.)

faces underlying tissue or rests on the basement membrane is the basal surface.

Epithelial cells are classified according to shape. Squamous cells are flat and platelike, cuboidal cells are of equal height and width, and columnar cells are higher than they are wide. Epithelium consisting of a single layer of cells is referred to as simple—simple squamous, simple cuboidal, or simple columnar. Endothelium is the special name given to the simple squamous layer that lines certain cavities. Epithelium consisting of several layers is referred to as **stratified** and is described by the shape of the surface layer of cells. Only the basal or deepest layer of cells is in contact with the basement membrane, and that layer usually consists of columnar cells.

Keratinized, stratified, squamous epithelium has a surface layer of squamous cells whose cytoplasm has

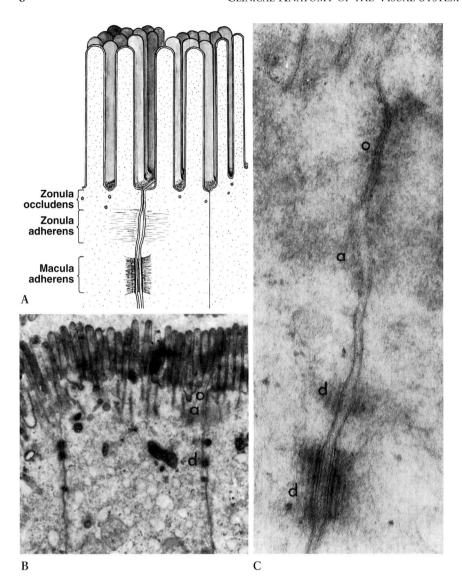

Zonula
occludens

Zonula
adherens

Macula
adherens

A

B

C

FIGURE 1-5. Junctional complex. (A) Appearance on electron microscopy of the apical cell interface between two epithelial cells with microvilli on the apical surfaces. (B) Electron micrograph shows the apical portion of one such cell (×18,000). (C) Electron micrograph shows the features of the junctional complex at high magnification (×105,000). (o = zonula occludens; a = zonula adherens; d = macula adherens or desmosome.) (Reprinted with permission from CR Leeson, ST Leeson. Histology. Philadelphia: Saunders, 1976;103.)

been transformed into a substance called **keratin**, a tough protective material that is relatively resistant to mechanical injury, bacterial invasion, and water loss. These keratinized surface cells constantly are sloughed off and are replaced from the layers below, where cell division takes place.

Glandular Epithelium

Many epithelial cells are adapted for secretion and, when gathered into groups, are referred to as **glands**. Glands can be classified according to the mechanism of secretion—exocrine glands secrete into a duct, whereas endocrine glands secrete directly into the bloodstream—or to the nature of their secretion—mucous, serous, or sebaceous. Holocrine gland secretions are composed of complete cells laden with the secretory material; apocrine glands secrete part of the cell cytoplasm in the secretion; and the secretion of merocrine glands is a product of the cell without loss of any cellular components.

Intercellular Junctions

Various intercellular junctions join epithelial cells to one another and to adjacent tissue. In a tight, or occluding, junction, the outer leaflet of the cell membrane of one cell comes into direct contact with its neighbor. These points of apposition are actually points along ridgelike elevations that fuse with complementary ridges on the surface of the neighboring cell.[2]

A tight junction that forms a zone or belt around the entire cell and joins it with each of the adjacent cells is called a **zonula occludens** (Figure 1-5). In these zones, there may be row on row of intertwining ridges that effectively occlude the intercellular space. For a substance to pass through a sheet of epithelium whose cells are joined by a zonula occludens, the substance must pass through the cell itself; it cannot pass between cells via the intercellular space. In some instances, ridges are fewer and are discontinuous, resulting in a so-called **leaky epithelium**.[2]

A **zonula adherens**, an intermediate junction, is a similar adhesion zone. However, the adjacent plasma membranes are separated by a narrow intercellular space that contains some mucoprotein-adhesive material. Adjacent to the adhering junction are fine microfilaments that extend from the membrane into the cytoplasm.[2] These produce relatively firm adhesion. A **terminal bar** consists of a zonula occludens and a zonula adherens side by side, with the tight junction lying nearest the cell apex.[1, 2]

Round, buttonlike intercellular junctions have been called **macula occludens** or **macula adherens**, depending on the type of adhesion.

A **desmosome** is a strong, spotlike attachment between cells. A dense plaque is present within the plasma membrane at the site of the adherence, and hairpin loops of cytoplasmic filaments called **tonofilaments** extend from the plaque into the cytoplasm. The intercellular space contains an acid-rich mucoprotein that acts as a strong adhesive.[2] A **hemidesmosome** attaches an epithelial cell to its basement membrane and the underlying connective tissue (see Figure 1-5). Bundles of filaments pass through the cell membrane and the adhesive joining the intracellular plaque to the underlying connective tissue.

A **gap junction**, or **communicating junction**, is macular in shape. The cells are separated by a thin, intercellular space through which small channels or pores pass, joining the cytoplasm of the two cells. These junctions allow for intercellular communication and exchange of ions from one cell to the next.[1, 2]

Connective Tissue

Connective tissue provides structure and support and is a "space-filler" for areas not occupied by other tissue. Connective tissue consists of cells, fibers, and ground substance. Ground substance and fibers collectively are called **matrix**. Connective tissue can be classified as loose or dense. Loose connective tissue has relatively fewer cells and fibers per area than does dense connective tissue, in which the cells and fibers are tightly packed. Dense connective tissue can be characterized as regular or irregular on the basis of fiber arrangement.

Among the cells that may be found in connective tissue are fibroblasts (flattened cells that produce and maintain the fibers and ground substance), macrophages (phagocytic cells), mast cells (which contain heparin and histamine), and fat cells. Connective tissue composed primarily of fat cells is called **adipose tissue**.

The fibers found in connective tissue include flexible collagen fibers with high tensile strength, delicate reticular fibers, and elastic fibers, which can undergo extensive stretching. Collagen fibers are a major component of much of the eye's connective tissue. These fibers are composed of protein macromolecules of tropocollagen having a coiled helix of three polypeptide chains. The individual polypeptide chains can differ in their amino acid sequences, and the tropocollagen has a banded pattern due to the sequence differences.[3] Collagen is separated into various types on the basis of such differences, and several types are components of ocular connective-tissue structures.

The amorphous ground substance, in which the cells and fibers are embedded, consists of water bound to glycosaminoglycans and long-chain carbohydrates.

Muscle Tissue

Muscle tissue is contractile tissue and can be classified as striated or smooth, voluntary or involuntary. Striated muscle has a regular pattern of light and dark bands and is subdivided into skeletal and cardiac muscle. Skeletal muscle is under voluntary control, whereas cardiac muscle is controlled involuntarily. The structure of skeletal muscle and the mechanism of its contraction are discussed in Chapter 10.

The smooth-muscle fiber is an elongated, slender cell with a single centrally located nucleus. The tissue is under the involuntary control of the autonomic nervous system.

Nervous Tissue

Nervous tissue contains two types of cells: neurons, which are cells specialized to react to a stimulus and conduct a nerve impulse; and neuroglia, which are cells that provide structure and metabolic support. The neuron cell body is the perikaryon, and it has several cytoplasmic projections. Those projections that conduct impulses *to* the cell body are dendrites (there usually are several), and the (usually single) projection that conducts impulses *away from* the cell body is an axon. These nerve fibers are either myelinated (enclosed in a lipoprotein material called **myelin**) or are unmyelinated; myelinization improves impulse conduction speed.[4] Both myelinated and unmyelinated fibers are surrounded by Schwann cell cytoplasm, and it is the Schwann cell that produces the myelin.

A nerve impulse passes between nerves at a specialized junction—the synapse. As the action potential reaches the presynaptic membrane of an axon, a neurotransmitter is released into the synaptic gap, influencing a response in the postsynaptic membrane. This response might be excitatory or inhibitory.

Neuroglial cells are more numerous than are neurons, outnumbering them by as much as 10–50 to 1, depending on location.[4] Neuroglial cells include astrocytes, oligodendrocytes, and microglia. Astrocytes provide a framework that gives structural support and contributes to the nutrition of neurons. Oligodendrocytes produce myelin in the central nervous system, where there are no Schwann cells. Microglia possess phagocytic properties and increase in number in areas of damage or disease.[4]

REFERENCES

1. Krause WJ, Cutts JH. Epithelium. In WJ Krause, JH Cutts (eds), Concise Text of Histology. Baltimore: Williams & Wilkins, 1981;27.

2. Copenhaver WM, Kelly DE, Wood RL. Epithelium. In WM Copenhaver, DE Kelly, RL Wood (eds), Bailey's Textbook of Histology (17th ed). Baltimore: Williams & Wilkins, 1978;103.

3. Copenhaver WM, Kelly DE, Wood RL. The Connective Tissues. In WM Copenhaver, DE Kelly, RL Wood (eds), Bailey's Textbook of Histology (17th ed). Baltimore: Williams & Wilkins, 1978;142.

4. Krause WJ, Cutts JH. Nervous Tissue. In WJ Krause, JH Cutts (eds), Concise Text of Histology. Baltimore: Williams & Wilkins, 1981;137.

The Cornea and Sclera

The outer connective-tissue coat of the eye has the appearance of two joined spheres. The smaller, anterior transparent sphere is the cornea and has a radius of curvature of approximately 8 mm. The larger, posterior opaque sphere is the sclera, which has a radius of approximately 12 mm (Figure 2-1A). The globe is not symmetric; its approximate diameters are 24 mm antero-posterior, 23 mm vertical, and 23.5 mm horizontal.[1]

CORNEA

Corneal Dimensions

All values given here are approximations. The transparent cornea appears, from the front, to be oval, as the sclera encroaches on the superior and inferior aspects. The anterior horizontal diameter is 12 mm, and the anterior vertical diameter is 11 mm.[1, 2] If viewed from behind, the cornea appears circular, with horizontal and vertical diameters of 11.7 mm (Figure 2-1B).[1, 3]

In profile, the cornea has an elliptic rather than a spheric shape, the curvature being steeper in the center and flatter near the periphery. The radius of curvature of the central cornea at the anterior surface is 7.8 mm and at the posterior surface is 6.5 mm.[1, 4] The central corneal thickness is 0.53 mm, whereas the corneal periphery is 0.71 mm thick (Figure 2-1C).[1, 4–6]

✍️ CLINICAL COMMENT: ASTIGMATISM

Astigmatism is a condition in which light rays coming from a point source are not imaged as a point. This is due to the unequal refraction of light by different meridians of the refracting elements. Since

the cornea is usually elliptic in profile, it contributes to astigmatism in the eye as it refracts light and helps to focus the rays onto the retina. The central optical area of the cornea (i.e., the central 3–4 mm) can be assessed by keratometric measurement to give a clinical assessment of the corneal contribution to astigmatism.

Regular astigmatism occurs when the longest radius of curvature and shortest radius of curvature lie 90 degrees apart. The usual corneal toricity occurs when the radius of curvature of the vertical meridian differs from that of the horizontal meridian. The most common situation, called with-the-rule astigmatism, occurs when the steepest curvature lies in the vertical meridian. Thus, the vertical meridian has the shortest radius of curvature. Against-the-rule astigmatism is not as common and occurs when the horizontal meridian is the steepest; the greatest refractive power is found in the horizontal meridian. If the meridians that contain the greatest differences are not along the 180- and 90-degree axes (± 30 degrees) but lie along the 45- and 135-degree axes (± 15 degrees), the astigmatism is called oblique. Irregular astigmatism is an uncommon finding in which the meridians corresponding to the greatest differences are not 90 degrees apart.

In addition to the cornea, the lens is a refractive element that focuses light rays and might contribute to astigmatism. In fact, the tendency of with-the-rule astigmatism to convert to against-the-rule astigmatism with aging is attributable primarily to the lens, which continues to grow throughout life.

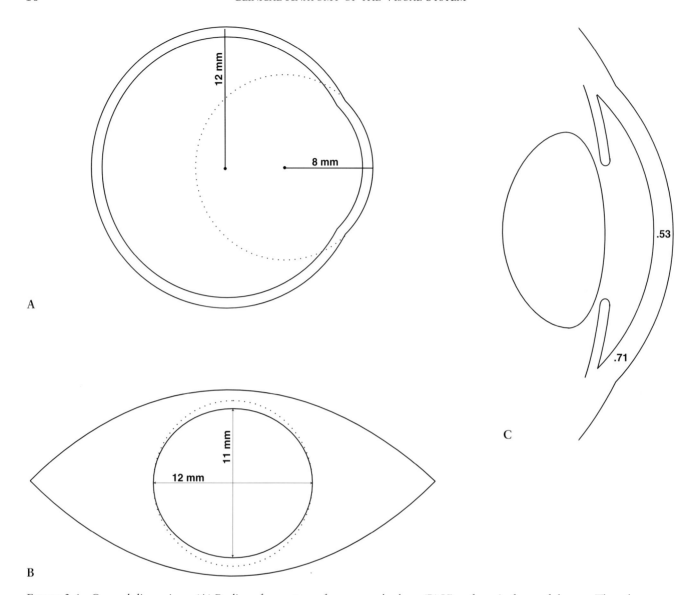

FIGURE 2-1. Corneal dimensions. (A) Radius of curvature of cornea and sclera. (B) View from in front of the eye. The sclera encroaches on the corneal periphery inferiorly and superiorly. Dotted lines show the extent of the cornea in the vertical dimension posteriorly. (C) Sagittal section of cornea showing central and peripheral thickness.

Corneal Histologic Features

The cornea is the principal refracting component of the eye. Its transparency and avascularity provide optimum light transmittance. The anterior surface of the cornea is covered by the tear film, and the posterior surface borders the aqueous-filled anterior chamber. At its periphery, the cornea is continuous with the conjunctiva and the sclera. From anterior to posterior, the five layers that compose the cornea are epithelium, Bowman's layer, stroma, Descemet's membrane, and endothelium (Figure 2-2).

Epithelium

The outermost layer of **stratified corneal epithelium** is five to six cells thick and measures approximately 50 µm.[1, 7]

The epithelium thickens in the periphery and is continuous with the conjunctival epithelium at the limbus.

The surface layer of corneal epithelium is two cells thick and displays a very smooth anterior surface. It consists of nonkeratinized squamous cells, each of which contains a flattened nucleus and fewer cellular organelles than do deeper cells. The plasma membrane of the surface epithelial cells is believed to secrete a glycocalyx component that adjoins the mucin layer of the tear film, changing a relatively hydrophobic surface to a hydrophilic surface. Many projections located on the apical surface of the outermost cells increase the surface area, thus enhancing the stability of the tear film. The finger-like projections are **microvilli,** and the ridgelike ones are **microplicae** (Figure 2-3).

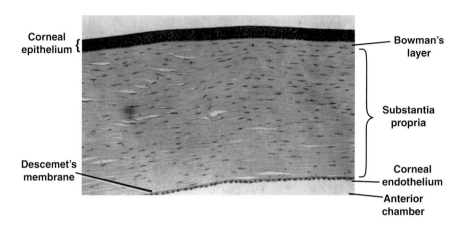

Corneal epithelium {

Bowman's layer

Substantia propria

Descemet's membrane

Corneal endothelium

Anterior chamber

FIGURE 2-2. Cornea (×100). (Reprinted with permission from WJ Krause, JH Cutts. Concise Text of Histology. Baltimore: Williams & Wilkins, 1981;175.)

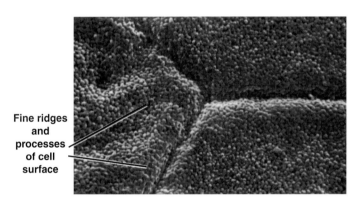

Fine ridges and processes of cell surface

FIGURE 2-3. Cornea: Junction of three superficial cells (scanning electron microscopy, ×5,000). (Reprinted with permission from WJ Krause, JH Cutts. Concise Text of Histology. Baltimore: Williams & Wilkins, 1981;175.)

Tight junctions (zonula occludens) join the surface cells along their lateral walls, near the apical surface. These junctures provide a barrier to intercellular movement of substances from the tear layer and prevent the uptake of excess fluid from the tear film. A highly effective, semipermeable membrane, which allows passage of fluid and molecules *through* the cells but not between them, is produced. Additional adhesion between the cells is provided by numerous desmosomes.

As the surface cells age, they lose their attachments and are sloughed off, being constantly replaced from the layers below. On scanning electron microscopy, the corneal surface is seen to consist of variously sized cells, ranging from small to large. The smaller, lighter cells are newer replacement cells, whereas the larger, darker cells are those that soon will be sloughed off.[8] The middle layer of the corneal epithelium is made up of two to three layers of wing cells, which are polyhedral and have convex anterior surfaces and concave posterior surfaces that fit over the basal cells (Figure 2-4). The name by which these cells commonly are called originates from the cells' winglike lateral processes. Desmosomes and gap junctions join wing cells to each other, and desmosomes join wing cells to surface and basal cells.

The innermost basal cell layer is a single layer of columnar cells (see Figures 2-4 and 2-5), which contain oval-shaped nuclei displaced toward the apex and oriented at right angles to the surface. The rounded, apical surface of each cell lies adjacent to the wing cells, and the basal surface attaches to the underlying basement membrane (basal lamina). The basal cells secrete this basement membrane, which attaches the cells to the underlying tissue via hemidesmosomes. Anchoring fibrils pass from these junctions through Bowman's layer into the stroma.[9] Desmosomes and gap junctions join the columnar cells (they are less numerous here than in the wing cell layer); interdigitations and desmosomes connect the basal cells with the adjacent layer of wing cells. The basal layer is the germinal layer where mitosis occurs.

The basal cells are joined to the basement membrane by hemidesmosomes. Opposite the plaque, fine anchoring fibrils form a complex branching and anastomosing network that runs from the basement membrane through Bowman's layer and penetrates the stroma approximately 1.5–2.0 μm.[9–14] The linkage between the hemidesmosome and the anchoring network is likely composed of basement membrane components.[5] The anchoring fibrils attach to anchoring plaques of extracellular matrix within the stroma.[12, 15]

Epithelial Replacement

Maintenance of the smooth corneal surface depends on replacement of the surface cells that constantly are being shed into the tear film. Cell proliferation occurs in the

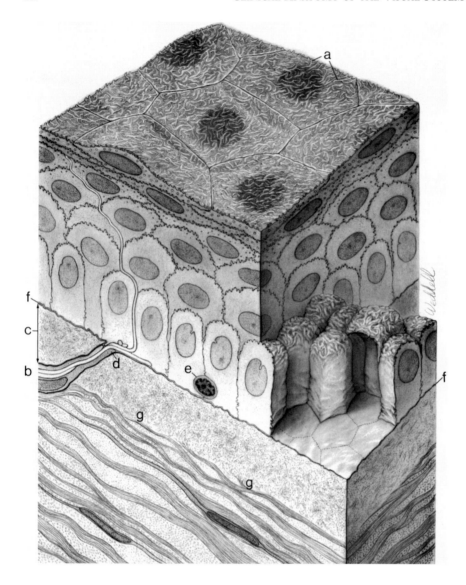

FIGURE 2-4. Three-dimensional drawing of corneal epithelium, in which the five layers of cells are evident. The polygonal shape of the basal and surface cells and their relative size are apparent. The wing cell processes fill the spaces formed by the dome-shaped apical surface of the basal cells. The turnover time for these cells is 7 days and, during this time, the columnar basal cell gradually is transformed into a wing cell and then into a thin, flat surface cell. During this transition, the cytoplasm changes and the Golgi apparatus becomes more prominent. Numerous vesicles develop in the superficial wing and surface layers, and glycogen appears in the surface cells. The intercellular space separating the outermost surface cells is closed by a zonula occludens, forming a barrier that prevents passage of the precorneal tear film into the corneal stroma. The cell surface shows an extensive net of microplicae (a) and microvilli that might be involved in the retention of the precorneal film. A corneal nerve (b) passes through Bowman's layer (c); the nerve loses its Schwann cell sheath near the basement membrane (d) of the basal epithelium. It then passes as a naked nerve between the epithelial cells toward the superficial layers. A lymphocyte (e) is seen between two basal epithelial cells. The basement membrane is seen at f. Some of the most superficial corneal stromal lamellae (g) are seen curving forward to merge with Bowman's layer. The regular arrangement of the corneal stromal collagen differs from the random disposition of that in Bowman's layer. (Reprinted with permission from MJ Hogan, JA Alvarado, JE Weddell. Histology of the Human Eye. Philadelphia: Saunders, 1971;84.)

basal layer, basal cells move up to become wing cells, and wing cells move up to become surface cells. Stem cells located in a 0.5- to 1.0-mm–wide band around the corneal periphery are the source for renewal of the corneal basal cell layer. A slow migration of basal cells occurs from the periphery toward the center of the cornea.[16, 17] Turnover time for the entire corneal epithelium is approximately 7 days, more rapid than for other epithelial tissues.[18, 19] Repair to corneal epithelial tissue proceeds quickly; minor abrasions heal within hours, and larger ones often heal overnight. However, if the basement membrane is damaged, complete healing with replacement basement membrane and hemidesmosomes can take months.[10, 11]

Despite the fact that cells constantly are being sloughed, the barrier function is maintained as the cell below moves into position to replace the one that has been shed. Tight junctions are present exclusively

FIGURE 2-5. Corneal epithelium. Light micrograph shows columnar basal cells, wing cells, and squamous surface cells of cornea. Bowman's layer and anterior stroma are also evident. (Courtesy of Patrick Caroline, Oregon Health Sciences University, Portland, OR.)

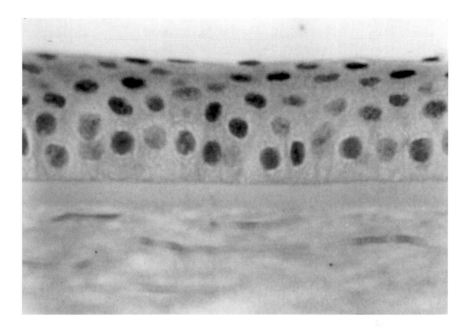

between the squamous cells that occupy the superficial position. The protein components necessary to form these junctions are not present in the basal cells but are increasingly present as the cells move up to the surface.[20]

The basal cell layer constantly is losing and reestablishing the hemidesmosome junctions as cells divide and move up into the wing cell layer. The plaque sites remain in the stroma for reattachment.[11]

✍ CLINICAL COMMENT: RECURRENT CORNEAL EROSION

Recurrent corneal erosion is a condition in which the corneal epithelium sloughs off either continually or periodically. This condition may occur because of either poor attachment between the epithelium and its basement membrane or poor attachment between the basement membrane and the underlying tissue. One cause of erosion is epithelial basement membrane dystrophy stemming from defective nutrition or metabolism.[5]

Age-related changes also can play a role in recurrent corneal erosion. Epithelium continues to secrete basement membrane throughout life; in the corneal epithelium, the thickness of the basement membrane doubles by 60 years of age. In addition, areas of reduplication of the membrane can occur with aging.[21] As the basement membrane thickens or as reduplication occurs, the thickness of the membrane can exceed the length of the anchoring fibrils, allowing sloughing of epithelial layers.

Corneal erosions are very painful because the dense network of sensory nerve endings in the epithelium is disrupted. A number of treatments may be used. Acute cases may be patched and

antibiotic ointment applied to allow healing of the surface without the shearing effect of opening and closing of the eyelids. Bandage soft contact lenses or collagen shields often are applied in chronic situations to alleviate pain.[21-24] For cases in which the suspected cause is a faulty basement membrane, treatment might include corneal puncture, whereby multiple perforations are made through the epithelial layers to induce new basement membrane formation and adhesion.[25-27] If reduplication is the cause of corneal erosion, the doubled membrane can be removed.[27]

Bowman's Layer

The second layer of the cornea, **Bowman's layer**, is approximately 8–14 μm thick.[1, 7, 28] It is a dense, fibrous sheet of interwoven collagen fibrils randomly arranged in a mucoprotein ground substance. The fibrils have a diameter of 20–25 nm, run in various directions, and are not ordered into bundles.[28] Bowman's layer sometimes is referred to as a membrane, but it is more correctly a transition layer to the stroma rather than a true membrane. It differs from the stroma in that it is acellular and contains collagen fibrils of a smaller diameter. The pattern of the anterior surface is irregular and reflects the contour of the bases of the basal cells of the epithelium.[28] Posteriorly, as the layer transitions into stroma, the fibrils gradually adopt a more orderly arrangement and begin to merge into bundles that intermingle with those of the stroma (Figure 2-6). The posterior surface is not clearly defined.[28]

Bowman's layer is produced prenatally by the epithelium and is not believed to regenerate. Therefore, if injured, the layer usually is replaced by epithelial

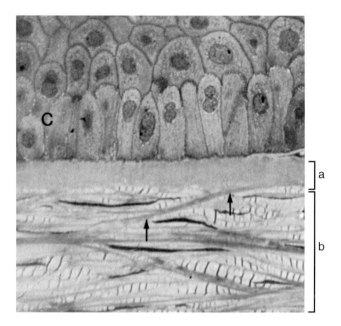

FIGURE 2-6. Light micrograph of Bowman's layer (*a*), the anterior stroma (*b*), and the corneal epithelium (*C*). There is a change in the direction of the superficial lamellae as they curve forward to merge with Bowman's layer (arrows; ×800). (Reprinted with permission from MJ Hogan, JA Alvarado, JE Weddell. Histology of the Human Eye. Philadelphia: Saunders, 1971;86.)

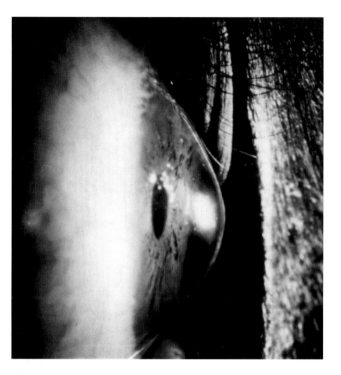

FIGURE 2-7. Keratoconus. (Courtesy of Patrick Caroline, Oregon Health Sciences University, Portland, OR.)

cells or stromal scar tissue. However, Bowman's layer is very resistant to damage by shearing, penetration, or infection.

As corneal nerves pass through Bowman's layer, they typically lose their Schwann cell covering and pass into the epithelium as naked nerves (see Figure 2-4). The layer tapers and ends at the corneal periphery and does not have a counterpart in either the conjunctiva or the sclera.

✍ CLINICAL COMMENT: KERATOCONUS

Keratoconus is a corneal dystrophy in which focal disruptions of basement membrane and Bowman's layer occur.[29, 30] Metabolic or nutritional disturbances are among the possible causes. The process usually begins in central cornea; the stroma eventually degenerates and thins, and the affected area projects outward in a cone shape owing to force that is exerted on the weakened areas by intraocular pressure (Figure 2-7). Folds occur in the posterior stroma and endothelium.[29, 30]

Spectacles may be used for a time for correction of refractive error but, with increasing irregular astigmatism, rigid gas-permeable contact lenses usually are necessary to achieve best corrected vision.[31] When contact lenses no longer correct vision, penetrating keratoplasty may be undertaken to replace the defective cornea with a donor cornea.

Stroma or Substantia Propria

The middle layer of the cornea, the **stroma** (**substantia propria**), is approximately 500 μm thick, or nine-tenths of the total corneal thickness (see Figure 2-2).[7] It is composed of collagen fibrils, fibroblasts (which in the cornea are called **keratocytes**), and intercellular ground substance.

The **collagen fibrils** have a uniform 25- to 35-nm diameter and run parallel to one another, forming flat bundles called **lamellae**.[28] The 200–300 lamellae are distributed throughout the stroma and lie parallel to the corneal surface. Each contains uniformly straight collagen fibrils arranged with regular spacing, sometimes described as a latticework. The fibrils, too, are oriented parallel to the corneal surface. Adjacent lamellae lie at angles to one another, but all fibrils within a lamella run in the same direction (Figure 2-8). Each lamella extends across the entire cornea, and each fibril runs from limbus to limbus. Some interweaving occurs between the lamellae.

The arrangement of the lamellae varies slightly within the stroma. In the anterior one-third of the stroma, the lamellae are thin (0.5–30.0 μm wide and 0.2–1.2 μm thick), and they branch and interweave more than they do in the deeper layers.[28, 32] In the posterior two-thirds of the stroma, the arrangement is more regular, and the lamellae become larger (100–200 μm wide and 1.0–2.5 μm thick).[28]

FIGURE 2-8. Corneal stroma. (A) A view of lamellae cut in three planes. The upper lamella (*a*) is cut obliquely, the next (*b*) is cut in cross section, and the third (*c*) is cut longitudinally. This lamella splits into two lamellae (arrow; ×28,000). (B) Cross-sectional (*a*) and longitudinal (*b*) views of the two lamellae. The fibrils measure 340–400 Å in diameter and are separated from each other by a space measuring 200–500 Å. A large, round granular mass (*c*) is observed within the lamella cut in cross section. Such masses are seen in most of the collagenous tissues of the eye and they may represent a stage in the formation of the mature fiber (×104,000). (Reprinted with permission from MJ Hogan, JA Alvarado, JE Weddell. Histology of the Human Eye. Philadelphia: Saunders, 1971;88.)

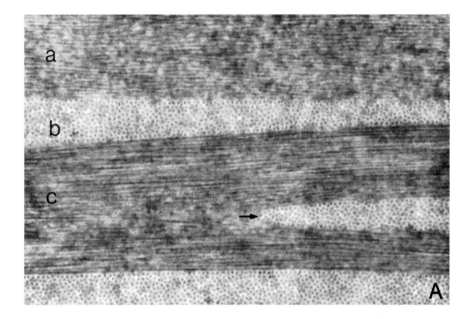

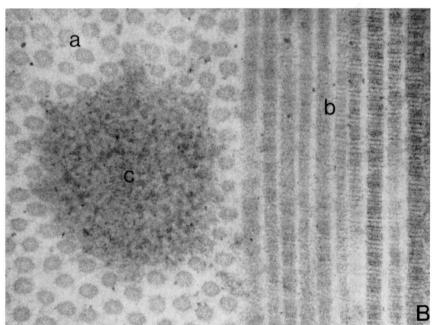

In the innermost layer, adjacent to Descemet's membrane, the fibrils interlace to form a thin collagenous sheet that contributes to the binding between stroma and Descemet's membrane.[28]

Corneal fibroblasts (keratocytes) are flattened cells that lie between, and occasionally within, the lamellae (Figure 2-9).[33] The cells have extensive branching processes that are joined by few intercellular junctions. Keratocytes produce the stromal components. Other cells may be found between lamellae, including white blood cells, lymphocytes, macrophages, and polymorphonuclear leukocytes, which may increase in number in pathologic conditions.

Ground substance fills the areas between fibrils, lamellae, and cells. It contains proteoglycans, a macromolecule with a carbohydrate glycosaminoglycan (GAG) portion. GAGs are hydrophilic, negatively charged carbohydrate molecules located at specific sites around each collagen fibril. They attract and bind with water, maintaining the precise spatial relationship between individual fibrils, and are one reason for the relatively high stromal hydration.[34]

The very regular lattice arrangement of the stromal components, specifically the fibrils, contributes to stromal transparency.[35] Studies have shown that the distance between areas of different refractive indices can affect

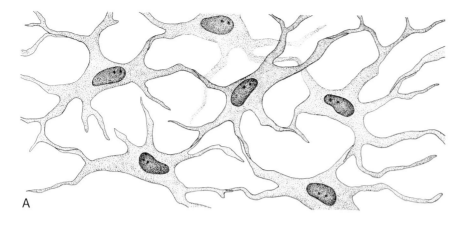

A

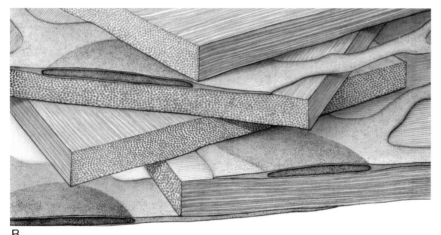

B

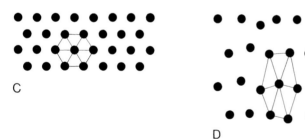

C

D

FIGURE 2-9. Summary diagram of the corneal stroma. (A) Fibroblasts. This diagram shows six fibroblasts lying between the stromal lamellae. The cells are thin and flat with long processes that contact fibroblast processes in other cells lying in the same plane. These cells once were believed to form a true syncytium, but electron microscopy has disproved this theory. There is almost always a 200-Å-wide intercellular space that separates the cells. Unlike fibroblasts elsewhere, these cells occasionally join one another at a macula occludens. (B) Lamellae. The cornea is composed of a very orderly, dense fibrous connective tissue. Its collagen, which is a very stable protein having an estimated half-life of 100 days, forms many lamellae. The collagen fibrils within a lamella are parallel to one another and run the full length of the cornea. Successive lamellae run across the cornea at an angle to one another. Three fibroblasts are seen between the lamellae. (C) Theoretic orientation of the corneal collagen fibrils. Each of the fibrils is separated from the others by an equal distance. Maurice[35] has explained the transparency of the cornea on the basis of this very exact equidistant separation. As a result of this arrangement, the stromal lamellae form a three-dimensional array of diffraction gratings. Scattered rays of light passing through such a system interact with one another in an organized way, resulting in the elimination of scattered light by destructive interference. The mucoproteins, glycoproteins, and other components of the ground substance are responsible for maintaining the proper position of the fibrils. (D) Orientation of the collagen fibrils in an opaque cornea. The diagram shows that the orderly positions of the fibrils has been disturbed. Because of this disarrangement, scattered light is not eliminated by destructive interference, and the cornea becomes hazy. Edema fluid in the ground substance also produces clouding of the cornea by disturbing the interfibrillar distance. (Reprinted with permission from MJ Hogan, JA Alvarado, JE Weddell. Histology of the Human Eye. Philadelphia: Saunders, 1971;92.)

FIGURE 2-10. Descemet's membrane. (A) The thickness of Descemet's membrane changes with increasing age. Eye of a 1½-year-old child. Light micrograph showing the endothelium (*e*) and Descemet's membrane (*d*), which are approximately the same thickness (×500). (B) Eye of a 50-year-old person. Descemet's membrane (*d*) is a little more than double the thickness of the endothelium (*e*) (×800). (Reprinted with permission from MJ Hogan, JA Alvarado, JE Weddell. Histology of the Human Eye. Philadelphia: Saunders, 1971;94.)

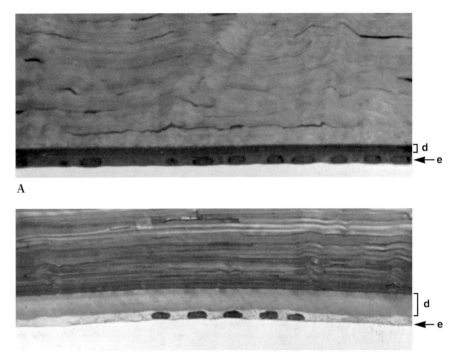

transparency. If the change in the index of refraction occurs across a distance that is less than one-half the wavelength of light, destructive interference occurs and light scattering is reduced significantly.[32, 36] In the stroma, the very specific spacing between the fibrils allows destructive interference of rays reflecting from adjacent fibers. Although the components of the epithelium, Bowman's layer, and Descemet's membrane are arranged irregularly, the scattering particles are separated by such small distances that light scattering is minimal in these layers.[32] The cornea scatters less than 1% of the light that enters it.[7]

Descemet's Membrane

Descemet's membrane is considered to be the basement membrane of the endothelium. It is produced constantly and, therefore, thickens throughout life, such that it has doubled by age 40.[21] In youth, it is 5 μm thick and will increase to approximately 15 μm over a lifetime (Figure 2-10).

Descemet's membrane consists of two laminae. The anterior one exhibits a banded appearance and is a latticework of collagen fibrils, secreted during embryonic development. This lamina is approximately 3 μm thick. The posterior lamina is nonbanded and homogeneous; it is secreted by the endothelium throughout life.[37]

Although no elastic fibers are present, the collagen fibrils are arranged in such a way that the membrane exhibits an elastic property; if torn, the membrane will curl into the anterior chamber. Descemet's membrane is very resistant to trauma, proteolytic enzymes, and some pathologic conditions, and can be regenerated if damaged. A thickened area of collagenous connective tissue sometimes is located at its termination in the limbus; this circular structure is called **Schwalbe's line** or **ring**.

The method of attachment between Descemet's membrane and the neighboring layers is poorly understood. Attachment sites between the stroma and Descemet's membrane are relatively weak as the membrane can be detached easily from posterior stroma.[15] The adhesions between Descemet's membrane and the endothelium are not the typical hemidesmosomes but some variation.

Endothelium

The innermost layer of the cornea, the **endothelium**, lies adjacent to the anterior chamber and is composed of a single layer of flattened cells. It normally is 5 μm thick.[7] The basal part of each cell rests on Descemet's membrane, and the apical surface, from which microvilli extend, lines the anterior chamber (Figure 2-11). Endothelial cells are polyhedral: Five- and seven-sided cells can be found in normal cornea, but 70–80% are hexagonal.[5, 38] The very regular arrangement of these cells is described as the **endothelial mosaic** (Figure 2-12).

Although Descemet's membrane is considered the basement membrane, no hemidesmosomes join it to the endothelium. Extensive interdigitations join the lateral walls of the cells, and gap junctions provide intercellular communication. Tight junctional complexes joining the endothe-

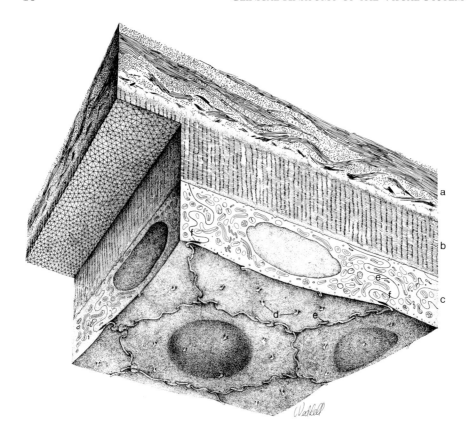

FIGURE 2-11. Three-dimensional drawing of the deep cornea showing the deepest corneal lamellae (*a*), Descemet's membrane (*b*), and the endothelium (*c*). The deeper stromal lamellae split, and some branches curve posteriorly to merge with Descemet's membrane. Descemet's membrane is seen in meridional and tangential planes. The collagenous lattice of this membrane has intersecting filaments that form nodes. The nodes are separated from one another by 100 Å and are exactly superimposed on one another to form a linear pattern in meridional sections. The endothelial cells are polygonal, measuring approximately 3.5 μm in thickness and 7–10 μm in length. Microvilli (*d*) protrude into the anterior chamber from the posterior cell, and the marginal folds (*e*) at intercellular junctions project into the anterior chamber. The intercellular space near the anterior chamber is closed by a tight junction (*f*). The cytoplasm contains an abundance of rod-shaped mitochondria. The nucleus is round and flattened in the anteroposterior axis. (Reprinted with permission from MJ Hogan, JA Alvarado, JE Weddell. Histology of the Human Eye. Philadelphia: Saunders, 1971;101.)

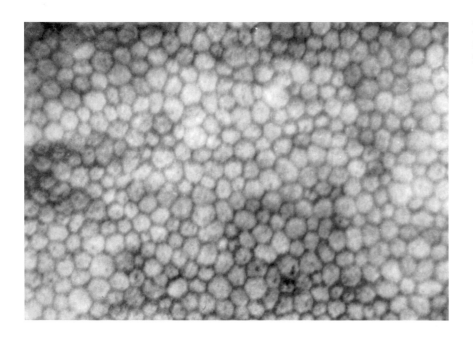

FIGURE 2-12. Endothelial mosaic. (Courtesy of Patrick Caroline, Oregon Health Sciences University, Portland, OR.)

lial cells are located near the cell apex and are a series of maculae occludens rather than zonulae occludens.[39]

The barrier formed by these adhesions has been shown to be slightly leaky as, in experiments, large molecules have penetrated the intercellular spaces.[40] This incomplete barrier allows the entrance of nutrients, including glucose and amino acids, from the aqueous humor. Excess water that accompanies these nutrients must be moved out of the cornea if proper hydration is to be maintained. An active mechanism, the **endothelial pump**, transports ions and water across the endothelial cell. This efficient metabolic pump maintains a balance between the fluid leak and the active transport of fluid. The endothelial cell is rich in cellular organelles; mitochondria reflect high metabolic activity and are more numerous in these cells than in any other cells of the eye except the retinal photoreceptor cells.[7]

Endothelial cells do not divide and replicate. Even in the young, cells migrate and spread out to cover a defect, with resultant cell thinning. The cell density (cells per unit area) of the endothelium decreases normally with aging, owing to cell disintegration: Density ranges from 3,000–4,000 cells/mm^2 in the young to 1,000–2,000 cells/mm^2 at age 80.[5, 39] The minimum cell density necessary for adequate function is in the range of 400–700 cells/mm^2.[41] Disruptions to the endothelial mosaic—endothelial cell loss or an increase in the variability of cell shape (pleomorphism) or size (polymegathism)—might affect corneal hydration (Figure 2-13). The active pump function can be affected by polymegathism or morphologic changes, but the endothelial barrier function is not compromised by a moderate loss of cells.[42]

✍ CLINICAL COMMENT: HASSALL-HENLE
  BODIES AND GUTTATA
  The endothelium can produce mounds of basement membrane material, which are seen as periodic thickenings in Descemet's membrane that bulge into the anterior chamber. Those located near the corneal periphery are called **Hassall-Henle bodies**. They are common, and their incidence increases with age. Such deposits of basement membrane in central cornea are called **corneal guttata** and are considered abnormal. The endothelium that covers these mounds is thinned and altered, and the endothelial barrier may be compromised. Both Hassall-Henle bodies and guttata are visible as dark areas when viewed with specular reflection on the biomicroscope, because the endothelium is displaced posteriorly from the plane of reflection (Figure 2-14).

✍ CLINICAL COMMENT: EFFECTS OF CONTACT
  LENSES ON ENDOTHELIUM
  Numerous studies have shown that contact lens wear can induce changes in the regularity of the endothelial mosaic.[43–47] Long-term contact lens wear (longer than 6 years) of rigid gas-permeable or soft contact lenses causes both pleomorphism and polymegathism, though cell density remains normal.

Corneal Function

The cornea has two primary functions—to refract light and to transmit light. Factors that affect the amount of corneal refraction include (1) the curvature of the anterior corneal surface, (2) the change in refractive index from air to cornea (actually the tear film), (3) corneal thickness, (4) the curvature of the posterior corneal surface, and (5) the change in refractive index from cornea to aqueous humor. The total refractive power of the eye focused at infinity is between 60 and 65 diopters (D), with 43–48 D attributable to the cornea.[5]

In the transmission of light through the cornea, it is important that there be minimal scattering and distortion. Scattering of incident light is minimized by the smooth optical surface formed by the corneal epithelium and its tear film covering. The very regular arrangement of the surface epithelial cells provides a relatively smooth surface, and the tear film fills in slight irregularities between cells. The absence of blood vessels and the maintenance of the correct spatial arrangement of components accounts for minimum scattering and distortion as light rays pass through the tissue. Because the stroma makes up 90% of the cornea, the regularity of spacing between the collagen fibrils is an important consideration in maintenance of corneal transparency. When the stroma is 75–80% water, the negatively charged molecules located around each collagen fibril maintain this precise arrangement by their bonds with the water molecules and corneal transparency is optimal.[5, 48]

Corneal Hydration

A number of factors help to maintain the correct amount of corneal hydration. The tight zonular junctions that join surface cells of the epithelium restrict the amount of fluid entering from the tear film; fluid must be transported across the cell. Tight junctions that join the endothelial cells provide an effective, if somewhat leaky, barrier to influx of water from the aqueous humor. Pumps in the epithelium and endothelium maintain the correct amount of hydration by moving water out of the stroma; the endothelial Na$^+$/K$^+$-ATPase pump system is the most important.

In the properly hydrated cornea, the endothelial tight junctions are leaky enough to permit circulation of water with no net flow (i.e., balance is maintained as nutrients pass into and waste moves out of the cornea).[49] Fluid that leaks into the stroma with the nutrients is balanced by active transport, which exchan-

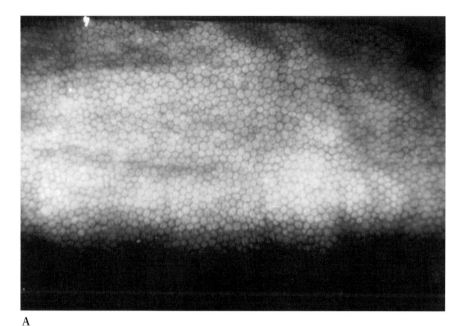

A

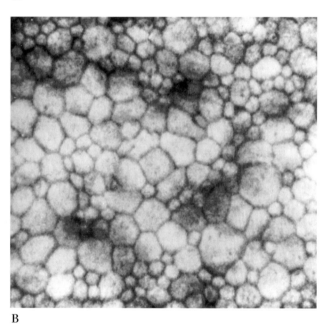

B

FIGURE 2-13. Endothelial integrity can be evaluated by determining the coefficient of variation (CV) of cell size. Normal endothelium has a CV of 0.25. (A) Endothelium of a 25-year-old healthy non–contact lens wearer. Endothelial cell density is 2,000 cells/mm^2, hexagonality is 69%, and CV is 0.25. (Courtesy of Dr. Scott MacRae, Oregon Health Sciences University, Portland, OR.) (B) Endothelium of a 40-year-old patient who has worn polymethyl methacrylate contact lenses for 23 years. Endothelial cell density is 1,676 cells/mm^2, hexagonality is 24%, and CV is 0.66. (Reprinted with permission from SM MacRae, M Matsuda, S Shellans, et al. The effects of hard and soft contact lenses on the corneal endothelium. Am J Ophthalmol 1986;102:50.)

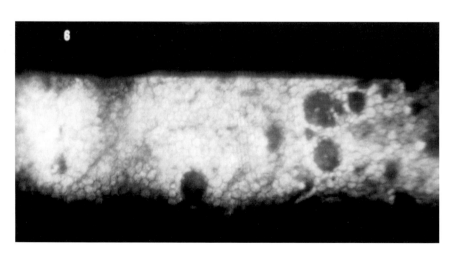

FIGURE 2-14. Guttata. Endothelium of a patient with Fuchs' endothelial dystrophy. Numerous guttata are evident by the dark areas; endothelial cell density is 1,600 cells/mm^2. (Courtesy of Dr. Scott MacRae, Oregon Health Sciences University, Portland, OR.)

ges ions and water via the Na$^+$/K$^+$-ATPase pump. Apparently, the pump operates at a constant rate, and the leak depends on the swelling pressure of the stroma; the rate of leakage is proportional to the pressure gradient across the endothelium.[50, 51] This is a self-adjusting, homeostatic mechanism.

If fluid is retained, the ground substance expands in stromal edema, thereby increasing the spacing between collagen fibrils. In an edematous stroma, fluid accumulates between and within the lamellae, causing loss of transparency.[32] The edema occurs in the spaces between fibrils, not within the fibrils themselves.

✍ CLINICAL COMMENT: CORNEAL EDEMA

Damage to either the epithelium or the endothelium can cause edema of the cornea, resulting in impaired visual acuity. Generally, with minor epithelial disruption, the edema is restricted to epithelium. With more extensive damage, however, the localized area of edema spreads into the stroma. Endothelial damage is more likely to cause generalized stromal edema. In an acute episode of high-pressure glaucoma, the intraocular pressure can overcome the transport activity of the endothelium and force fluid from the aqueous humor into the stroma.

An increase in fluid retention thickens the stroma and pushes Descemet's membrane posteriorly. Then, the posterior stroma and Descemet's membrane buckle, producing vertical lines called **striae**, which can be seen with the biomicroscope.[52]

Corneal Wound Healing

Damaged corneal epithelium regenerates quickly. Basal cells initially migrate over the damaged area and, as healing progresses, the cells are replaced. Hemidesmosomes in the basal cell layer disappear near the wound edge, and the cells flatten and are transformed into motile cells migrating across the defect, covering it with a one–cell-thick layer.[10, 11, 53, 54] A concomitant increase in the cell volume increases the surface area of the individual cell, and the columnar appearance of the cell is lost. After the defect is covered, cell proliferation fills in the defect, and tight adhesions are established once again. If the basement membrane is intact, this healing takes only days, but if the basement membrane is damaged, several weeks will be needed for recovery.[13]

Bowman's layer will not regenerate if damaged but will be replaced either by stromalike fibrous tissue or by epithelium. The characteristics of the replacement tissue, when the stroma is damaged, are slightly different from those of the original tissue, and so a scar may result. The diameter of regenerated corneal stromal collagen is larger than normal, comparable to that found in the sclera.[7] The fibrils across the defect are not as well organized,

and the tensile strength of the collagen fibrils in the repaired cornea is diminished.[55]

Descemet's membrane is a very strong and resistant membrane and, if damaged, can be regenerated by the endothelial cells that secrete it. Endothelial cells are not replaced when damaged but migrate to cover the area, causing the cells to thin and the cell density to decrease.

The biomolecular factors that influence the healing processes in the cornea are not fully understood, especially considering that the cornea lacks a vascular supply. Factors identified thus far include fibronectin, which promotes epithelial cell adhesion and motility, and epidermal growth factor, which enhances epithelial and endothelial healing.[56–63]

Corneal Physiologic Properties

The cornea is very metabolically active and depends on oxygen derived primarily from the atmosphere and absorbed through the tear film; small amounts also are absorbed from the aqueous humor and limbal capillaries.[64, 65] Nutrients are obtained from limbal capillaries and the aqueous humor. For details of the complexities of corneal physiology, the reader is referred to a text that deals specifically with physiology of the eye such as *Adler's Physiology of the Eye* (WM Hart Jr [ed]) or *Physiology of the Eye* (I Fatt, BA Weissman).

Corneal Blood Supply

The cornea is avascular and obtains its nourishment by diffusion from the aqueous humor in the anterior chamber and from the conjunctival and episcleral capillary networks located in the limbus. Absence of blood vessels is a contributing factor in corneal transparency, and vessel growth into the stroma may be impeded because of the stroma's compact composition. Studies are ongoing to determine whether an antiangiogenic substance inhibiting the ingrowth of vessels is present in corneal tissue.[66]

✍ CLINICAL COMMENT: CORNEAL NEOVASCULARIZATION

In response to oxygen deprivation, the body may produce new blood vessels in an attempt to supply the oxygen-depleted area. This growth of abnormal blood vessels is termed **neovascularization**. In a contact lens wearer, neovascularization is usually an indication that the cornea is not receiving enough oxygen. It can be a sign of a poorly fit or poorly moving lens, or a thick edge. The incidence of neovascularization is higher in soft contact lens wearers than in those wearing rigid gas-permeable lenses and increases in those who wear their lenses for extended periods.

New vessels extend from the conjunctival loops into the cornea (Figure 2-15). Careful monitoring

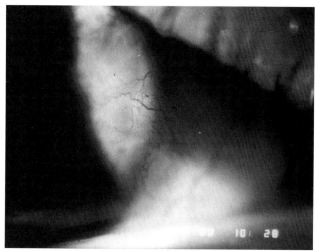

A

FIGURE 2-15. (A) Grade 2+ neovascularization. (Courtesy of Family Vision Center, Pacific University, Forest Grove, OR.) (B) Grade 3+ neovascularization. (Courtesy of Dr. Christina Schnider.) (C) Grade 4+ neovascularization. (Courtesy of Dr. Christina Schnider, Menicon USA, Inc., Clovis, CA.)

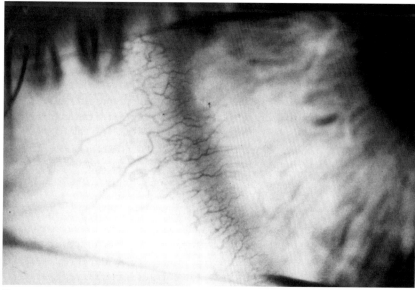

B

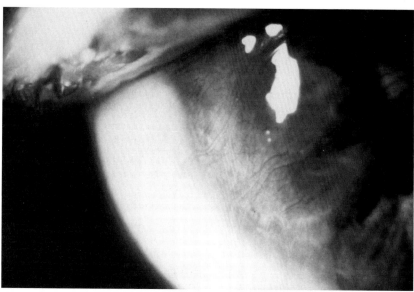

C

of patients with neovascularization and elimination of the causative factor may prevent extensive neo-vascularization. When the oxygen supply to the cornea resumes, the vessels will no longer carry blood but the structures will remain and atrophy. These are known as **ghost vessels** and appear, on viewing with the biomicroscope, as fine white lines.

Corneal infections also may induce neovascularization in the body's attempt to increase blood supply to the affected area.

Corneal Innervation

The cornea is densely innervated with sensory fibers. Seventy to 80 large nerves, branches of the anterior ciliary and short ciliary nerves, enter the peripheral stroma. Approximately 2–3 mm after they pass into the cornea, the nerves lose their myelin sheath, but the covering from the Schwann cell remains.[67] Considerable branching occurs, and three nerve networks are formed. One is located in midstroma, and a subepithelial network is located in the region of Bowman's layer and anterior stroma. Branches from this second network enter the epithelium, where the final nerve network is located (see Figure 12-2).

As the nerves pass through Bowman's layer, the Schwann cell covering is lost and the fibers terminate as naked nerve endings between the tightly packed epithelial cells.[7] No nerve endings are located in Descemet's membrane or the endothelium. Any abrasion of the cornea, even a superficial one, is quite painful because of the density of this sensory innervation.

SCLERA

The **sclera** forms the posterior five-sixths of the connective-tissue coat of the globe and is composed of an outer layer (the episclera) and an inner layer (the scleral stroma), between which there is no clear boundary. The sclera maintains the shape of the globe, offering resistance to internal and external forces, and provides an attachment for the extraocular muscle insertions. The thickness of the sclera varies from 1.0 mm at the posterior pole to 0.3 mm just behind the rectus muscle insertions.[1, 68, 69]

Scleral Histologic Features

Episclera

The **episclera** is composed of loose, vascularized, connective tissue. The larger episcleral vessels are visible through the conjunctiva. Branches of the anterior ciliary arteries form a capillary network in the episclera just anterior to the rectus muscle insertions and surrounding the peripheral cornea. The episclera, which is joined to Tenon's capsule by strands of connective tissue, becomes thinner toward the back of the eye.

✍ CLINICAL COMMENT: CILIARY INJECTION

The episcleral network becomes congested in ciliary injection, giving the limbus a light purple-rose coloration in serious corneal inflammations or diseases of the iris or ciliary body.

Scleral Stroma

The **scleral stroma** is a thick, dense connective-tissue layer that is continuous with the corneal stroma at the limbus. The diameter of the collagen fibrils in this tissue varies from 25 to 230 nm. These fibrils are arranged in irregular bundles that branch and interlace.[28, 70] Bundle widths and thicknesses vary, the external bundles being narrower and thinner than the deeper ones. The orientation of the bundles is very irregular as compared to bundles in the cornea: The bundles in the outer regions of the sclera run approximately parallel to the surface, with interweaving between the bundles, whereas in the inner regions the bundles run in all directions.[28] This random arrangement and the amount of interweaving may contribute to the strength and flexibility of the eye. Generally, the fibrils parallel the limbus anteriorly, and the pattern becomes meridional near the rectus muscle insertions and circular around the optic nerve exit. The collagen of the muscle tendon at its insertion merges and interweaves with the fibrils of the sclera.[71]

Elastic fibers are found occasionally in the sclera between, and sometimes within, bundles.[28] Fibroblasts also are present, although they are less numerous than in the cornea. The stromal ground substance is similar to the corneal ground substance but contains fewer GAGs.[48]

The innermost aspect of the sclera merges with the choroidal tissue in the suprachoroid layer.

Scleral Spur

The **scleral spur** is a region of circularly oriented collagen bundles that extends from the inner aspect of the sclera.[1] In its entirety it is actually a ring, though on cross-section it appears wedge-shaped, resembling a spur (Figure 2-16). At the spur's posterior edge, its fibers blend with the more obliquely arranged scleral fibers.[1] The posterior scleral spur is the origin of the longitudinal ciliary muscle fibers, and most of the trabecular meshwork sheets attach to its anterior aspect, such that the collagen of the spur is continuous with that from the trabeculae.

Scleral Opacity

The opacity of the sclera depends on a number of factors, including the number of GAGs, the amount of

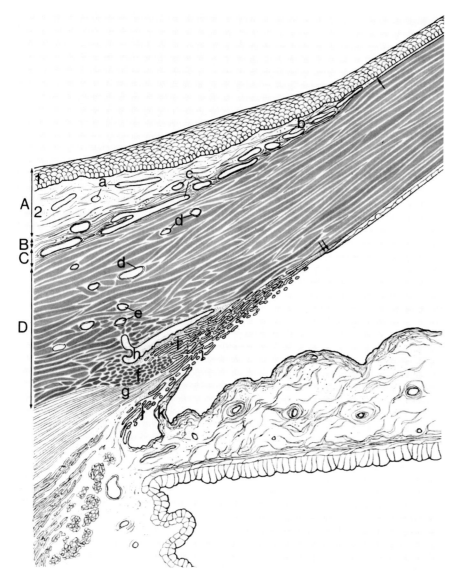

FIGURE 2-16. Limbus. The limbal conjunctiva (A) is formed by an epithelium (1) and a loose connective tissue stroma (2). Tenon's capsule (B) forms a thin, somewhat ill-defined connective tissue layer over the episclera (C). The limbal stroma occupies the area (D) and is composed of the scleral and corneal tissues that merge in this region. The conjunctival stromal vessels are seen at (a). They form the peripheral corneal arcades (b), which extend anteriorly to the termination of Bowman's layer (arrow). The episcleral vessels (c) are cut in different planes. Vessels forming the intrascleral (d) and deep scleral plexus (e) are shown within the limbal stroma. The scleral spur, with its coarse and dense collagen fibers, is shown (f). The anterior part of the longitudinal portion of the ciliary muscle (g) merges with the scleral spur and the trabecular meshwork. The lumen of Schlemm's canal (h) and the loose tissues of its wall are seen clearly. The sheets of the trabecular meshwork (i) are internal to the cords of the uveal meshwork (j). An iris process (k) is seen to arise from the iris surface and to join the trabecular meshwork at the level of the anterior portion of the scleral spur. Descemet's membrane terminates (double arrows) within the anterior portion of the triangle, outlining the aqueous outflow system. (Reprinted with permission from MJ Hogan, JA Alvarado, JE Weddell. Histology of the Human Eye. Philadelphia: Saunders, 1971;127.)

water, and the size and distribution of the collagen fibrils. The sclera contains one-fourth the number of GAGs that are present in the cornea[69] and, as a probable consequence, the sclera is relatively dehydrated (68%) as compared to the cornea. The greater variation in fibril size and the irregular spacing between scleral components induces light scattering, which renders the sclera opaque.[28]

Scleral Color

The anterior sclera is visible through the conjunctiva and, if healthy, is white but may appear colored as a result of age or disease. In the newborn, the sclera will have a bluish tint, as the sclera is almost transparent and the underlying vascular pigmented uvea shows through. The sclera also may appear blue in connective-tissue diseases that cause scleral thinning. The sclera might appear yellow in the presence of fatty deposits, which can occur with age. Likewise, in liver disease, the sclera may appear yellow owing to buildup of metabolic wastes.

Scleral Foramina and Canals

The sclera contains a number of foramina and canals. The anterior scleral foramen is the area occupied by the cornea. The optic nerve passes through the posterior scleral foramen, which is bridged by a network of scleral tissue called the **lamina cribrosa**. It is similar to a sieve, with interwoven collagen fibrils forming canals

FIGURE 2-17. Posterior sclera. Posterior of globe showing the optic nerve passing through the posterior scleral foramen, the long and short ciliary arteries and nerves passing through the posterior apertures, and the vortex veins passing through the middle apertures.

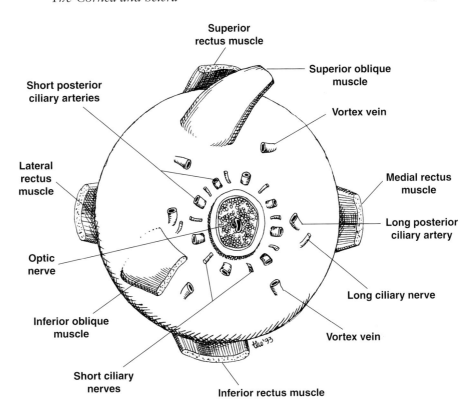

through which the optic nerve bundles pass.[71, 72] The lamina cribrosa is the weakest area of the outer connective-tissue tunic.[1]

✍ CLINICAL COMMENT: OPTIC NERVE CUPPING

Because it is the weakest area of the outer connective-tissue layer, the lamina cribrosa is the area that will most likely be affected by increased pressure inside the eye. A cupping out or ectasia of the center area of the optic nerve head may be evident in patients with elevated intraocular pressure and is one of the clinical signs sometimes noted in glaucoma.

The canals that pass through the sclera carry nerves and vessels and are possible routes by which disease can exit or enter the eye. The canals are designated by their location. The posterior apertures are located around the posterior scleral foramen and are the passages for the posterior ciliary arteries and nerves. The middle apertures lie approximately 4 mm posterior to the equator and carry the vortex veins (Figure 2-17). The anterior apertures are near the limbus at the muscle insertions and are the passages for the anterior ciliary vessels, which are branches from the muscular arteries.

Scleral Blood Supply

Because it is relatively inactive metabolically, the sclera has a minimal blood supply. A number of vessels pass through the sclera to other tissues, but the sclera is considered avascular as it contains no capillary beds. Nourishment is furnished by small branches from the episcleral and choroidal vessels and branches of the long posterior ciliary arteries.[69]

Scleral Innervation

Sensory innervation is supplied to the posterior sclera by branches of the short ciliary nerves; the remainder of the sclera is served by branches of the long ciliary nerves.[69]

LIMBUS

The **limbus**, located at the corneoscleral junction, is a band approximately 1.5–2 mm wide that encircles the periphery of the cornea. The radius of curvature abruptly changes at this junction of cornea and sclera, creating a shallow, narrow furrow, the **external scleral sulcus**. Internally at this juncture, there is a larger furrow—the **internal sclera sulcus**—that has a scooped-out appearance.

Histologically, the anterior boundary of the limbus consists of a plane connecting the termination of Bowman's layer and the termination of Descemet's membrane. The posterior boundary is a plane perpendicular to the surface of the globe and passing through the posterior edge of the scleral spur (see Figure 2-16).[73] These boundaries will be used in this discussion, although clinically the boundaries are not as specific.

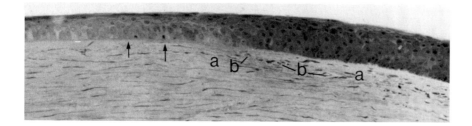

FIGURE 2-18. Light micrograph demonstrating corneolimbal transition. The corneal epithelium is at left; it gradually thickens as it becomes the limbal epithelium. Bowman's layer tapers until it finally disappears (arrows) in the conjunctival stroma. The conjunctival stroma (*a*) is denser in this region than further posteriorly. A few vessels of the peripheral corneal arcades (*b*) are seen in cross section (×190). (Reprinted with permission from MJ Hogan, JA Alvarado, JE Weddell. Histology of the Human Eye. Philadelphia: Saunders, 1971;128.)

The limbus is the transitional zone between cornea and conjunctiva and between cornea and sclera. Some layers of the cornea continue into the limbal area, and others terminate (see Figure 2-16). In the limbus, (1) the very regular squamous corneal epithelium becomes the thicker columnar conjunctival epithelium, (2) the very regular corneal stroma becomes the irregularly arranged scleral stroma, (3) the corneal endothelial sheet becomes discontinuous to wrap around the strands of the trabecular meshwork, (4) Bowman's layer and Descemet's membrane terminate at the anterior border, and (5) the conjunctival stroma, episclera, and Tenon's capsule begin within the limbal area.

Limbal Histologic Features

At the limbus, the corneal epithelium increases from a layer 5 cells thick to a layer 10–15 cells thick (Figure 2-18).[1, 73] Melanocytes may be present in the basal layer, and pigmentation may be evident in the limbus and conjunctiva, especially in darker-skinned persons. Bowman's layer tapers and terminates. Its fibers become indistinguishable from those of the anterior sclera (see Figure 2-18).[15]

The limbus contains the transition from the very regular corneal lamellae to the irregular and random organization of collagen bundles in the sclera. This change is gradual such that, as the transparent cornea merges into the opaque sclera, no line of demarcation can be identified. The scleral fibers extend further anteriorly on the external than on the internal side of the limbus.[2]

Descemet's membrane tapers at the anterior limbal boundary, and the posterior nonbanded portion becomes interlaced with the connective tissue of the anterior sheets of the trabecular meshwork. The corneal endothelium continues into the anterior chamber angle as the endothelial covering of the sheets of the trabecular meshwork.[15, 39]

The conjunctival submucosa begins in the limbus and has no counterpart in the cornea. This stromal tissue forms mounds that project toward the surface epithelium at the limbus, giving an undulating appearance. The basal layer of the epithelium follows these ridges, called **papillae**, which are found also near the eyelid margin. Papillae give the inner aspect of the epithelium a wavy appearance, though the surface remains smooth.

Tenon's capsule lies just inner to the conjunctival submucosa and the episclera is inner to Tenon's capsule. Both begin in the limbus but do not continue into the cornea. Tenon's capsule, the episclera, and the conjunctival stroma fuse in the limbal area.[2]

Palisades of Vogt

The **palisades of Vogt** are radial projections of limbal epithelium and stroma that extend into the cornea in spokelike fashion.[12] On biomicroscopy, they appear as thin gray pegs approximately 0.5 mm wide and 2–4 mm long.[73] The surface of the limbal area remains flat where these projections occur. The epithelium in this area is the suspected site of stem cell origin, the source of corneal epithelial cell replication.

Limbal Blood Vessels and Lymphatics

Capillary loops from conjunctival and episcleral vessels form networks in the limbus, which surround the cornea and provide nourishment to the avascular corneal tissue. Limbal veins collect blood from the anterior conjunctival veins and drain into the radial episcleral veins, which then empty into the anterior ciliary veins.[74] Lymphatic channels located in the limbal area do not enter the cornea.

Cell Replacement

In the limbal basal epithelial layer, a cell has been identified that is smaller and darker-staining than the usual epithelial cells. It has histochemical features suggestive of stem cell characteristics, with the capacity for corneal epithelial cell proliferation.[75–79] Centripetal movement from the limbal area is responsible for the migration and replacement of corneal epithelial cells in both normal cell replacement and wound healing.[11]

Limbal Physiologic Features

The limbus has two functions—to provide nutrients to adjacent tissue and to provide a pathway for the drainage of aqueous humor from the eye. The vessels that loop in the conjunctival and episcleral tissue of the limbus provide some metabolites for the peripheral cornea. The structures in the internal scleral sulcus, the trabecular meshwork, and the canal of Schlemm that provide the major route for drainage of the aqueous humor are discussed in Chapter 6.

REFERENCES

1. Warwick R. Eugene Wolff's Anatomy of the Eye and Orbit (7th ed). Philadelphia: Saunders, 1976;30.

2. Van Buskirk EM. The anatomy of the limbus. Eye 1989;3:101.

3. Duke-Elder WS. Textbook of Ophthalmology. St. Louis: Mosby, 1946;40.

4. Martola E, Baun J. Central and peripheral corneal thickness. Arch Ophthalmol 1968;79:28.

5. Pepose JS, Ubels JL. The Cornea. In WM Hart Jr (ed), Adler's Physiology of the Eye (9th ed). St. Louis: Mosby, 1992;29.

6. Siu A, Herse P. The effect of age on human corneal thickness. Statistical implications of power analysis. Acta Ophthalmol (Copenh) 1993;71(1):51.

7. Hogan MJ, Alvarado JA. The Cornea. In MJ Hogan, JA Alvarado (eds), Histology of the Human Eye. Philadelphia: Saunders, 1971;55.

8. Pfister RR. The normal surface of corneal epithelium: a scanning electron microscope study. Invest Ophthalmol 1973;12:654.

9. Gipson IK, Spurr-Michaud SJ, Tisdale AS. Anchoring fibrils form a complex network in human and rabbit cornea. Invest Ophthalmol Vis Sci 1987;28(2):212.

10. Gipson IK, Spurr-Michaud S, Tisdale A, et al. Reassembly of the anchoring structures of the corneal epithelium during wound repair in the rabbit. Invest Ophthalmol Vis Sci 1989;30:425.

11. Gipson IK, Spurr-Michaud SJ, Tisdale AS. Hemidesmosome and anchoring fibril collagen appears synchronously during development and wound healing. Dev Biol 1988;126:253.

12. Gipson IK. The epithelial basement membrane zone of the limbus. Eye 1989;3:132.

13. Khodadoust AA, Silverstein AM, Kenyon KR, et al. Adhesion of regenerating epithelium. Am J Ophthalmol 1968;65(3):339.

14. Tisdale AS, Spurr-Michaud SJ, Rodrigues M, et al. Development of the anchoring structures of the epithelium in rabbit and human fetal corneas. Invest Ophthalmol Vis Sci 1988;29(5):727.

15. Binder PS, Rock ME, Schmidt KC, et al. High-voltage electron microscopy of normal human cornea. Invest Ophthalmol Vis Sci 1991;32:2234.

16. Throft R. The X,Y,Z hypothesis of corneal epithelial maintenance. Invest Ophthalmol Vis Sci 1983;24(10):1442.

17. Tseng SCG. Concept and application of limbal stem cells. Eye 1989;3:141.

18. Hanna C, O'Brien JE. Cell production and migration in the epithelial layer of the cornea. Arch Ophthalmol 1960;64:536.

19. Hanna C, Bicknell BA, O'Brien JE. Cell turnover in the adult human eye. Arch Ophthalmol 1961;65:695.

20. McCartney ND, Cantu-Crouch D. Rabbit corneal epithelial wound repair; tight junction reformation. Curr Eye Res 1991;11:15.

21. Alvarado J, Murphy C, Juster R. Age-related changes in the basement membrane of the human corneal epithelium. Invest Ophthalmol Vis Sci 1983;24(8):1015.

22. Bartlett JD, Jaanus SD. Clinical Ocular Pharmacology (2nd ed). Boston: Butterworth, 1989;379.

23. Susicky P. Use of soft contact lenses in the treatment of recurrent corneal erosions [abstract]. Cesk Oftalmol 1990;46(5):381.

24. Robin JB, Keys CK, Kaminski LA, et al. The effect of collagen shields on rabbit corneal reepithelialization after chemical debridement. Invest Ophthalmol Vis Sci 1990;31(7):1294.

25. Geggel HS. Successful treatment of recurrent corneal erosion with Nd:YAG anterior stromal puncture. Am J Ophthalmol 1990;110(4):404.

26. Katsev DA, Kincaid MC, Fouraker BD, et al. Recurrent corneal erosion: pathology of corneal puncture. Cornea 1991;10(5):418.

27. Pfister RR. Clinical measures to promote corneal epithelial healing. Acta Ophthalmol Suppl 1992;202:73.

28. Komai Y, Ushiki T. The three-dimensional organization of collagen fibrils in the human cornea and sclera. Invest Ophthalmol Vis Sci 1991;32:2244.

29. Bron AJ. Keratoconus. Cornea 1988;7(3):163.

30. Chi HH, Katzin HM, Teng CC. Histopathology of keratoconus. Am J Ophthalmol 1956;42:847.

31. Astin C. Contact lens fitting after anterior segment disease. Contact Lens J 1992;20(5):11.

32. Goldman J, Benedek G, Dohlman C, et al. Structural alterations affecting transparency in swollen human corneas. Invest Ophthalmol 1968;7(5):501.

33. Poole CA, Brookes NH, Clover GM. Keratocyte networks visualized in the living cornea using vital dyes. J Cell Sci 1993;106:685.

34. Scott JE, Haigh M. "Small" proteoglycan: collagen interactions. Keratin sulfate proteoglycan associates with rabbit corneal collagen fibrils at the "a" and "c" bands. Biosci Rep 1965;5:765.

35. Maurice DM. The structure and transparency of the cornea. J Physiol 1957;136:263.

36. Farrell RA, McCally RL, Tatham PER. Wavelength dependencies of light scattering in normal and cold swollen rabbit corneas and their structural implications. J Physiol 1973;233:589.

37. Johnson DG, Bourne WM, Campbell RJ. The ultrastructure of Descemet's membrane. Arch Ophthalmol 1982;100:1942.

38. Doughty MJ. Toward a quantitative analysis of corneal endothelial cell morphology: a review of techniques and their application. Optom Vis Sci 1989; 66:626.

39. Waring GO, Bourne WM, Edelhauser HF, et al. The corneal endothelium: normal and pathologic structure and function. Ophthalmology 1982;89(6):531.

40. Kaye GI, Sibley RC, Hoefle FB. Recent studies on the nature and function of the corneal endothelial layer. Exp Eye Res 1973;15:585.

41. Bourne WM, McCarey BE, Kaufman HE. Specular microscopy of the human corneal endothelium in vivo. Am J Ophthalmol 1976;81:319.

42. Bergmanson JPG. Histopathological analysis of corneal endothelial polymegethism. Cornea 1992; 11:133.

43. Connor CG, Zagrod ME. Contact lens–induced corneal endothelial polymegethism: functional significance and possible mechanisms. Am J Optom Physiol Opt 1986;63:539.

44. Holden BA, Sweeney DF, Vannas A, et al. Effects of long term extended contact lens wear on the human cornea. Invest Ophthalmol Vis Sci 1985; 26:1489.

45. Holden BA, Vannas A, Nolsson L, et al. Epithelial and endothelial effects from the extended wear of contact lenses. Curr Eye Res 1985;4:739.

46. Matsuda M, Inaba M, Suda T. Corneal endothelial changes associated with aphakic extended contact lens wear. Arch Ophthalmol 1988;106:70.

47. MacCrae SM, Matsuda M, Shellans S, et al. The effects of hard and soft contact lenses on the corneal endothelium. Am J Ophthalmol 1986;102:50.

48. McCulley JP. The circulation of fluid at the limbus (flow and diffusion at the limbus). Eye 1989;3:114.

49. Liebovitch LS, Weinbaum S. A model of epithelial water transport: the corneal endothelium. Biophys J 1981;35:315.

50. Baum JP, Maurice DM, McCarey BE. The active and passive transport of water across the corneal endothelium. Exp Eye Res 1984;39:335.

51. O'Neal MR, Polse KA. In vivo assessment of mechanisms controlling corneal hydration. Invest Ophthalmol Vis Sci 1985;26:849.

52. Wechsler S. Striate corneal lines. Am J Optom Physiol Opt 1974;51:852.

53. Crosson CE, Klyce SD, Beuerman RW. Corneal epithelial wound closure. Invest Ophthalmol Vis Sci 1986;27(4):464.

54. Tervo T, van Setten G-B, Paällysaho T, et al. Wound healing of the ocular surface. Ann Med 1992;24:19.

55. Davison PF, Galbary EJ. Connective-tissue remodeling in corneal and scleral wounds. Invest Ophthalmol Vis Sci 1986;27(10):1478.

56. Brazzell RK, Stern ME, Aquavella JV, et al. Human recombinant epidermal growth factor in experimental corneal wound healing. Invest Ophthalmol Vis Sci 1991;32(2):336.

57. Hoppenreijs VP, Pels E, Vrensen GF, et al. Effects of human growth factor on endothelial wound healing of human corneas. Invest Ophthalmol Vis Sci 1992;33(6):1946.

58. Hoppenreijs VP, Pels E, Vrensen GF, et al. Platelet-derived growth factor: receptor expression in corneas and effects on corneal cells. Invest Ophthalmol Vis Sci 1993;34(3):637.

59. Kim LS, Oh JS, Kim IS, et al. Clinical efficacy of topical homologous fibronectin in persistent corneal epithelial disorders. Korean J Ophthalmol 1992;6(1):12.

60. Mooradian DL, McCarthy JB, Skubitz AP, et al. Characterization of FM-C/H-V, a novel synthetic peptide from fibronectin that promotes rabbit corneal epithelial cell adhesion, spreading, and motility. Invest Ophthalmol Vis Sci 1993;34(1):153.

61. Pastor JC, Calonge M. Epidermal growth factor and corneal wound healing. Cornea 1992;11(4):311.

62. Rieck P, Hartmann C, Jacob C, et al. Human recombinant bFGF stimulates corneal endothelial wound healing in rabbits. Curr Eye Res 1992;11(12):1161.

63. Schultz G, Chegini N, Grant M, et al. Effects of growth factors on corneal wound healing. Acta Ophthalmol Suppl 1992;202:60.

64. Hill RM, Fatt I. How dependent is the cornea on the atmosphere? J Am Optom Assoc 1964;5:873.

65. Smelser GK, Ozanics V. Importance of atmospheric oxygen for maintenance of the optical properties of the human cornea. Science 1952;115:140.

66. Klintworth GK, Burger PC. Neovascularization of the cornea: current concepts of its pathogenesis. Int Ophthalmol Clin 1981;23(1):27.

67. Lawrenson JG, Ruskell GL. The structure of corpuscular nerve endings in the limbal conjunctiva of the human eye. J Anat 1991;177:75.

68. Meyer E, Ludatscher RN, Miller B, et al. Connective tissue of the orbital cavity in retinal detachment: an ultrastructural study. Ophthalmic Res 1992;24:365.

69. Hogan MJ, Alvarado JA. The Sclera. In MJ Hogan, JA Alvarado. Histology of the Human Eye. Philadelphia: Saunders, 1971;183.

70. Quantock AJ, Meek KM. Axial electron density of human sclera. Biophys J 1988;54:159.

71. Thale A, Tillmann B. The collagen architecture of the sclera—SEM and immunohistochemical studies. Anat Anz 1993;175:215.

72. Elkington AR, Inman CB, Steart PV, et al. The structure of the lamina cribrosa of the human eye: an immunocytochemical and electron microscopical study. Eye 1990;4:42.

73. Hogan MJ, Alvarado JA. The Limbus. In MJ Hogan, JA Alvarado. Histology of the Human Eye. Philadelphia: Saunders, 1971;112.

74. Meyer PAR. The circulation of the human limbus. Eye 1989;3:121.

75. Cotsarelis G, Cheng SZ, Dong E, et al. Existence of slow-cycling limbal epithelial basal cells that can be preferentially stimulated to proliferate. Cell 1989; 57:201.

76. Ebato B, Friend J, Throft RA. Comparison of central and peripheral human corneal epithelium in tissue culture. Invest Ophthalmol Vis Sci 1987; 28:1450.

77. Lauweryns R, van den Oord JJ, De Vos R, et al. A new epithelial cell type in the human cornea. Invest Ophthalmol Vis Sci 1993;34(6):1983.

78. Thoft RA, Wiley LA, Sundarraj N. The multipotential cells of the limbus. Eye 1989;3:109.

79. Zieske JD, Bukusoglu G, Yankauckas MA. Characterization of a potential marker of corneal epithelial stem cells. Invest Ophthalmol Vis Sci 1992; 33(1):143.

The Uvea

The middle layer of the eye, the **uvea** (**uveal tract**), is composed of three regions. From front to back, they are the iris, the ciliary body, and the choroid. The uvea sometimes is called the **vascular layer** because its largest structure, the choroid, is composed mainly of blood vessels, which supply the outer retinal layers.

IRIS

The **iris** is a thin, circular structure located anterior to the lens, often compared to a diaphragm of an optical system. The center aperture, the **pupil**, actually is located slightly nasal and inferior to the iris center.[1] Pupil size regulates retinal illumination. The diameter can vary from 1 mm to 8 mm according to lighting conditions. The pupil is very small (miotic) in brightly lit conditions and fairly large (mydriatic) in dim illumination. The average diameter of the iris is 12 mm, and its thickness varies. It is thickest in the region of the **collarette**, a circular ridge approximately 1.5 mm from the pupillary margin. This slightly raised jagged ridge was the attachment for the fetal pupillary membrane during embryologic development.[1, 2] The collarette divides the iris into the **pupillary zone**, which encircles the pupil, and the **ciliary zone**, which extends from the collarette to the iris periphery (Figure 3-1). The color of these two zones often differs.

The pupillary margin of the iris rests on the anterior surface of the lens and, in profile, the iris has a truncated cone shape such that the pupillary margin lies anterior to its peripheral termination, the **iris root** (Figure 3-2). The root, being approximately 0.5 mm thick, is the thinnest part of the iris and joins the iris to the anterior aspect of the ciliary body.[1] The iris divides the anterior segment of the globe into anterior and posterior chambers, and the pupil allows the aqueous humor to flow from the posterior into the anterior chamber with no resistance.

✍ CLINICAL COMMENT: OCULAR OR HEAD TRAUMA

With trauma to the eye or head, the thin root may tear away from the ciliary body, creating a condition called **iridodialysis**, which can result in damaged blood vessels and nerves. Blood may hemorrhage into either the anterior or the posterior chamber, or both, and nerve damage may cause sector paralysis of the iris muscles.

Histologic Features of the Iris

The iris can be divided into four layers: the anterior border layer, the stroma and sphincter muscle, the anterior epithelium and dilator muscle, and the posterior epithelium.

Anterior Border Layer

The surface layer of the iris, the **anterior border layer**, is a thin condensation of the stroma. In fact, some do not consider this to be a separate layer. It is composed of fibroblasts, pigmented melanocytes, and collagen fibrils. The highly branching processes of the cells interweave to form a meshwork in which the fibroblasts are on the surface and the melanocytes are located below (Figure 3-3).[1, 2] The thickness of the melanocyte layer may vary throughout the iris, with accumulations of melanocytes forming elevated frecklelike masses, evident in the anterior border layer.[1] The density and arrangement of the meshwork

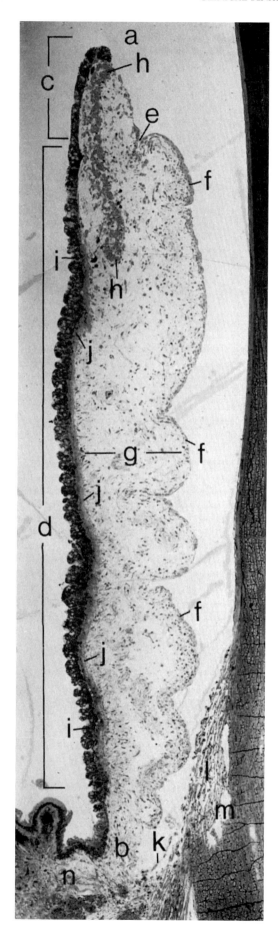

differ among irises and are contributing factors in iris color. The collagen fibrils are arranged in radial columns that in light-colored irises are seen easily as white fibers.[3]

The anterior border layer is absent at the oval-shaped iris crypts. Near the root, extensions of this layer form iris processes that can attach to the trabecular meshwork. The number of these processes varies, but they usually do not impede aqueous outflow. The anterior border layer ends at the root.

Iris Stroma and Sphincter Muscle

The connective-tissue **stroma** is composed of pigmented and nonpigmented cells, collagen fibrils, and extensive ground substance. The pigmented cells include melanocytes and clump cells, whereas the nonpigmented cells are fibroblasts, lymphocytes, macrophages, and mast cells.[1] Though melanocytes and fibroblasts have many branching processes, the cells are widely spaced in the stroma, and so their branches do not form a meshwork. **Clump cells** are large, round, darkly pigmented cells and are variously described as displaced neuroectodermal cells or (more likely) altered macrophages.[1, 3] They usually are located in the pupillary portion of the stroma, often near the sphincter muscle.

The iris blood vessels are branches of the circular vessel, the major circle of the iris, located in the ciliary body near the iris root, and usually follow a radial course from the iris root to the pupil margin. Iris blood vessels, even arteries, have an especially thick collagen tunica adventitia and often are referred to as **thick-walled blood vessels**.[1–3] An incomplete circular vessel, the minor circle of the iris, is located in the iris stroma in the region of the

FIGURE 3-1. Light micrograph of the iris and anterior chamber. The cornea, anterior chamber angle, trabecular meshwork, canal of Schlemm, and part of the ciliary body are included. The anterior and posterior iris contraction furrows are accentuated by the slight dilatation of the pupil. The pupil and the pupillary ruff are at *a*, and the iris root is at *b*. The pupillary portion of the iris is at *c*, and the ciliary portion at *d*. The collarette (*e*) and minor arterial circle of the iris lie at the junction of these two portions. The cellular anterior border layer (*f*) is distinct from the very loosely arranged stromal tissue (*g*). The sphincter muscle lies in the stroma (*h*). The posterior iris shows a posterior (*i*) and anterior (*j*) epithelium; the latter forms the dilator muscle. The anterior chamber angle shows part of a uveal band (*k*). The trabecular meshwork (*l*) and canal of Schlemm (*m*) lie external to the chamber angle. The ciliary body and its muscle are posterior to the iris (*n*) (×60). (Reprinted with permission from MJ Hogan, JA Alvarado, JE Weddell. Histology of the Human Eye. Philadelphia: Saunders, 1971;210.)

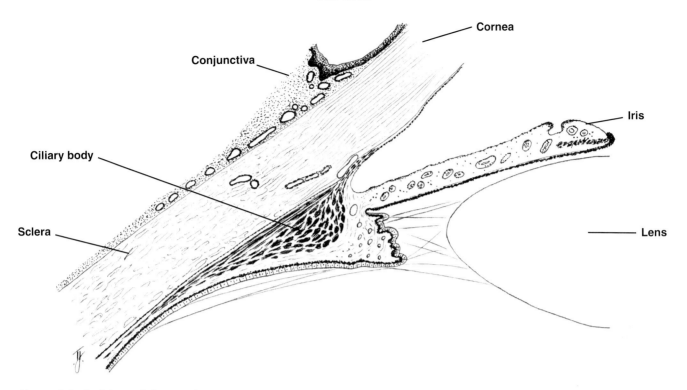

FIGURE 3-2. Periphery of the anterior segment.

FIGURE 3-3. Anterior layers of the iris. The anterior border layer is covered by a single layer of fibroblasts (*a*), the long, branching processes of which interconnect. The branching processes of the fibroblasts form variably-sized openings on the iris surface. Beneath the layer of fibroblasts is a fairly dense aggregation of melanocytes and a few fibroblasts. The superficial layer of fibroblasts has been removed at (*b*) to show these cells. The number of cells in the anterior border layer is greater than that in the underlying stroma. The iris stroma contains a number of capillaries (*c*) that sometimes are quite close to the surface. (Reprinted with permission from MJ Hogan, JA Alvarado, JE Weddell. Histology of the Human Eye. Philadelphia: Saunders, 1971;217.)

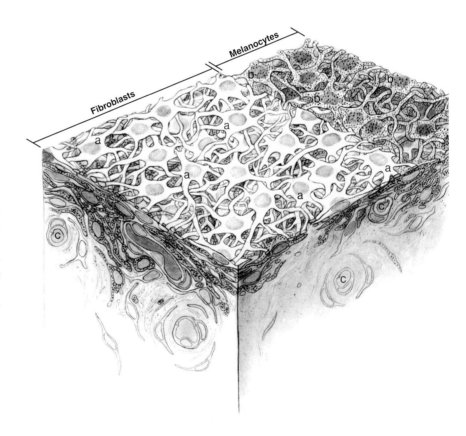

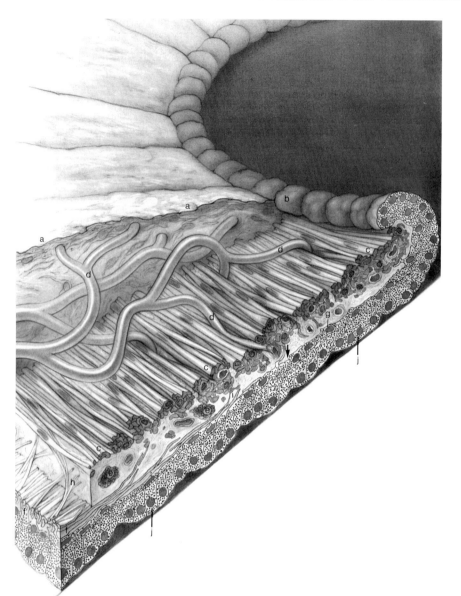

FIGURE 3-4. Pupillary portion of the iris. The dense, cellular anterior border layer (*a*) terminates at the pigment ruff (*b*) in the pupillary margin. The sphincter muscle is at (*c*). The arcades (*d*) from the minor circle extend toward the pupil and through the sphincter muscle. The sphincter muscle and the iris epithelium are close to each other at the pupillary margin. Capillaries, nerves, melanocytes, and clump cells (*e*) are found within and around the muscles. The three to five layers of dilator muscle (*f*) gradually diminish in number until they terminate behind the midportion of the sphincter muscle (arrow), leaving low, cuboidal epithelial cells (*g*) to form the anterior epithelium of the pupillary margin. Spurlike extensions from the dilator muscle form Michel's spur (*h*) and Fuchs' spur (*i*), which extend anteriorly to blend with the sphincter muscle. The posterior epithelium (*j*) is formed by tall columnar cells with basally located nuclei. Its apical surface is contiguous with the apical surface of the anterior epithelium. (Reprinted with permission from MJ Hogan, JA Alvarado, JE Weddell. Histology of the Human Eye. Philadelphia: Saunders, 1971;231.)

collarette and is a remnant of embryologic development. The iris capillaries are not fenestrated and form part of the blood-aqueous barrier.[1] The iris stroma is continuous with the stroma of the ciliary body.

The **sphincter muscle** lies within the stroma (see Figure 3-1) and is composed of smooth-muscle cells joined by tight junctions.[1] It is, as its name implies, a circular muscle 0.75–1 mm wide, encircling the pupil and located in the pupillary zone of the stroma (Figure 3-4).[1, 2] The sphincter muscle is anchored firmly to adjacent stroma and retains its function even if severed radially.[1] Contraction of the sphincter causes the pupil to constrict in **miosis**. The muscle is innervated by the parasympathetic system.

✐ CLINICAL COMMENT: IRIDECTOMY

In some cases of glaucoma, to facilitate the movement of aqueous from the posterior chamber to the anterior chamber, an iridectomy is performed. Via this surgical procedure, a wedge-shaped, full-thickness section of tissue is removed from the iris. If the sphincter muscle is cut during this procedure, the ability of the muscle to contract is not lost. Iridotomy, a similar procedure in which an opening is made in the iris without excising tissue, often is accomplished using a laser, and the muscle usually is not involved.

Anterior Epithelium and Dilator Muscle

Posterior to the stroma are two layers of epithelium. The first of these, the epithelial layer lying nearest to the stroma, is the **anterior iris epithelium**, which is composed of the unique myoepithelial cell. The apical portion is pigmented cuboidal epithelium joined by tight junctions and desmosomes, whereas the basal portion is composed of elongated, contractile, smooth-muscle processes (Figure 3-5). The muscle fibers extend into the stroma,

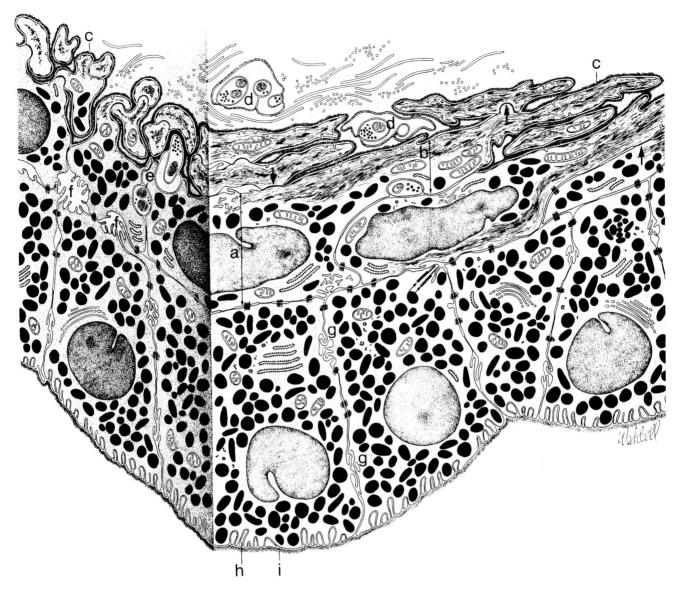

FIGURE 3-5. Posterior epithelial layers. The anterior iris epithelium has two morphologically distinct portions: an apical epithelial portion (*a*) and a basal muscular portion (*b*). The cytoplasm of the basal portion is filled with myofibrils and a moderate number of mitochondria. The tongue-like muscular processes overlap, creating three to five layers. Tight junctions (arrows), such as those in the sphincter muscle, are found between the dilator muscle cells. A basement membrane (*c*) surrounds the muscle processes. Unmyelinated nerves and their associated Schwann cells (*d*), as well as a few naked axons, innervate the muscle. The axon (*e*) is in close contact with the anterior epithelium, being separated from it by a space measuring 200 Å wide. The cytoplasm of the epithelial portions contains cell organelles, melanin granules, the nucleus, and bundles of myofilaments. Most of the intercellular junctions present here are maculae occludentes, and only a few desmosomes are present; desmosomes are not found in the muscular portion. The apical surface of the anterior epithelium is contiguous with that of the posterior epithelium. Desmosomes and tight junctions join the two layers, but there are some areas of separation (*f*) between the cells. The spaces so formed are filled with microvilli, and an occasional cilium also is found here (double arrows). The posterior pigmented iris epithelium shows lateral interdigitations (*g*) and areas of infolding along its basal surface (*h*). A typical basement membrane is found also on the basal side (*i*). Numerous tight junctions and desmosomes occur along the lateral and apical walls. The cytoplasm of this epithelium contains numerous melanin granules measuring approximately 0.8 μm in cross section and up to 2.5 μm in length. Stacks of cisternae of the rough-surfaced endoplasmic reticulum, clustered unattached ribosomes, mitochondria, and a Golgi apparatus commonly are observed. (Reprinted with permission from MJ Hogan, JA Alvarado, JE Weddell. Histology of the Human Eye. Philadelphia: Saunders, 1971;255.)

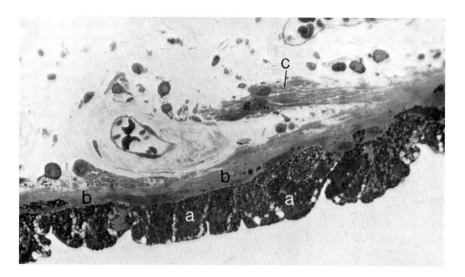

FIGURE 3-6. Posterior iris epithelium (*a*) and dilator muscle (*b*) in the pupillary region. A spur of dilator muscle tissue extends into the stroma toward the sphincter (*c*) (×640). (Reprinted with permission from MJ Hogan, JA Alvarado, JE Weddell. Histology of the Human Eye. Philadelphia: Saunders, 1971;245.)

forming three to five layers of dilator muscle joined by tight junctions.

The **dilator muscle** is present from the iris root to a point in the stroma below the midpoint of the sphincter.[1] Near the termination of the dilator muscle, small projections insert into the stroma or, more accurately, into the sphincter (Figure 3-6).[1,2] Because the fibers are arranged radially, contraction of the dilator muscle pulls the pupillary portion toward the root, thereby enlarging the pupil in **mydriasis**. The dilator is sympathetically innervated.

The anterior epithelium continues to the pupillary margin as cuboidal epithelial cells, and the epithelium continues posteriorly as the pigmented epithelium of the ciliary body.

Posterior Epithelium

The second epithelial layer posterior to the stroma is the **posterior iris epithelium**, a single layer of heavily pigmented, approximately columnar cells joined by tight junctions and desmosomes.[2,3] In the periphery, the posterior iris epithelium begins to lose its pigment as it continues into the ciliary body as the nonpigmented epithelium. A thin basement membrane covers the basal aspect of this cellular layer, lining the posterior chamber.

The anterior and posterior iris epithelial layers are positioned apex to apex, a result of events during embryologic development. Apical microvilli extend from both surfaces, and desmosomes join the two apical surfaces. The epithelial cells curl around from the posterior iris to the anterior surface at the pupillary margin, forming the pigmented **pupillary ruff** or frill, which encircles the pupil; this normally has a serrated appearance (see Figure 3-4).[1]

✍ CLINICAL COMMENT: IRIS SYNECHIAE

An **iris synechia** is an abnormal attachment between the iris surface and another structure. In a **posterior** synechia, the posterior iris surface is adherent to the anterior lens surface. In an **anterior synechia**, the anterior iris surface is adherent to the corneal endothelium or the trabecular meshwork. Synechiae can occur as a result of a sharp blow to the head or a whiplash-type movement that brings the two structures forcefully together. Alternatively, cells and debris from a uveal infection that are circulating in the aqueous humor can make the surfaces "sticky" and so cause synechiae.[4]

If a posterior synechia involves a large portion of the pupillary margin, aqueous will accumulate in the posterior chamber. Continual production of aqueous causes the pressure in the posterior chamber to increase, which in turn causes the iris to bow forward in a configuration called **iris bombé**. This can push the peripheral iris against the trabecular meshwork, setting the stage for a dramatic increase of intraocular pressure (IOP). A drug-induced dilation usually will break a posterior synechia. The break usually occurs between the epithelial layers, leaving remnants of the posterior epithelium on the anterior surface of the lens.

An anterior synechia usually occurs at the iris periphery and involves the meshwork. It is called a **peripheral anterior synechia** (PAS). Aqueous outflow will be impeded by a PAS, causing an increase in IOP if the adhesion occupies a considerable amount of the trabecular meshwork.

Anterior Iris Surface

Thin, radial, collagenous columns or trabeculae are evident on the anterior surface of lightly pigmented irises. Thicker, radially oriented, branching trabeculae encircle depressions or openings in the surface called **crypts**.[3] Crypts are located on both sides of the collarette (**Fuchs'** crypts) and near the root (**peripheral crypts**). They allow the aqueous quick exit and entrance into spaces in the iris stroma as the volume of the iris changes with iris dilation and contraction.

Circular contraction folds, evident on the anterior surface of the ciliary zone, are caused as the tissue moves toward the iris root during pupillary dilation. Plate 3-1 shows the topography of the anterior and posterior iris surfaces.

Posterior Iris Surface

The posterior surface of the iris is fairly smooth but, when viewed with magnification, small circular furrows are evident near the pupil.[2] **Radial contraction furrows (of Schwalbe)** are located in the pupillary zone, and the deeper **structural furrows (of Schwalbe)** run throughout the ciliary zone and continue into the ciliary body as the valleys between the ciliary processes.[1–3] Also found on the posterior surface are **circular contraction folds** similar to those seen on the anterior surface.

Iris Color

Iris color depends on the cell and pigment density and on the collagen arrangement and density in the anterior border layer and stroma.[3] If the iris is heavily pigmented, the anterior surface appears brown and smooth, even velvety, whereas in a lighter iris, the collagen trabeculae are evident and the color ranges from grays to blues to greens depending on density of pigment and collagen. A **freckle** or a **nevus** is an area of hyperpigmentation, an accumulation of melanocytes, and frequently is seen in the anterior layer. In all colored irises, the two epithelial layers are heavily pigmented. Only in the albino iris do the epithelial layers lack pigment.[3]

✍ CLINICAL COMMENT: PIGMENTARY
　　DISPERSION SYNDROME
　　In pigmentary dispersion syndrome, pigment granules are shed from the posterior iris surface and are dispersed into the anterior chamber. They can be deposited on the iris, lens, or corneal endothelium, or in the trabecular meshwork, where they might compromise aqueous outflow.[4] Significant pigment loss will be evident on transillumination of the iris when the red fundus reflex shows through in the depigmented areas.

✍ CLINICAL COMMENT: HETEROCHROMIA
　　Heterochromia of the iris is a condition in which one iris differs in color from the other or portions of one iris differ in color from the rest of the iris. This can be either congenital or a sign of uveal inflammation. A history regarding iris coloration should be elicited.[5]

CILIARY BODY

When viewed from the front of the eye, the **ciliary body** is a ring-shaped structure. Its width is approximately 5.9 mm on the nasal side and 6.7 mm on the temporal side.[2] The posterior area of the ciliary body, which terminates at the ora serrata, appears fairly flat, but the anterior ciliary body contains numerous folds or processes that extend into the posterior chamber. In sagittal section, the ciliary body has a triangular shape, the base of which is located anteriorly; one corner of the base lies at the scleral spur, the iris root extends from the approximate center of the base, and a portion of the base borders the anterior chamber. The outer side of the triangle lies against the sclera, and the inner side lines the posterior chamber and a small portion of the vitreous cavity. The apex is located at the ora serrata (Figure 3-7).

The ciliary body can be divided into two parts: the pars plicata (corona ciliaris) and the pars plana (orbicularis ciliaris). The **pars plicata** is the wider, anterior portion containing the ciliary processes (see Figure 3-7). Approximately 70–80 ciliary processes extend into the posterior chamber, and the regions between them are called **valleys (of Kuhnt)**. A ciliary process measures approximately 2 mm in length, 0.5 mm in width, and 1 mm in height, but there are significant variations in all measurements.[1]

The **pars plana** is the flatter region of the ciliary body. It extends from the posterior of the pars plicata to the **ora serrata**, which is the transition between ciliary body and choroid. The ora serrata has a serrated pattern, the forward-pointing apices of which are called **teeth** or **dentate processes**. The rounded portions that lie between the teeth are called **bays** (Figure 3-8A). The dentate processes are elongations of retinal tissue into the region of the pars plana.

The zonule fibers course from the ciliary body to the lens. Some of these fibers insert into the internal limiting membrane of the pars plana region and travel forward through the valleys between the ciliary processes. Some attach to the internal limiting membrane of the valleys of the pars plicata (Figure 3-8B). The attachment to the vitreous, the vitreous base, extends forward approximately 2 mm over the posterior pars plana.[1]

Supraciliaris (Supraciliary Lamina)

The **supraciliaris** is the outermost layer of the ciliary body adjacent to the sclera. Its loose connective tissue is arranged in ribbonlike layers containing pigmented melanocytes, fibroblasts, and collagen bands.[1] The arrangement of these bands allows the ciliary body to slide against the sclera without detaching from or stretching the tissue. The arrangement of the supraciliaris allows for the accumulation of fluid within its spaces, which

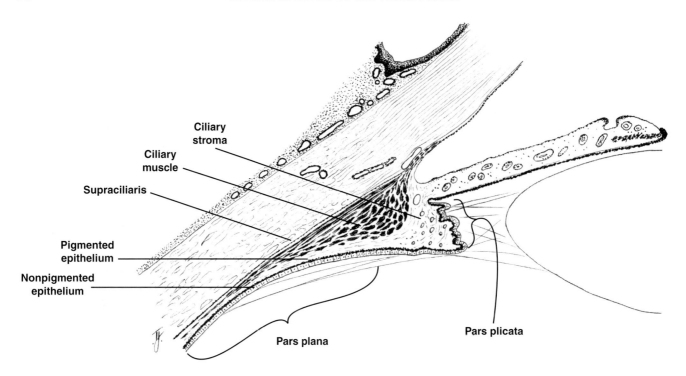

FIGURE 3-7. Partitions and layers of ciliary body.

may cause a displacement of the ciliary body from the sclera. Damage to the layer due to trauma may result in a ciliary body detachment.

Ciliary Muscle

The **ciliary muscle** is composed of smooth-muscle fibers oriented in longitudinal, radial, and circular directions. Interweaving occurs between fiber bundles and from layer to layer, such that various amounts of connective tissue are found among the muscle bundles.[1] The **longitudinal muscle fibers (of Brucke)** lie adjacent to the supraciliaris and parallel to the sclera. Each muscle bundle resembles a long narrow V, the base of which is at the scleral spur, whereas the apex is in the choroid. The tendon of origin attaches the muscle fibers to the scleral spur and to adjacent trabecular meshwork sheets. The insertion of the ciliary muscle is in the anterior one-third of the suprachoroid in the form of stellate-shaped terminations or "muscle stars."[1,2] Below the longitudinal muscle fibers, the **radially oriented fibers** form wider, shorter interdigitating Vs that originate at the scleral spur and insert into the connective tissue near the base of the ciliary processes.[1] This layer is a transition from the longitudinally oriented fibers to the circular fibers.

The innermost region of ciliary muscle, **(Müller's) annular muscle**, is formed of circular muscle bundles with a sphincter-type action. These fibers are located near the major circle of the iris. Figure 3-9 shows the relationship between these regions of the ciliary muscle and surrounding structures.

The ciliary muscle is dually innervated by the autonomic nervous system. Parasympathetic stimulation activates the muscle for contraction, whereas sympathetic innervation likely has an inhibitory effect that is a function of the level of parasympathetic activity.[6–8]

Ciliary Stroma

The highly vascularized, loose connective-tissue **stroma** of the ciliary body lies between the muscle and the epithelial layers and forms the core of each of the ciliary processes; it is continuous with the connective tissue that separates the bundles of ciliary muscle. Anteriorly, the stroma is continuous with iris stroma. It thins in the pars plana, where it continues posteriorly as choroidal stroma. The major arterial circle of the iris is located in the ciliary stroma anterior to the circular muscle and near the iris root. This circular artery is formed by the anastomosis of the long posterior ciliary arteries and the anterior ciliary arteries. The stromal capillaries are large and fenestrated, particularly in the ciliary processes, and most are located near the pigmented epithelium.[1]

Figure 3-8. (A) Inner aspect of the ciliary body shows the pars plicata (*a*) and the pars plana (*b*). The ora serrata is at *c* and, posterior to it, the retina exhibits cystoid degeneration (*d*). The bays (*e*) and dentate processes (*f*) of the ora are shown; linear ridges or striae (*g*) project forward from the dentate processes across the pars plana to enter the valleys between the ciliary processes. The zonular fibers arise from the pars plana beginning 1.5 mm from the ora serrata. They curve forward from the sides of the dentate ridges into the ciliary valleys, then from the valleys to the lens capsule. Zonules coming from the valleys on either side of a ciliary process have a common point of attachment on the lens. The zonules attach up to 1 mm from the equator posteriorly and up to 1.5 mm from the equator anteriorly. At the equatorial border, the attaching zonules give a crenated appearance to the lens. The ciliary processes vary in size and shape and often are separated from one another by lesser processes. The radial (*h*) and circular furrows (*i*) of the peripheral iris are shown.

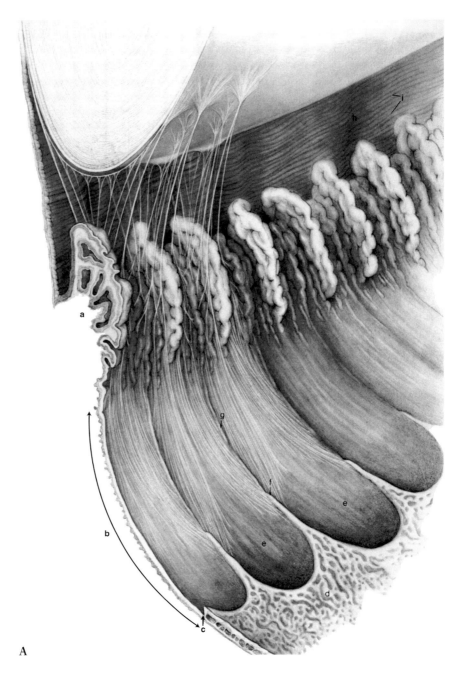

A

Ciliary Epithelium

Two layers of epithelium, positioned apex to apex, cover the ciliary body and line the posterior chamber and part of the vitreous chamber. Both epithelial layers contain cellular components characteristic of cells actively involved in secretion.[9]

The outer layer (i.e., the one next to the stroma) is pigmented and cuboidal, and the cells are joined by desmosomes and gap junctions.[1, 10, 11] Anteriorly, the **pigmented ciliary epithelium** is continuous with the anterior iris epithelium and, posteriorly, it is continuous with the retinal pigment epithelium (RPE). A basement membrane attaches the pigment epithelium to the stroma. This base-

ment membrane is continuous anteriorly with the basement membrane of the anterior iris epithelium and posteriorly with the inner basement membrane portion of Bruch's membrane of the choroid.[1]

The inner epithelial layer (i.e., the one lining the posterior chamber) is nonpigmented and is composed of columnar cells in the pars plana and cuboidal cells in the pars plicata.[1] The lateral walls of the cells contain extensive interdigitations and are joined, near their apices, by desmosomes, gap junctions, and zonula occludens, which form one site of the blood-aqueous barrier.[3, 10–12] The **nonpigmented ciliary epithelium** is continuous anteriorly with the posterior iris epithelium (Figure 3-10) and posteriorly at the ora serrata, where it undergoes significant

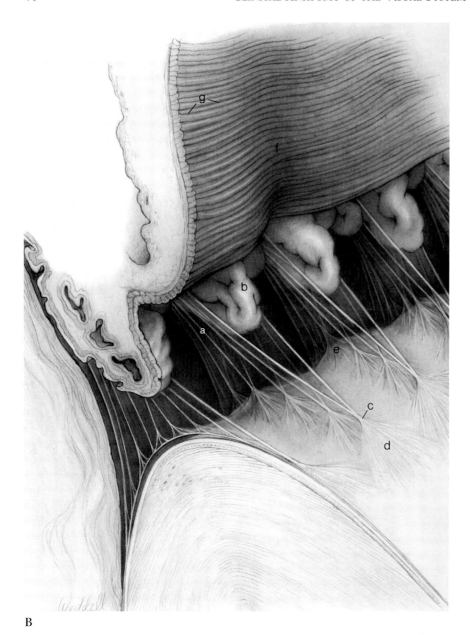

FIGURE 3-8. (*continued*) (B) Anterior view of the ciliary processes showing the zonules attaching to the lens. Zonules form columns (*a*) on either side of the ciliary processes (*b*), which meet on a single site (*c*) as they attach to the lens. These two columns form a triangle, the base of which is on the ciliary body and the apex of which is on the lens. The zonules form a tentlike structure (*d*) as they become attached to the lens capsule. The equatorial surface of the lens is crenated (*e*) by the attachment of the zonule. The iris is pulled upward, revealing its posterior surface, with the radial (*f*) folds and the circular furrows (*g*). (Reprinted with permission from MJ Hogan, JA Alvarado, JE Weddell. Histology of the Human Eye. Philadelphia: Saunders, 1971;272.)

B

transformation, becomes neural retina. The metabolically active nonpigmented epithelial cells are involved in active secretion of aqueous humor components and serve as a diffusion barrier between blood and aqueous.[13]

The two epithelial layers are positioned apex to apex because of invagination of the neural ectoderm in forming the optic cup (see Chapter 7). Intercellular junctions, desmosomes, and tight junctions connect the two layers.[1] Gap junctions between the apical surfaces provide a means of cellular communication between the layers and probably are important in the formation of aqueous.[10–12, 14]

The basement membrane covering the nonpigmented epithelium, the internal limiting membrane of the ciliary body, lines the posterior chamber, is continuous with the internal limiting membrane of the retina, and is the attachment site for the zonular fibers as well as the fibers of the vitreous base. The basal aspect of the nonpigmented cell has numerous infoldings, into which the basement membrane extends.[1, 3]

CHOROID

The **choroid** extends from the ora serrata to the optic nerve and is located between the sclera and the retina, providing nutrients to outer retinal layers. It is made up primarily of blood vessels. However, a thin connective-tissue layer lies on each side of the stromal vessel layer (Figure 3-11).

FIGURE 3-9. Ciliary body, including the ciliary muscle and its components. The cornea and sclera have been dissected away, but the trabecular meshwork (*a*), Schlemm's canal (*b*), and two external collectors (*c*), as well as the scleral spur (*d*), have been left undisturbed. The three components of the ciliary muscle are shown separately, viewed from the outside and sectioned meridionally. Section *1* shows the longitudinal ciliary muscle. In section *2*, the longitudinal ciliary muscle has been dissected away to show the radial ciliary muscle. In section *3*, only the innermost circular ciliary muscle is shown. According to Calasans,[34] the ciliary muscle originates in the ciliary tendon, which includes the scleral spur (*d*) and the adjacent connective tissue. The cells originate as paired V-shaped bundles. The longitudinal muscle forms long V-shaped trellises (*e*) that terminate in the epichoroidal stars (*f*). The arms of the V-shaped bundles formed by the radial muscle meet at wide angles (*g*) and terminate in the ciliary processes. The V-shaped bundles of the circular muscle originate at such distant points in the ciliary tendon that their arms meet at a very wide angle (*h*). The iridic portion is shown at (*i*) joining the circular muscle cells. (Reprinted with permission from MJ Hogan, JA Alvarado, JE Weddell. Histology of the Human Eye. Philadelphia: Saunders, 1971;309.)

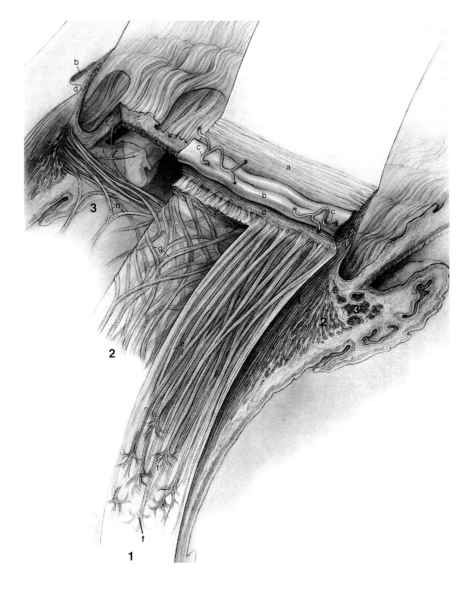

Suprachoroid Lamina (Lamina Fusca)

Thin, pigmented, ribbonlike branching bands of connective tissue, the **suprachoroid lamina** or **lamina fusca**, traverse a potential space, the suprachoroidal or perichoroidal space, between the sclera and the choroidal vessels.[1, 3] This layer contains components from both sclera (collagen bands and fibroblasts) and choroidal stroma (melanocytes).[1] If the choroid separates from the sclera, part of the suprachoroid will adhere to the sclera and part will remain attached to the choroid.[2] The looseness of the tissue allows the vascular net to swell without causing detachment. The anterior suprachoroidal lamina is the site of the muscle-star insertions of the longitudinal muscle fibers from the ciliary body. The suprachoroidal space carries the long posterior ciliary arteries and nerves from the posterior to the anterior portion of the globe.

Choroidal Stroma

The **choroidal stroma** is a pigmented, vascularized, loose connective-tissue layer containing melanocytes, fibroblasts, macrophages, lymphocytes, and mast cells. Collagen fibrils are arranged circularly around the vessels, which are branches of the short, posterior ciliary arteries. These vessels are organized into tiers, those with larger lumina occupying the outer layer (**Haller's layer**). They branch as they pass inward, forming the medium-sized vessels (**Sattler's layer**), which continue branching to form a capillary bed (Plate 3-2). The venules join to become veins that gather in a characteristic vortex pattern in each quadrant of the eye and exit the choroid as four (occasionally five) large vortex veins. Choroidal veins are unusual in that they contain no valves.[2]

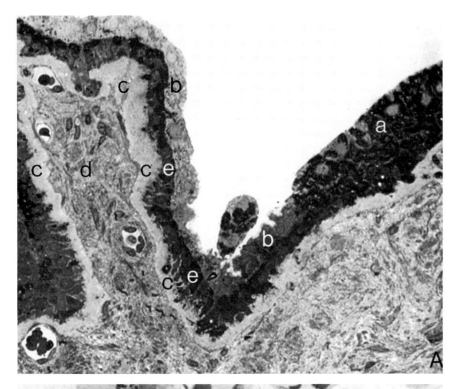

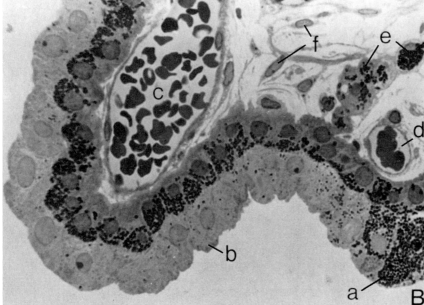

FIGURE 3-10. (A) Light micrograph of the ciliary body of an elderly person. The transition of the pigmented iris epithelium (*a*) into the nonpigmented ciliary epithelium (*b*) is shown. Note the basement membrane-like strip (*c*) interposed between the dense collagenous connective tissue layers of this ciliary process (*d*) and the pigmented epithelium (*e*) (×500). (B) Light micrograph of the ciliary body of a young person, showing the transition of the nonpigmented ciliary body epithelium (*b*) into the pigmented iris epithelium. The epithelium reveals increasing numbers of melanin granules until some of the cells become filled with pigment (*a*). A large vein (*c*) and a capillary (*d*) lie in the stroma close to the pigmented epithelium. Compare the stroma of the young eye with that shown in (A). Some melanocytes (*e*) and fibroblasts (*f*) are seen (×640). (Reprinted with permission from MJ Hogan, JA Alvarado, JE Weddell. Histology of the Human Eye. Philadelphia: Saunders, 1971;275.)

The choroidal vessels are innervated by the autonomic nervous system. Sympathetic stimulation causes vasoconstriction. The effect of the parasympathetic system is less clear.[15]

Choriocapillaris

The specialized capillary bed is called the **choriocapillaris**. It forms a single layer of anastomosing, fenestrated capillaries having wide lumina. In each, the lumen is approximately three to four times that of ordinary capillaries, such that two or three red blood cells can pass through the capillary abreast, whereas in ordinary capillaries the cells usually course single file (see Figure 3-11B).[1] Occasional pericytes (Rouget's cells), which may have a contractile function, are found around the capillary wall.[1, 3] The choriocapillaris is densest in the macular area, where it is the sole blood

FIGURE 3-11. (A) Photomicrograph of a section through the full thickness of the eye. Retina (*R*), choroid (*C*), sclera (*S*), and muscle (*M*) fibers of an extraocular muscle are seen (×50). (B) Pigment epithelium (×1,000). (Part A reprinted with permission from CR Leeson, ST Leeson. Histology. Philadelphia: Saunders, 1976;557. Part B reprinted with permission from WJ Krause, JH Cutts. Concise Text of Histology. Baltimore: Williams & Wilkins, 1981;181.)

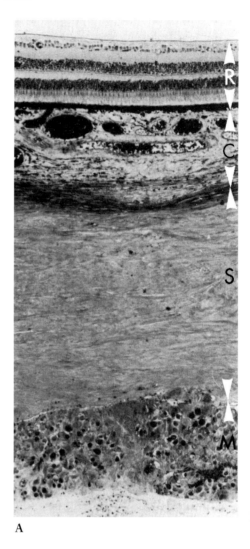

A

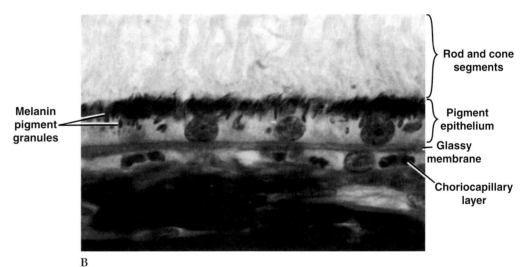

Rod and cone segments

Pigment epithelium

Glassy membrane

Choriocapillary layer

Melanin pigment granules

B

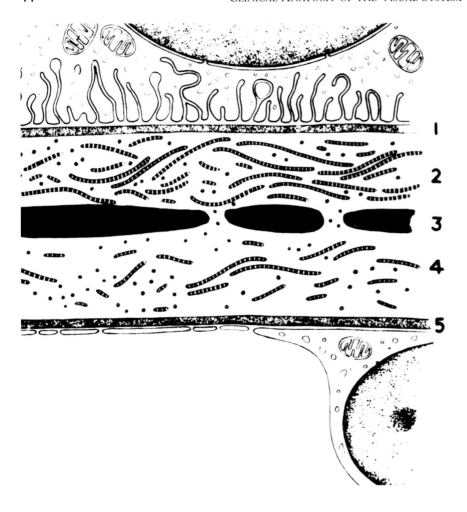

FIGURE 3-12. The layers of Bruch's membrane, delineated on the basis of electron-microscopic studies: (1) the basement membrane of the retinal pigment epithelial cells, (2) the inner collagenous zone, (3) the elastic layer, (4) the outer collagenous zone, and (5) the interrupted basement membrane of the choriocapillaris. (Reprinted with permission from MJ Hogan, JA Alvarado, JE Weddell. Histology of the Human Eye. Philadelphia: Saunders, 1971;331.)

supply for a small region of retina. The choriocapillaris is unique to the choroid and does not continue into the ciliary body.

Bruch's Membrane (Basal Lamina)

The innermost layer of the choroid, **Bruch's membrane**, unites with the retina. It runs from the optic nerve to the ora serrata, where it undergoes some modification before continuing into the ciliary body.[1] Bruch's membrane (or the **basal lamina**) is a multilaminated sheet containing a center layer of elastic fibers. At the electron-microscopic level, the membrane components, from outer to inner, are (1) the interrupted basement membrane of the choriocapillaris, (2) the outer collagenous zone, (3) the elastic layer, (4) the inner collagenous zone, and (5) the basement membrane of the RPE cells (Figure 3-12).[1, 2] Fine filaments from the basement membrane of the RPE merge with the fibrils of the inner collagenous zone, contributing to the tight adhesion between choroid and the outer pigmented layer of the retina.

At the ora serrata, the basement membrane of the RPE is continuous with the basement membrane of the pigmented epithelium of the ciliary body, the collagenous and elastic layers disappear into the ciliary stroma, and the basement membrane of the choriocapillaris continues as the basement membrane of the ciliary body capillaries.

FUNCTIONS OF THE UVEA

Functions of the Iris

The iris acts as a diaphragm to regulate the amount of light entering the eye. The two iris muscles are innervated separately: The parasympathetically innervated sphincter muscle is responsible for constriction of the pupil, and the sympathetically innervated dilator muscle causes pupillary enlargement.

Functions of the Ciliary Body

The ciliary body produces and secretes the aqueous humor. Its musculature causes accommodation and can affect aqueous outflow.

✍ CLINICAL COMMENT: ACCOMMODATION
The ability of the eye to change power and bring near objects into focus on the retina is called **accommodation**. It is accomplished by increasing

the power of the lens. Contraction of the ciliary muscle decreases the diameter of the ring formed by the ciliary body, releasing tension on the zonule fibers and allowing the lens capsule to adopt a more spherical shape. The lens thickens, and the anterior surface curve increases. These changes result in an increase in refractive power, or accommodation. When the ciliary muscle is relaxed, the eye is said to be at rest and is used for distance vision. During accommodation, the iris sphincter also contracts, restricting incoming light rays and decreasing spherical aberration.

Ciliary muscle contraction can change the configuration of the trabecular meshwork because some of the longitudinal fibers are attached to trabecular meshwork sheets. This altered configuration can facilitate aqueous movement through the anterior chamber angle structures.[16] Accommodation has been found to cause a decrease in IOP.[17] Accommodation is discussed further in Chapter 5.

✎ CLINICAL COMMENT: PRESBYOPIA
Presbyopia is the loss of the ability to accommodate, a normal age-related change and the subject of continuing research. In rhesus monkeys, the tendon that attaches the ciliary muscle to the scleral spur shows extensive age-related structural changes: It thickens with age, and becomes surrounded by a dense layer of collagen, thus losing its elasticity. This loss of elasticity restricts muscle movement and hampers accommodation.[18] A similar mechanism may be a component of human presbyopia, along with changes involving the lens itself; these are discussed in Chapter 5.

Aqueous Production

Both the ciliary body capillaries and the epithelial layers are active in the production and secretion of aqueous. The large capillaries of the ciliary body have numerous fenestrations, which facilitate the movement of substances into and out of the blood.[1] Active transport and secretion move substances from the stroma through the epithelium. The nonpigmented epithelium, in particular, actively secretes components of the aqueous humor into the posterior chamber.[1, 2]

Blood-Aqueous Barrier

The **blood-aqueous barrier** selectively controls the substance that is secreted as the aqueous humor. The fenestrated ciliary body capillaries permit large molecules to exit the blood. However, the tight zonular junctions of the nonpigmented epithelium prevent the molecules from passing between the cells, forcing them instead to pass through the cell to enter the posterior chamber. One of

the substances thus controlled is protein. The protein content of aqueous humor is very small when compared to that of blood.[19] Proteins pass easily out of the ciliary vessels through the fenestrations but are not secreted into the posterior chamber owing to the tight junction barrier of the nonpigmented epithelium.[11, 20, 21]

The iris is freely permeated by the aqueous humor, which readily enters the stroma via the surface crypts.[1] To prevent large molecules from leaking out of the iris blood vessels and altering the content of the aqueous fluid, the iris capillaries have no fenestrations, and their endothelial cells maintain the barrier function via the zonula occludens junctions.[22]

Functions of the Choroid

The vascular choroid provides nutrients to the outer retina and is an egress for catabolites from the retina, which diffuse through Bruch's membrane into the choriocapillaris. The darkly pigmented choroid absorbs excess light that passes through the RPE layer. The suprachoroidal space provides a pathway for the posterior vessels and nerves that supply the anterior segment.

With aging, excessive basement membrane (basal lamina) material is deposited in the collagenous zones of Bruch's membrane.[23–25] These deposits in the inner collagenous zone, called **drusen**, can be seen as small, pinhead-sized, yellow-white spots in the fundus. The drusen, which contain cellular fragments and an accumulation of basal laminar material, are located below the RPE basement membrane and displace the retina inward.[26]

✎ CLINICAL COMMENT: AGE-RELATED
MACULAR DEGENERATION
Degenerative processes involving the choroid-retina interface in the macular area often are manifested as **age-related macular degeneration** (ARMD). ARMD is the most common cause of blindness in Western countries.[27] It is multifaceted in origin and involves the presence of multiple or confluent drusen, a thick layer of basal laminar deposit, and detachment or atrophy of the RPE and photoreceptors. Subretinal neovascularization with subsequent formation of disciform scars also may occur.[26, 28]

Metabolites from the choriocapillaris and waste products from the retina must pass through Bruch's membrane. As a person ages, phospholipids accumulate in the membrane, probably owing to defective mechanisms in the dephosphorylation process.[24, 29–31] The accumulation of lipids in Bruch's membrane with increasing age appears to be greater in the central fundus than in the periphery.[32] Bruch's membrane becomes hydrophobic and presents a barrier to water movement, thereby inhibiting the passage of metabolites and catabo-

Young

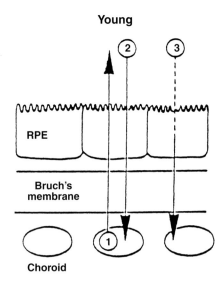

Old

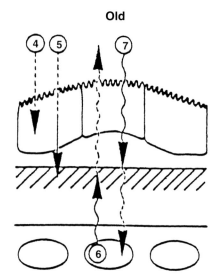

FIGURE 3-13. Summary of the implications of lipid accumulation in Bruch's membrane for transport systems operating across the retinal pigment epithelium (RPE). In the youngest age group, (1) metabolites pass from the choroid through Bruch's membrane across the RPE to the neural retina; (2) water moves predominantly from the neural retina to the choroid; (3) the progress of catabolism results in accumulation of waste products that are predominantly cleared via the choroid. In the older age group, (4) with increasing age, catabolism results in accumulation within the RPE, namely lipofuscin; (5) waste products rich in lipid begin to accumulate within Bruch's membrane; (6) the accumulation of lipid-rich debris within Bruch's membrane may inhibit metabolic input to the neural retina; and (7) the presence of a hydrophobic barrier within Bruch's membrane will impede the passage of water and may result in detachment of the RPE. (Reprinted with permission from D Pauliekhoff, CA Harper, J Marshall, et al. Aging changes in Bruch's membrane. A histochemical and morphological study. Ophthalmology 1990;97[2]:171.)

lites. If water accumulates between the RPE and Bruch's membrane, displacement and detachment of the retina may occur.[31] This process is represented diagrammatically in Figure 3-13.

Loss of nutrients to the highly metabolic retina can cause two responses: atrophy of the RPE and photoreceptors or the development of a neovascular membrane in an attempt to compensate for the loss of nutrients. The new vessels branch from the choriocapillaris and penetrate Bruch's membrane. However, they are fragile, leak, and tend to hemorrhage into retinal tissue.[31, 33] Visual loss in ARMD results from detachment of the RPE due to water accumulation, atrophy of the RPE and photoreceptors, or the presence of a subretinal neovascular membrane.[24, 29]

BLOOD SUPPLY TO THE UVEAL TRACT

The short posterior ciliary arteries enter the globe in a circle around the optic nerve, and their branches form the choroidal vessels. The long posterior ciliary arteries and the anterior ciliary arteries join to form the major circle of the iris, which supplies vessels to the iris and cil-

iary body. The venous return for most of the uvea is via the vortex veins.[1, 2] See Chapter 11 for more information on these vessels.

UVEAL INNERVATION

Sensory innervation of the uvea is via the nasociliary branch from the trigeminal nerve. Sympathetic fibers from the superior cervical ganglion via the ophthalmic and short ciliary nerves innervate the choroidal blood vessels, and sympathetic fibers from the superior cervical ganglion via the long ciliary nerves innervate the iris dilator and ciliary muscle. Parasympathetic fibers from the ciliary ganglion innervate the ciliary muscle, the iris sphincter, and the choroidal vessels.

REFERENCES

1. Hogan MJ, Alvarado JA. Histology of the Human Eye. Philadelphia: Saunders, 1971;202.

2. Warwick R. Wolff's Anatomy of the Eye and Orbit (7th ed). Philadelphia: Saunders, 1976;61.

3. Fine BS, Yanoff M. Ocular Histology. Hagerstown, MD: Harper & Row, 1979;195.

4. Bartlett JD, Jaanus SD. Clinical Ocular Pharmacology (3rd ed). Boston: Butterworth–Heinemann, 1995;776, 915.

5. Catania LJ. Primary Care of the Anterior Segment. East Norwalk, CT: Appleton & Lange, 1988;211.

6. Gilmartin B. A review of the role of sympathetic innervation of the ciliary muscle in ocular accommodation. Ophthalmic Physiol Opt 1986;6(1):23.

7. Rosenfield M, Gilmartin B. Oculomotor consequences of beta-adrenoreceptor antagonism during sustained near vision. Ophthalmic Physiol Opt 1987; 7(2):127.

8. Gilmartin B, Bullimore MA, Rosenfield M, et al. Pharmacological effects on accommodative adaptation. Optom Vis Sci 1992;69(4):276.

9. Eichhorn M, Inada K, Lutjen-Drecoll E. Human ciliary body in organ culture. Curr Eye Res 1991;19(4):277.

10. Raviola G, Raviola E. Intercellular junctions in the ciliary epithelium. Invest Ophthalmol Vis Sci 1978;17:958.

11. Caprioli J. The Ciliary Epithelia and Aqueous Humor. In WM Hart Jr (ed), Adler's Physiology of the Eye (9th ed). St. Louis: Mosby–Year Book, 1992;228.

12. Raviola G. The structural basis of the blood-ocular barriers. Exp Eye Res 1977;25(Suppl):27.

13. Shiose Y. Electron microscopic studies on blood-retinal and blood-aqueous barriers [abstract]. Jpn J Ophthalmol 1970;14:73.

14. Takats K, Kasahara T, Kasahara M, et al. Ultracytochemical localization of the erythrocyte/HepG2–type glucose transporter (GLUT1) in the ciliary body and iris of the rat eye. Invest Ophthalmol Vis Sci 1991; 32(5):1659.

15. Ruskell G. Facial parasympathetic innervation of the choroidal blood vessels in monkeys. Exp Eye Res 1971;12:166.

16. Ebersberger A, Flugel C, Lutjen-Drecoll E. Ultrastructural and enzyme histochemical studies of regional structural differences within the ciliary muscle in various species [abstract]. Klin Monatsbl Augenheilkd 1993;203(1):53.

17. Mauger RR, Likens CP, Applebaum M. Effects of accommodation and repeated applanation tonometry on intraocular pressure. Am J Optom Physiol Opt 1984;61(1):28.

18. Tamm E, Lutjen-Drecoll E, Rohen JW, et al. Posterior attachment of ciliary muscle in young, accommodating, old, presbyopic monkeys. Invest Ophthalmol Vis Sci 1991;32:1678.

19. Krause U, Raunio V. Proteins of the normal human aqueous humor. Ophthalmologica 1970;160: 280.

20. Smith RS. Ultrastructural studies of the blood-aqueous barrier: I. Transport of an electron dense tracer in the iris and ciliary body of the mouse. Am J Ophthalmol 1971;71:1066.

21. Varma SD, Reddy DVN. Phospholipid composition of aqueous humor plasma and lens in normal and alloxam diabetic rabbits. Exp Eye Res 1972; 13:120.

22. Waitzman MB, Jackson RT. Effects of topically administered ouabain on aqueous humor dynamics. Exp Eye Res 1965;4:135.

23. Sarks SH. Aging and degeneration in the macular region: a clinico-pathological study. Br J Ophthalmol 1976;60:324.

24. van der Schaft TL, Mooy CM, deBrujin WC, et al. Histological features of the early stages of age-related macular degeneration: a statistical analysis. Ophthalmology 1992;99:278.

25. van der Schaft TL, Mooy CM, deBrujin WC, et al. Immunohistochemical light and electron microscopy of basal laminar deposit. Graefes Arch Clin Exp Ophthalmol 1994;232(1):40.

26. Ramrattan RS, van der Schaft TL, Mooy CM, et al. Morphometric analysis of Bruch's membrane, the choriocapillaris, and the choroid in aging. Invest Ophthalmol Vis Sci 1994;35(6):2857.

27. Leibowitz HM, Kruegar DE, Maunde LR, et al. The Framingham eye study monograph: an ophthalmological and epidemiological study of cataract, glaucoma, diabetic retinopathy, macular degeneration, and visual acuity in a general population of 2631 adults. Surv Ophthalmol 1980;24:335.

28. Bressler NM, Bressler B, Fine SL. Age-related macular degeneration. Surv Ophthalmol 1988;32: 375.

29. Sheraidah G, Steinmetz R, Maguire J, et al. Correlation between lipids extracted from Bruch's membrane and age. Ophthalmology 1993;100(1):47.

30. Pauleikhoff D. Drusen in Bruch's membrane. Their significance for the pathogenesis and therapy of age-associated macular degeneration [abstract]. Ophthalmologe 1992;89(5):363.

31. Pauleikhoff D, Harper CA, Marshall J, et al. Aging changes in Bruch's membrane. A histochemical and morphological study. Ophthalmology 1990; 97(2):171.

32. Holz FG, Shersidah G, Pauleikhoff D, et al. Analysis of lipid deposits extracted from human macular and peripheral Bruch's membrane. Arch Ophthalmol 1994;112(3):402.

33. Bailey RN. The surgical removal of a subfoveal choroidal neovascular membrane: an alternative treatment to laser photocoagulation. J Am Optom Assoc 1993;64(2):104.

34. Calasans OM. The architecture of the ciliary muscle of man. Ann Fam Med Univ Sao Paolo 1953; 27:3.

CHAPTER

4

The Retina

The innermost coat of the eye is a neural layer, the retina, located between the choroid and the vitreous. It includes the macula, the area at the posterior pole used for sharpest acuity and color vision. The retina extends from the circular edge of the optic disc, where the nerve fibers exit the eye, to the ora serrata. It is continuous with the epithelial layers of the ciliary body with which it shares embryologic origin. The retina is derived from neural ectoderm and consists of an outer pigmented layer, derived from the outer layer of the optic cup, and the neural retina, derived from the inner layer of the optic cup (see Chapter 7). The pigmented layer is tightly adherent to the choroid throughout, but the neural retina is attached only to the pigmented epithelium and thus to the choroid in a peripapillary ring around the disc and at the ora serrata. Although it contains millions of cell bodies and their processes, the neural retina has the appearance of a thin, transparent membrane.

The retina is the site of transformation of light energy into a neural signal and contains the first three types of cells in the visual pathway, the route by which visual information from the environment reaches the central nervous system for interpretation. Those three types of cells are the photoreceptor, the bipolar, and the ganglion cells. Photoreceptor cells transform photons of light into a neural signal and transfer this signal to bipolar cells, which in turn synapse with ganglion cells that transmit the signal from the eye. Other retinal cells—horizontal cells, amacrine cells, and interplexiform neurons—modify and integrate the signal before it leaves the eye. These cells and the detailed anatomy of the retina are discussed in this chapter. The remainder of the visual pathway is described in Chapter 14.

RETINAL HISTOLOGIC FEATURES

Under light microscopy, the retina has a laminar appearance in which 10 layers are evident (Figure 4-1). On closer examination, it can be seen that these are not all true layers but rather a single layer of pigmented epithelium and three layers of neuronal cell bodies between which lie their processes and synapses. The epithelial layer and the types and functions of the neural cells are described first, followed by a discussion of the components of each of the 10 so called retinal layers.

Retinal Pigment Epithelium

The **retinal pigment epithelium (RPE)**, the outermost retinal layer, is a single cell thick and consists of pigmented hexagonal cells. These cells are columnar in the area of the posterior pole and are even longer, narrower, and more densely pigmented in the macular area.[1] The cells become larger and more cuboidal as the layer nears the ora serrata, where the transition to the pigmented epithelium of the ciliary body is located. Owing to the orientation of the embryologic cells, the basal aspect of the cells is adjacent to the choroid, and the apical surface faces neural retina. The basal aspect contains numerous infoldings and is adherent to its basement membrane, which forms a part of Bruch's membrane of the choroid; therefore, its attachment to the choroid is strong. Despite its close association with the choroid, the RPE is considered a part of the retina as it is from the same embryologic germ-cell layer—namely, neural ectoderm.

The RPE cells contain numerous melanosomes, pigment granules that extend from the basal area into the

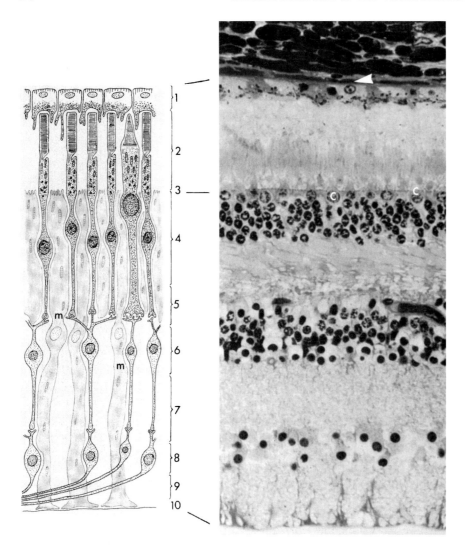

FIGURE 4-1. (Left) Layers of the retina. (1) Retinal pigment epithelial layer; (2) photoreceptor layer; (3) external limiting membrane; (4) outer nuclear layer; (5) outer plexiform layer; (6) inner nuclear layer; (7) inner plexiform layer; (8) ganglion cell layer; (9) nerve fiber layer; (10) internal limiting membrane. Only photoreceptors (rods and one cone), bipolar cells, ganglion cells, and the fibers of Müller (m) are illustrated. The numbers refer to the layers as listed in the text. (Right) Photomicrograph of same area (×400). At top is the inner portion of the choroid with choriocapillaris (dark, arrow). Cone nuclei are indicated (c). (Reprinted with permission from CR Leeson, ST Leeson. Histology. Philadelphia: Saunders, 1976;556.)

middle portion of the cell and somewhat obscure the nucleus, which is located in the basal region. Pigment density differs in various parts of the retina and in individual cells, which might give the fundus a mottled appearance when viewed with the ophthalmoscope. Other pigmented bodies, lipofuscin granules, contain degradation products of phagocytosis and increase in number with age.[1–5] The cell cytoplasm also contains smooth and rough endoplasmic reticulum, Golgi apparatus, and numerous lysosomes.

The apical portion of an RPE cell consists of microvilli that extend into the layer of photoreceptors, enveloping the specialized outer segment tips (Figure 4-2). However, no intercellular junctions connect the RPE and photoreceptor layers. A potential space separates the epithelial cell and the photoreceptor.[1] This is the subretinal space[6] and is a remnant of the gap formed between the two layers of the optic cup on invagination of the optic vesicle (see Chapter 7).

Terminal bars consisting of zonula occludens and zonula adherens join the RPE cells near their apices.[1] Gap junctions between the cells allow for electrical cou-

pling, providing a low-resistance pathway for the passage of ions and metabolites.[7]

Photoreceptor Cells

Photoreceptor cells, the rods and cones, are special sense cells containing photopigments that absorb photons of light. The cells originally were named for their shapes, but more important in the designation of rods or cones is the level of illumination in which each is active; the name does not always reflect the shape, particularly in the cone population. Rods are more active in dim illumination, and cones are active in well-lit conditions. Visual pigments in the photoreceptors are activated on excitation by light.

Retinal Pigment Epithelium–Neuroretinal Interface

Several factors are involved in maintaining the close approximation between the photoreceptor cell layer and the RPE layer. Passive forces, such as intraocular pres-

FIGURE 4-2. Three-dimensional drawing of the relation of the outer segments of the rods to the retinal pigment epithelial cells. Thick sheaths (*a*) of the pigment epithelium enclose the external portions of the rod outer segments (*b*). Numerous fingerlike villous processes (*c*) are found between the photoreceptors; they contain pigment granules (*d*). The apical portion of the pigment epithelial layer of cells is seen at the bottom. It contains numerous pigment granules (*e*); mitochondria (*f*); a well-developed, smooth-surfaced endoplasmic reticulum (*g*); a poorly developed, rough-surfaced endoplasmic reticulum (*h*); and scattered free ribosomes. The stacks of the rod outer segment discs are depicted in meridional section (*i*) and in cross section (*j*). There is scalloping of the periphery of the discs (*k*). Microtubules originating in the basal body of the rod cilium extend externally into the outer segment; one such microtubule is shown in cross section (*l*). (Reprinted with permission from MJ Hogan, JA Alvarado, JE Weddell. Histology of the Human Eye. Philadelphia: Saunders, 1971;414.)

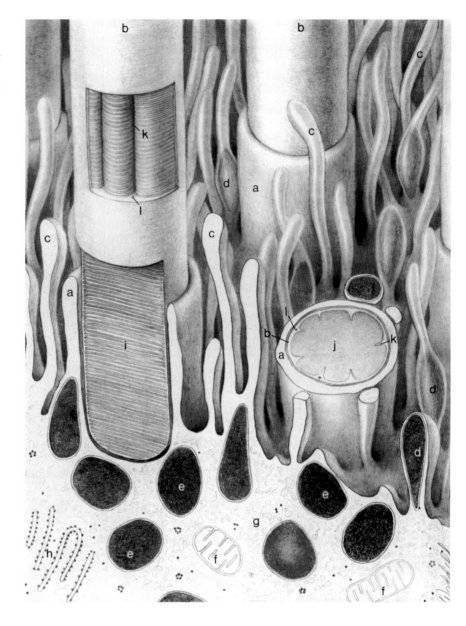

sure (IOP), osmotic pressure,[8–10] fluid transport across the RPE,[11, 12] and the presence of the vitreous[13] help preserve the position of the neural retina. Interdigitations between the RPE microvilli and the rod and cone outer segments provide a physical closeness between the two entities,[1] and the material that occupies the extracellular space between the two layers likely provides adhesive forces.[14–16]

The extracellular space between the RPE cells and the photoreceptors and surrounding outer and inner segments of the photoreceptors was once believed to be occupied by an unstructured, amorphous material. More recent studies have described an organized honeycomblike structure, the **interphotoreceptor matrix (IPM)**.[17] The outer segments are surrounded completely by the IPM and extend through openings in the meshwork. The constituents of the IPM domains around the rods differ from those around the cones; those surrounding the cones are described as a matrix sheath.[17, 18] The domains are believed to be bound together laterally, forming a highly coherent structural unit.[17] The IPM constituents are bound tightly to both the epithelial cells and the photoreceptor cells and may exceed the strength of the RPE cells. In laboratory experiments, a forceful separation between these two layers often ruptures the RPE cell, leaving remnants of pigment attached to the photoreceptors.[2, 19] The adhesive mechanism is attributed to molecular bonds within this extracellular material.[14, 16, 19–21]

The IPM provides a means for the exchange of metabolites[22] and for interactions between the two layers.[23] In addition, it may be partly responsible for orienting the photoreceptor outer segments for optimum light capture.[15] Despite these apparent forces, the interface between the RPE and the photoreceptor layer is the common location of separation in a retinal detachment.

✏ CLINICAL COMMENT: RETINAL DETACHMENT
When a retinal detachment occurs, the separation usually lies between the RPE cells and the photoreceptors as there are no intercellular junctions joining them. The RPE cells remain attached to the choroid and cannot be separated from it without difficulty. Retinal detachment separates the photoreceptors from their blood supply and, if the layers are not repositioned quickly, the affected area of photoreceptor cells will necrose. An argon laser often is used to photocoagulate the edges of the detachment, producing scar tissue. This photocoagulation prevents the detachment from enlarging and facilitates the repositioning of the photoreceptors.

Composition of Rods and Cones

Rods and cones are composed of several parts, starting nearest the RPE: the outer segment, containing the visual pigment for the conversion of light into a neural signal; a connecting stalk, the cilium; the inner segment, containing the metabolic apparatus; and the outer fiber, cell body, and inner fiber, which ends in a synaptic terminal (Figure 4-3).

Outer Segment.   The **outer segment** is made up of a stack of membranous discs and is enclosed by the plasmalemma of the cell. Each disc is a flattened membrane sac with a narrow intradisc space; the discs are stacked on top of one another and are separated by an extradisc space. Visual pigment molecules are located within the disc membranes. A biochemical change is initiated within these molecules when they are activated by a photon of light. The tip of the outer segment is oriented toward the RPE, and the base toward the inner segment.

Cilium.   A **connecting stalk**, or **cilium**, extends from the innermost disc, joining the outer segment with the inner segment and acting as a conduit between them (Figure 4-4). It is a modified cilium, consisting of a series of nine pairs of tubules from which the central pair (which usually is present in motile cilia) is missing. The plasmalemma around the outer segment is continuous across the cilium with that of the inner segment.

Inner Segment.   The **inner segment** contains cellular structures and can be divided into two parts. The **ellipsoid** is nearer the outer segment and contains numerous mitochondria. The part closer to the cell body, which sometimes is called the **myoid**, contains other cellular organelles, such as the endoplasmic reticulum and Golgi apparatus; protein synthesis is concentrated in this area.[24]

The term myoid, however, is derived from a similar area in amphibians that contains a contractile structure that produces orientational movements of the outer segments of cones.[25] The human myoid does not have contractile properties,[26] though the axis of the inner and outer segments is oriented toward the exit pupil of the eye, maximizing the ability of the photoreceptor to capture light. The radial orientation becomes more evident in cells located further away from the macula.[6, 27, 28]

Outer Fiber, Cell Body, and Inner Fiber.   The **outer fiber** extends from the inner segment to the **cell body**, the portion containing the nucleus. The **inner fiber** is an axonal process containing microtubules and runs inward from the cell body, ending in specialized synaptic terminals that contain synaptic vesicles. The photoreceptor nerve endings synapse with bipolar and horizontal cells.

Rod and Cone Morphology

Rods.   The plasmalemma, enclosing the rod outer segment, is separate from the disc membrane except for a small region at the base where invaginations of the plasmalemma form discs, whose intradisc space is continuous with the extracellular space (see Figure 4-3A). The remainder of the discs form sacs that are closed at both ends and are free of attachment to the surrounding membrane and adjacent discs.[6, 29] The discs are fairly uniform in width, and the photosensitive pigment rhodopsin is located within the disc membrane.

In work by Young,[24] radiolabeled amino acids were incorporated into rhodopsin and observed to move from the inner segment, where protein is synthesized, into newly assembled discs in the outer segment. The labeled discs moved from the base to the tip, and the label finally was seen in phagosomes of the RPE cells. This study established that components of disc membranes are produced in the inner segment and move along the connecting stalk to be incorporated into discs at the outer segment base.[24] The discs gradually are displaced outward by the formation of new discs and, as they reach the tip, are sloughed off, taken up by the RPE cells, and phagocytosed.[30, 31] This process, the rod outer segment renewal system, appears to involve active processes in both the RPE and the outer segment.[24, 32] The discs apparently are shed regularly, with most of the shedding occurring in the early morning.[33–36]

The rod inner and outer segments are approximately the same width. The inner segment is joined to the cell body by the relatively long and narrow outer fiber. The inner fiber extends from the cell body and terminates in a rounded, pear-shaped structure called a **spherule** (see Figure 4-3A). The internal surface of the spherule is invaginated to form a synaptic complex that contains bipolar dendrites and horizontal cell processes.

FIGURE 4-3. (A) Photoreceptor cells. Portions of Müller cells (dotted lines) are shown adjoining the rods and cones. (B) Retina (×1,000). (Part B reprinted with permission from WJ Krause, JH Cutts. Concise Text of Histology. Baltimore: Williams & Wilkins, 1981;180.)

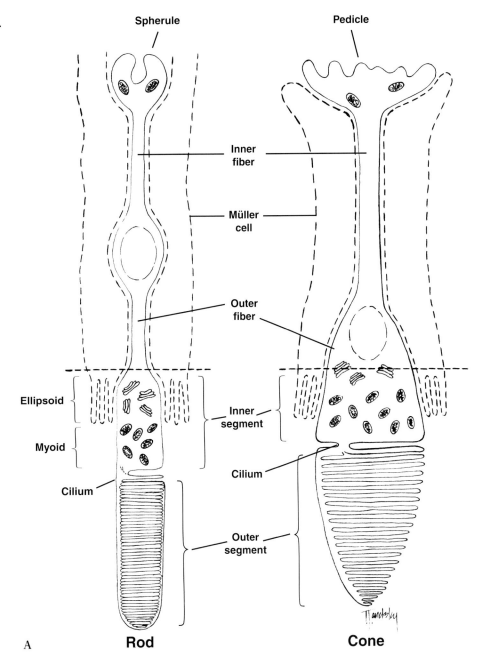

A

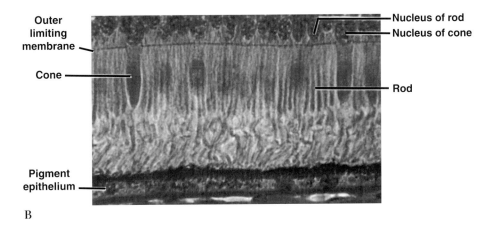

B

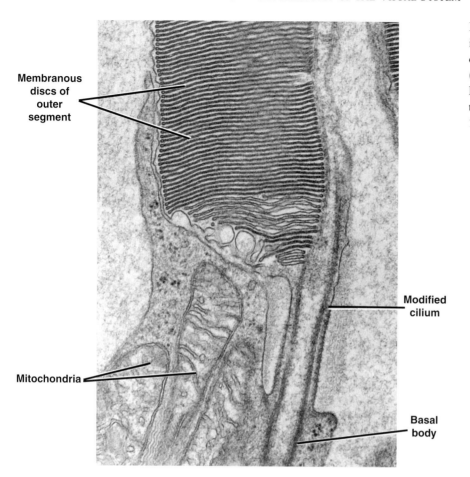

FIGURE 4-4. Junction of outer and inner segment of rod. (Transmission electron microscope, ×45,000.) (Reprinted with permission from WJ Krause, JH Cutts. Concise Text of Histology. Baltimore: Williams & Wilkins, 1981;182.)

Each rod spherule synapses with from one to four bipolar cells.[37]

Cones. As it is in the rod, the outer segment of the cone is enclosed by a plasmalemma, but in this case the plasmalemma is continuous with the membranes forming many of the discs, and the discs are not separated easily from one another (Figure 4-5).[38] In many cones, the discs at the base are wider than those at the tip, giving the characteristic cone shape, although some cone outer segments have a shape similar to the rod.

The cone outer segment is shorter than that of the rod and may not reach the RPE layer. However, tubular processes have been identified that protrude from the apical surface of the epithelial cell to surround the cone outer segment.[39] One of three visual pigments, called **iodopsins**, are contained within the disc membrane, and each is activated and absorbs light in a specific area in the color spectrum.

It has been theorized from early studies of cone outer segment renewal that the formation of discs at the cone base was not very uniform and sequential, as radio-labeled protein appeared to be distributed throughout the outer segment membrane, not merely in the disc membranes.[31, 40] More recent electron-microscopic studies suggest that formation of new discs does occur at the base but, owing to the more extensive connections with the surrounding plasmalemma, the labeled molecules are able to diffuse throughout the cone outer segment membrane rather than being confined to discs, as occurs in the rods.[38] Investigations continue into the mechanism by which the discs become narrower as they approach the tip.[41] Cone discs too are shed periodically, often at the end of the day, and are phagocytosed by the RPE.[36, 38, 42, 43] The factors that regulate the cycle of disc shedding still are under investigation.

The shape of the inner segment also contributes to the cone shape: The ellipsoid area of the cone is wider and contains more mitochondria than the rod.[1] The outer fiber is short and stout in the cone; thus, cone nuclei lie outer to rod nuclei. The inner fiber terminates in a broad, flattened structure called a **pedicle** that has within its flattened surface several invaginated areas (see Figure 4-3A). Inter-receptor contacts between lateral expansions of the pedicle to adjacent rods or cones have

FIGURE 4-5. Cone outer segment. (Transmission electron microscope, ×56,000.) (Reprinted with permission from WJ Krause, JH Cutts. Concise Text of Histology. Baltimore: Williams & Wilkins, 1981;182.)

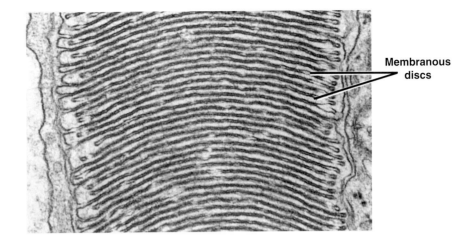

Membranous discs

been identified as gap junctions, which may permit electrical communication between photoreceptors.[6, 44]

Bipolar Cells

The **bipolar cell** is the first-order neuron in the visual pathway. The nucleus of the bipolar cell is large and contains little cell body cytoplasm. Its dendrite synapses with photoreceptor and horizontal cells, and its axon synapses with ganglion and amacrine cells. Bipolar cells relay information from photoreceptors to horizontal and ganglion cells and receive extensive synaptic feedback from amacrine cells.[45] Nine types of bipolar cells have been classified by Kolb et al.[46] on the basis of morphology, physiology, and dendritic contacts with photoreceptors; all types except the rod bipolar cell are associated with the cone.

Only one type of **rod (mop) bipolar cell** has been identified. It has a relatively large body and several spiky dendrites, usually arising from a single thick process. Rod bipolar cells begin to appear 1 mm from the fovea and continue into the periphery. They are the only bipolar cells that contact rods.[1, 46] The expanse of the dendritic tree widens and the reach of the axonal terminals increases in the rod bipolar cells located in peripheral retina as compared to those in central retina. The dendrites of a single rod bipolar cell contact 30–35 rods in central retina and 40–45 rods in the periphery, improving light sensitivity.[46, 47] These dendritic processes are the central element within the spherule invagination. The axon is large and unbranched and synapses with amacrine processes and up to four ganglion cell bodies or their dendrites.[1]

The **midget bipolar cell** has a relatively small body and can be either flat or invaginating. The **flat midget bipolar cell** has small dendritic "bouquets," each of which is the size of a single cone pedicle in the central retina. In the periphery, the cell has two or three dendritic clusters to contact two or three neighboring cones.[46, 48] Dendritic terminals of flat midget bipolar cells end in a flat expansion and make contact with only the flat area of the cone pedicle. In contrast, the axon has many endings and synapses with ganglion cells of all types.[1]

The **invaginating midget bipolar cell** is similar to the flat midget bipolar cell. Its dendritic terminals make contact with cone pedicles only as the central element in special junctions called **triads** (Figure 4-6). Triads consist of an invagination in the pedicle containing two horizontal cell processes and a bipolar dendrite.[6, 48] In central retina, the dendritic bouquet of an invaginating midget bipolar cell is the size of a single cone pedicle (which can have 12 triads), implying that each cone is innervated by only one bipolar cell. In the periphery, the bipolar cell may have up to three such dendritic expansions, with the capacity to contact several pedicles.[46] The axon of the invaginating midget bipolar cell synapses with the dendrite of a single midget ganglion cell and with amacrine processes.[1]

The two types of **diffuse cone bipolar cells** are designated type a (called **flat bipolars** by Polyak[49]) and type b (called **brush bipolars** by Polyak). In the central retina, the diffuse cone bipolar cell contacts approximately five neighboring cones and, in the periphery, each contacts between 10 and 15 neighboring cones. The location of the axon terminal differentiates the two types.[46]

The **blue cone bipolar cell** has been identified as an ON-center type; a cell suspected to be a blue cone bipolar OFF-center cell also has been found.[50] These neurons innervate more than one cone pedicle and differ from diffuse cone bipolar cells in that they contact widely spaced rather than neighboring cones.[46]

The **giant cone bipolar cell** is so called owing to the extent of its dendritic tree. The major dendrite branches into three trees, and then clusters of processes branch

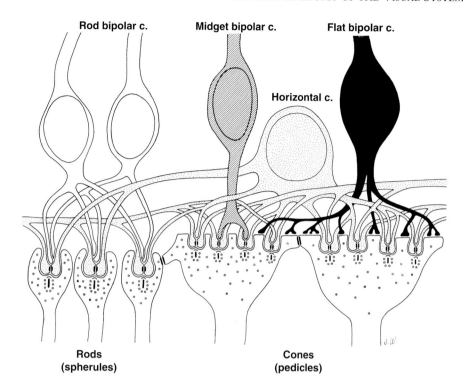

Rod bipolar c.   **Midget bipolar c.**   **Flat bipolar c.**

Horizontal c.

Rods
(spherules)

Cones
(pedicles)

FIGURE 4-6. Rod spherule and cone pedicle and their synapses. Rod and cone bipolar cells show extensive contacts. The horizontal cells also make synapses with both the rods and the cones. Interconnections are shown between rod spherules and cone pedicles. (Reprinted with permission from MJ Hogan, JA Alvarado, JE Weddell. Histology of the Human Eye. Philadelphia: Saunders, 1971;456.)

from these, each group being the size of a cone pedicle. The two types, designated **diffuse** and **bistratified**, differ only in the location of their axon terminations.[46, 51] Figure 4-7 shows several of the bipolar cell types.

Ganglion Cells

The next cell in the pathway is the **ganglion cell**, the second-order neuron. Ganglion cells can be bipolar (e.g., a single dendrite) or multipolar.[52] Cell size varies greatly, some being very large (28–36 μm).[46] Classifications can be made on the basis of the branching pattern of the dendrite, which may be either stratified, with horizontal branches arranged in one to three layers, or diffuse, branching like a tree. Eighteen types of ganglion cells have been identified.[46]

The **midget ganglion cell**, called **P1**, is the most common. This relatively small cell has a single dendrite and can be differentiated into two types, according to the stratification of the dendritic branching.[46] Certain of the P1 midget cells are connected to only one midget bipolar cell, invaginating or flat, which in turn might be linked to a single cone receptor,[53] providing a channel that processes high-contrast detail and color resolution. This situation is likely to occur in the fovea. A convergent pathway occurs in a number of P1 cells that receive input from two bipolar axons. The P1 cell is so named because it projects to the parvocellular layer of the lateral geniculate body.[46]

The **P2 ganglion cell** also terminates in the parvocellular layer but has a densely branched, compact den-

dritic tree that spreads horizontally. These cells can be differentiated into two types depending on the location of the dendrite termination.[46]

The **M-type ganglion cell** projects to the magnocellular layer of the lateral geniculate body. The M cell has coarse dendrites with spiny features, and the dendritic tree enlarges from central retina to the periphery.[46]

The remainder of the ganglion cell types are designated G3 to G23 (not all numbers are represented), and they vary by cell body size, branching characteristics, termination location of dendrites, and diameter of fiber and dendritic tree.[46] Figure 4-8 shows several types of ganglion cells, both central and peripheral.

Each ganglion cell has a single axon, which emerges from the cell body and turns to run parallel to the inner surface of the retina. These fibers come together to leave the eye as the optic nerve. The termination for many of these axons is the lateral geniculate body; others project to various areas of the midbrain.[46]

The photoreceptor, bipolar, and ganglion cells carry the neural signal in a three-step pathway through the retina. The neural signal is modified within the retina by other cells that create intraretinal cross-connections, provide feedback information, or integrate retinal function.[1]

Horizontal Cells

The **horizontal cell** transfers information in a horizontal direction parallel to the retinal surface. It has one long process or axon and several short dendrites with branching terminals; the processes spread out parallel to the retinal surface (Figure 4-9). The processes may be bidirectional and so the terms **axon** and **dendrite** might not apply in this case. Horizontal cells synapse with photoreceptors, bipolar cells, and other horizontal cells. One type of horizontal cell synapses only within a cone pedicle in the special triad junction. It is believed that horizontal cells contact bipolar cells lying some distance from the photoreceptor that activated the horizontal cell. It then releases an inhibitory transmitter, thus playing a role in the complex process of visual integration.[51, 54]

Three types of horizontal cells have been differentiated: HI, HII, and HIII. **HI** cells have dendrites that synapse with seven to nine cone pedicles and a large thick axon ending in a fan-shaped terminal to contact rod spherules. All the **HII** processes apparently contact cones and might be sensitive for blue cones.[46] **HIII** cells have a very large dendritic tree that synapses with a large number of cones, not all of them neighboring; there is some evidence that these horizontal cells avoid blue cones, thus being selective for red and green.[46, 55] The termination of the axon has not yet been determined.

Amacrine Cells

The **amacrine cell** has a large cell body, a lobulated nucleus, and a single process with extensive branches that extend toward the vitreous. The process, which has both dendritic and axonal characteristics and carries information horizontally, forms complex synapses with axons of bipolar cells, dendrites, and soma of ganglion cells, with processes of interplexiform neurons, and with other amacrine processes.[1, 56] The amacrine cell plays an important role in modulating the information that reaches the ganglion cells, owing to the extremely broad spread of its process.[51]

Three groups of amacrine cells—small-field amacrines, medium-field amacrines, and large-field amacrines—have been described according to the extent of the field covered by the intertwined branching process (Figure 4-10). Each of these groups can be subdivided into eight different types according to morphology, dendritic tree size and branching pattern, and stratification level of nerve endings.[46]

Amacrine cells, because they can have both presynaptic and postsynaptic endings, might be part of the inhibitory feedback system.[6] Some cells have been found to combine information from rod and cone pathways before innervating a ganglion cell.[46]

Interplexiform Neurons

Recently, a type of **interplexiform neuron** was identified. It has a large cell body and is found among the layer of amacrine cells. The processes extend into both of the synaptic layers (Figure 4-11) and convey infor-

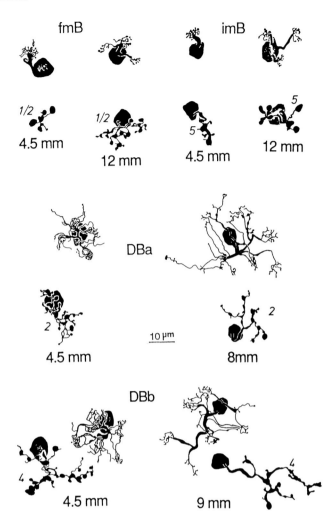

FIGURE 4-7. Camera lucida drawings of cone bipolar cells of the human retina as seen in whole-mount Golgi preparations. Each cell is drawn at two levels: the dendritic tree in the outer plexiform layer (OPL) (top) and the axon terminal in the inner plexiform layer (IPL) (bottom). The stratification of the axon terminal in whichever of the five strata of the IPL is applicable is given by the adjacent italicized number. Positions on the retina in millimeters of eccentricity are indicated for each cell illustrated. Midget bipolar cells, fmB and imB varieties, are indicated above the diffuse small-field bipolar types, DBa and DBb. See text for further detailed descriptions. Scale bar = 10 μm. (Reprinted with permission from H Kolb, KA Linberg, SK Fisher. Neurons of the human retina: a Golgi study. J Comp Neurol 1992;318:150.)

mation between these layers, apparently providing feedback from inner retinal layers to the photoreceptors.[46, 51] The nerve endings are both presynaptic and postsynaptic to amacrine processes or amacrine cell bodies. They also synapse on processes entering photoreceptor terminals, which may be from either bipolar or horizontal cells.[6, 57]

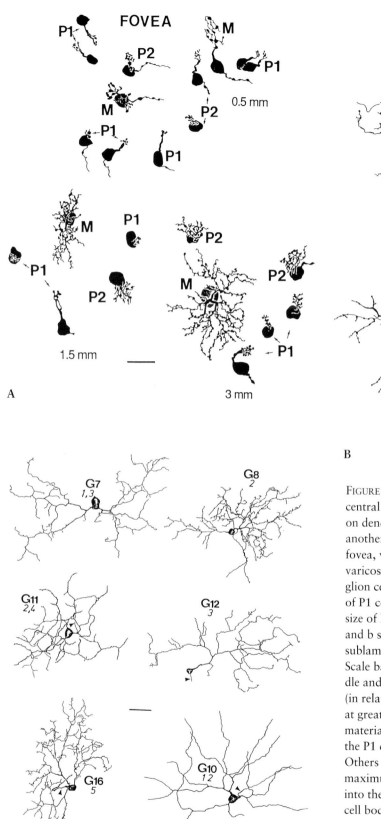

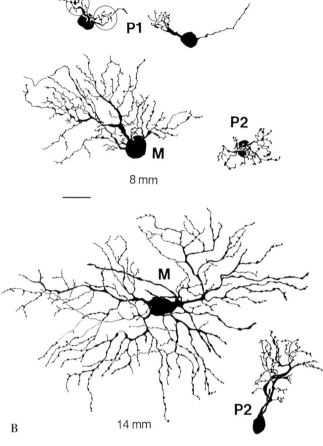

FIGURE 4-8. (A) P1, P2, and M ganglion cells of foveal and central human retina. The three types can be distinguished on dendritic tree size when they occur adjacent to one another. P1 ganglion cells have a minute dendritic tree at the fovea, which expands to be no more than a small bouquet of varicosities 9–12 μm across ×3 mm of eccentricity. P2 ganglion cells have dendritic trees approximately double the size of P1 cells. M ganglion cells are, on average, three times the size of P2 cells in dendritic extent. All three types occur as a and b subtypes, dependent on levels of their dendritic trees in sublamina a or sublamina b of the inner plexiform layer. Scale bar = 25 μm. (B) P1, P2, and M ganglion cells of middle and far peripheral retina. These cells exhibit continuation (in relation to part A) of their increasing dendritic tree sizes at greater eccentricities. P1 cells have not been seen in our material much past midperipheral retina (10 mm). Many of the P1 cells in this region have two dendritic heads (circled). Others are normal, single-headed P1 cells, which reach a maximum dendritic tree size of 25 μm. P2 and M cells occur into the far periphery and are distinguished clearly by both cell body size and dendritic tree size. Scale bar = 25 μm. (C) Small-field ganglion cell varieties of the human retina. All have rather bushy dendritic trees except G10, but the dendrites all are of fine caliber and are delicate. Scale bar = 50 μm. (Reprinted with permission from H Kolb, KA Linberg, SK Fisher. Neurons of the human retina: a Golgi study. J Comp Neurol 1992;318:147.)

Neuroglial Cells

Neuroglial cells, though not actively involved in the transfer of neural signals, provide structure and support and play a role in the neural tissue reaction to injury or infection. Several types of neuroglial cells are found in the retina.

Müller Cells

Müller cells are large neuroglial cells that extend throughout much of the retina. They play a supportive role, providing structure. The apex of the cell is in the photoreceptor layer, whereas the basal aspect is at the inner retinal surface. Cellular processes form a reticulum among the retinal cell bodies and fill in most of the space of the retina not occupied by neuronal elements (Figure 4-12).

Park et al.[47] described the neuronal cell bodies and their processes as appearing to reside in tunnels within the Müller cell. Delicate apical villi, **fiber baskets (of Schultze)**, terminate between the inner segments of the photoreceptors.[1, 25] On light microscopy, Müller cell processes can be seen passing through the layer containing the nerve fibers of the ganglion cells, perpendicular to the retinal surface. Expanded processes along the basal aspect of the Müller cell contribute to the membrane separating the retina from the vitreous, and extensions of Müller cells wrap around portions of blood vessels.[1] The pervasiveness of the Müller cell results in very little extracellular space in the retina, as is illustrated in Figure 4-12. The Müller cell is involved in glycogen metabolism and has a high glycogen content, thereby contributing to retinal nutrition.[58–60]

Microglial Cells and Astrocytes

Microglial cells are wandering phagocytic cells and might be found anywhere in the retina. Their number increases in response to tissue inflammation and injury.

Astrocytes are star-shaped fibrous cells found in inner retina. These perivascular cells form an irregular supportive network that encircle nerve fibers and retinal capillaries.[1]

TEN RETINAL LAYERS

The 10-layered arrangement of the retina, mentioned previously, is actually a remarkable organization of alternate groupings of the retinal neurons just described and of their processes. Traditionally, descriptive names were given to these so-called layers, and these designations still are in use today (Figure 4-13).

1. RPE layer
2. Photoreceptor layer
3. External limiting membrane
4. Outer nuclear layer (ONL)
5. Outer plexiform layer (OPL)
6. Inner nuclear layer (INL)
7. Inner plexiform layer (IPL)
8. Ganglion cell layer
9. Nerve fiber layer (NFL)
10. Internal limiting membrane

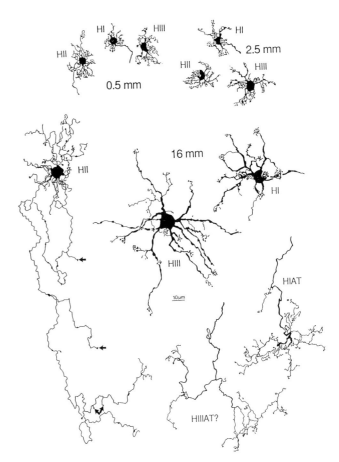

FIGURE 4-9. Whole-mount views of the horizontal cells of the human retina. Cells of the fovea (0.5 mm) are small and difficult to distinguish into the three types but nevertheless are recognizable to the trained eye. By 2.5 mm eccentricity, HI, HII, and HIII types are discernible from one another. In peripheral retina (16 mm), HIII is clearly a bigger cell than is HI and has an asymmetric dendritic field. HII cells have a woolly appearance that distinguishes them readily from HI and HIII cells. The short, curled axon of the HII type gives rise to occasional terminals (arrow). The HI axon terminal ends as a fan-shaped structure with many "lollipop" terminals (*HIAT*), whereas a finer, more loosely clustered terminal is putatively assigned to the HIII horizontal cell type HIIIAT. Scale bar = 10 μm. (Reprinted with permission from H Kolb, KA Linberg, SK Fisher. Neurons of the human retina: a Golgi study. J Comp Neurol 1992;318:147.)

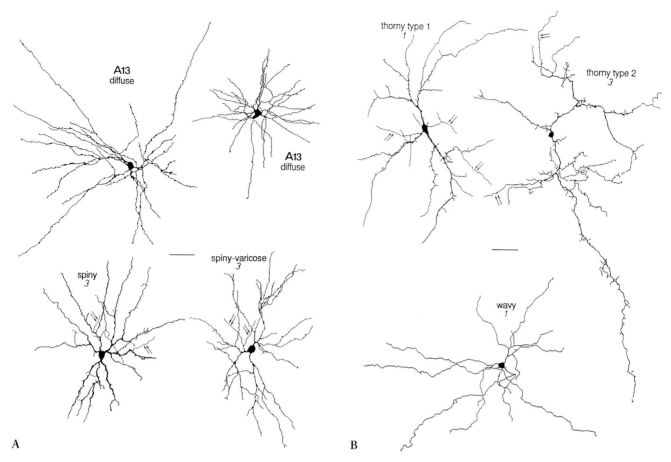

FIGURE 4-10. (A) Medium-field amacrine cells of the human retina. A13 amacrines are similar to cat A13s. In central retina (top right), these cells have a considerably smaller dendritic field than in peripheral retina (top left). A13 cells have particularly large cell bodies. The spiny and spiny-varicose amacrine cells have been described in monkey retina. They have axonlike processes (double arrows) arising from the primary dendrites that have not been impregnated to their full extent. See text for more details. Scale bar = 50 μm. (B) Large-field, amacrine cells of the human retina. Thorny types 1 and 2 are subvarieties of the same type that branch at different levels of the inner plexiform layer. Both are "axon-bearing" types, although in our examples the axons (double arrows) are impregnated only for a short distance. The wavy cell has not been reported before in primate retina. See text for further details. Scale bar = 50 μm. (Reprinted with permission from H Kolb, KA Linberg, SK Fisher. Neurons of the human retina: a Golgi study. J Comp Neurol 1992;318:147.)

Retinal Pigment Epithelium

The RPE consists of a single layer of pigmented cells, as previously discussed. The RPE is an active area having several functions: First, the zonulae occludens of the RPE are an important part of the blood-retinal barrier, which selectively controls movement of substances from the choriocapillaris into the retina. (In this regard, the RPE is analogous to the epithelium of the choroid plexus, in the ventricles of the brain.) Second, cellular lysosomes within the cells enable the cells to phagocytose fragments from the continual shedding of the photoreceptor outer segment discs. Third, the RPE metabolizes and stores vitamin A, which is used in the formation of photopigment molecules[61, 62] and is the site for some of the biochemical processes necessary for the renewal of these molecules.[6] Fourth, the pigment granules within the cells absorb light, thereby reducing excess scattering. Fifth, the cells contribute to the formation of the intercellular complex between the RPE layer and the photoreceptors.[63, 64]

Photoreceptor Cell Layer

The **photoreceptor cell layer** is composed of the outer and inner segments of rods and cones. Projections from the apical surface of Müller cells separate the inner segments.

External Limiting Membrane

The **external limiting membrane** is not a true membrane but actually consists of intercellular junctions between

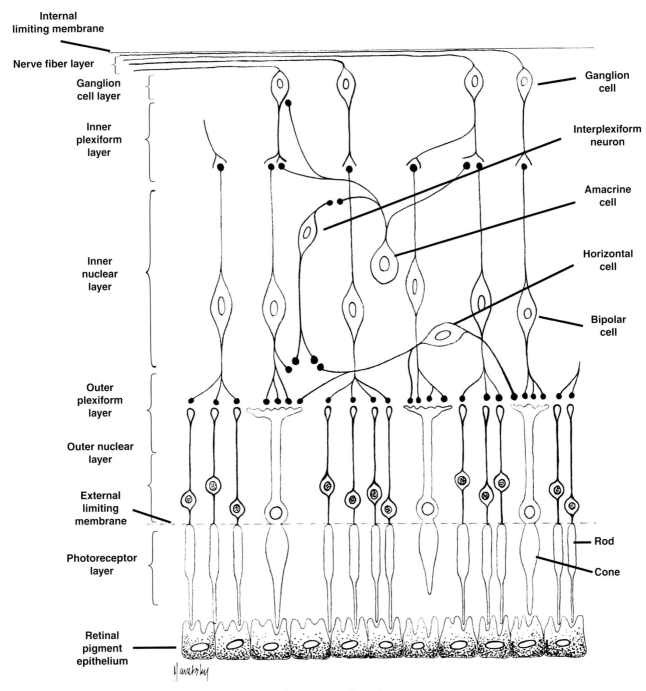

FIGURE 4-11. Retinal cells and synapses. The 10 retinal layers are indicated.

photoreceptor cells, and between photoreceptor and Müller cells at the level of the inner segments. On light microscopy, the so-called membrane looks like a series of dashes, giving the appearance of a fenestrated sheet through which processes of the rods and cones pass. This band of zonula adherens has the potential to act as a metabolic barrier to the passage of some large molecules.[6, 63]

Outer Nuclear Layer

The **ONL** contains the rod and cone cell bodies; the cone cell body and nucleus are larger than those of the rod. Cone outer fibers are very short and, for this reason, cone nuclei lie in a single layer close to the external limiting membrane; cell bodies of the rods are arranged in several rows inner to them.

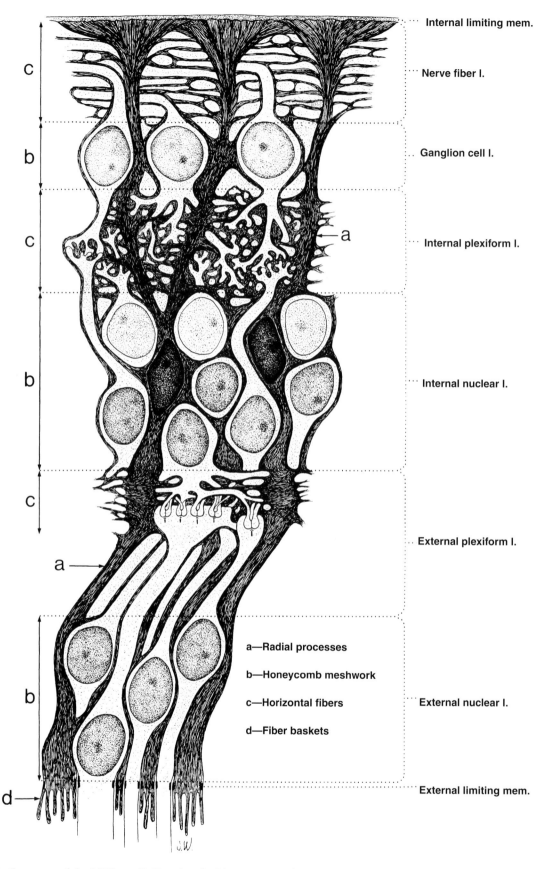

Internal limiting mem.

Nerve fiber l.

Ganglion cell l.

Internal plexiform l.

Internal nuclear l.

External plexiform l.

a—Radial processes

b—Honeycomb meshwork

c—Horizontal fibers

d—Fiber baskets

External nuclear l.

External limiting mem.

FIGURE 4-12. Structure of the Müller cell. (Reprinted with permission from MJ Hogan, JA Alvarado, JE Weddell. Histology of the Human Eye. Philadelphia: Saunders, 1971;465.)

FIGURE 4-13. Light micrograph of a plastic-embedded, thin section of the full-thickness of the retina. The layers are identified by numbers: (*1*) retinal pigment epithelial layer; (*2*) photoreceptor layer; (*3*) external limiting membrane; (*4*) outer nuclear layer; (*5*) outer plexiform layer; (*6*) inner nuclear layer; (*7*) inner plexiform layer; (*8*) ganglion cell layer; (*9*) nerve fiber layer; (*10*) internal limiting membrane. (×720.) (Reprinted with permission from MJ Hogan, JA Alvarado, JE Weddell. Histology of the Human Eye. Philadelphia: Saunders, 1971;465.)

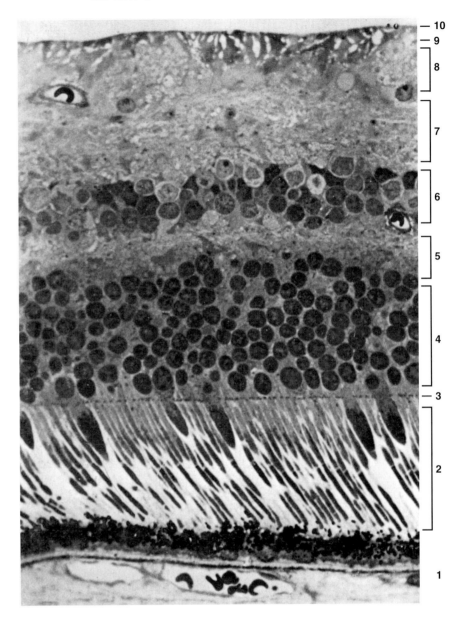

Outer Plexiform Layer (Outer Synaptic Layer)

The **OPL** has a wide external band, composed of inner fibers of rods and cones, and a narrower inner band, consisting of synapses between photoreceptor cells and cells from the INL. Rod spherules and cone pedicles synapse with bipolar and horizontal cells. Many of these synapses consist of invaginations in the photoreceptor terminal; the invaginations are deep in the spherule but more superficial in the pedicle.[6] In these junctures, the presynaptic element contains a membranous plate, the synaptic ribbon (Figure 4-14).[6, 53] Rods have invaginating synapses with multiple postsynaptic elements (sometimes more than three). Invaginating synapses in cone pedicles that consist of two postsynaptic horizontal cell processes flanking a bipolar dendrite are termed **triads** (see Figure 4-6). Invaginating midget bipolar cells are involved in cone triads, and all cones have at least one invaginating midget bipolar and one flat midget bipolar contact.[6]

Synaptic contacts also occur outside invaginating synapses. Horizontal cells make synaptic contact with bipolar dendrites or other horizontal cell processes. Bipolar dendrites synapse with photoreceptor cell endings; a single photoreceptor can have contact with more than one bipolar dendrite. The relatively long axon of the interplexiform neuron makes numerous synaptic connections with processes entering receptor terminals.[57, 65]

Desmosomelike attachments called **synaptic densities** are located within the arrangement of interwoven, branching, bipolar dendrites and horizontal cell processes. These synaptic densities are seen as a series of

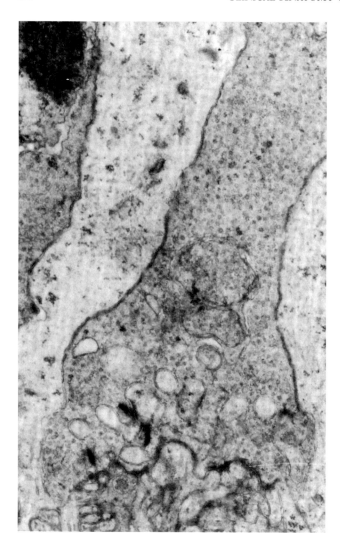

FIGURE 4-14. Electron micrograph of cone pedicle. Note the dark linear bodies (synaptic ribbons) in the pedicle (×20,000). (Reprinted with permission from CR Leeson, ST Leeson. Histology. Philadelphia: Saunders, 1976;563.)

dashed lines when viewed by light microscopy and resemble a discontinuous membrane that has been termed the **middle limiting membrane**. This "membrane" demarcates the extent of the retinal vasculature[25] and may retard exudates and hemorrhages from spreading through the outer retinal layers.[47]

Inner Nuclear Layer

The **INL** consists of the cell bodies of horizontal neurons, bipolar neurons, amacrine neurons, interplexiform neurons, Müller cells, and some displaced ganglion cells. The nuclei of the horizontal cells are located next to the OPL, where their processes synapse. The nuclei of the amacrine cells are located next to the IPL, where their processes terminate. The bipolar cell has its dendrite in the OPL and its axon in the IPL (Figure 4-15). The interplexiform

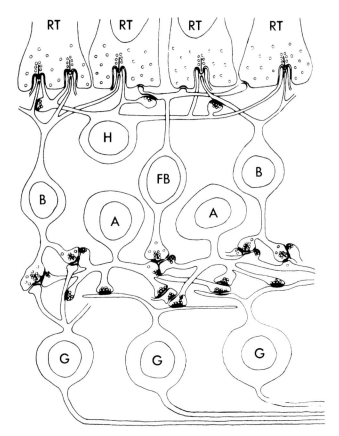

FIGURE 4-15. Arrangements of synaptic contacts found in vertebrate retinas. In outer synaptic layer, processes from bipolar (*B*) and horizontal cells (*H*) penetrate into invaginations in receptor terminals (*RT*) and terminate near synaptic ribbons (lamellae) of receptor. Processes of flat bipolar cells (*FB*) make superficial contacts on bases of some receptor terminals. Horizontal cells make conventional synaptic contacts onto bipolar dendrites and other horizontal cell processes (not shown). Because horizontal cells usually extend farther laterally in the outer synaptic layer than do bipolar dendrites, distant receptors presumably can influence bipolar cells via horizontal cells. In the inner synaptic layer, two basic synaptic pathways are suggested. Bipolar terminals may contact one ganglion cell dendrite and one amacrine process at ribbon synapses (left side of diagram) or two amacrine cell (*A*) processes (right). When the latter arrangement predominates in a retina, numerous conventional synapses between amacrine processes (serial synapses) are observed, and ganglion cells (*G*) are contacted mainly by amacrine processes (right). Amacrine processes in all retinas make synapses of conventional type back onto bipolar terminals (reciprocal synapses). (Reprinted with permission from JE Dowling. Organization of vertebrate retinas. Invest Ophthalmol 1970;9:655.)

neuron also has processes in both synaptic layers and is thought to receive input in the IPL and project to the OPL.[57] The retinal vasculature of the deep capillary network is located in the INL.

Inner Plexiform Layer (Inner Synaptic Layer)

The **IPL** consists of synaptic connections between axons of bipolar cells and dendrites of ganglion cells. The IPL contains the synapse between the first-order and second-order neuron in the visual pathway (see Figure 4-15). Generally, the axon of the invaginating midget bipolar cell ends in the inner half of the IPL, and the axon of the flat midget bipolar cell ends in the outer half of the IPL.[46, 48] The IPL also is the site of synapses between amacrine processes and bipolar axons; between amacrine processes and ganglion cell bodies and dendrites; between amacrine cells; and between amacrine cells and interplexiform neurons (Figure 4-16).

The ribbon synapses in this layer involve contact among a bipolar axon, an amacrine process, and a ganglion dendrite.[6, 66] A reciprocal synapse, thought to be inhibitory, involves the second contact of an amacrine process with a bipolar axon, providing negative feedback.[47] Some displaced amacrine and ganglion cell bodies may be located in the IPL.

Ganglion Cell Layer

The **ganglion cell layer** is generally a single cell thick except near the macula, where it might be 8–10 cells thick, and at the temporal side of the optic disc, where it is two cells thick. Displaced amacrine cells, which send their processes outward, may be found in this layer, as may some displaced Müller cell bodies and astroglial cells.[6] Toward the ora serrata, the number of ganglion cells diminishes and the NFL thins.

Nerve Fiber Layer

The **NFL** (**stratum opticum**) consists of the ganglion cell axons. Their course runs parallel to the retinal surface; the fibers proceed to the optic disc, turn at a right angle, and exit the eye through the lamina cribrosa as the optic nerve. The fibers generally are unmyelinated within the retina. The NFL is thickest at the margins of the optic disc, where all the fibers accumulate. The group of fibers that radiate to the disc from the macular area is called the **papillomacular bundle**. This is the most important grouping of fibers as it carries the information that determines visual acuity.

The retinal vessels, including the superficial capillary network, are located primarily in the NFL but may lie in part in the ganglion cell layer. Processes of Müller cells are common in the NFL where they ensheathe vessels and nerve fibers.

✍ CLINICAL COMMENT: FLAME-SHAPED HEMORRHAGES
Hemorrhages from the vasculature in the NFL have a characteristic shape. Because of the arrangement of the nerve fibers, the blood pools in feathered patterns called **flame-shaped hemorrhages**, and the shape is indicative of the NFL location (Figure 4-17). Hemorrhages in deeper retinal layers usually appear rounded and often are called **dot** or **blot hemorrhages**.

Internal Limiting Membrane

The **internal limiting membrane** forms the innermost boundary of the retina. The outer retinal surface of this membrane is uneven and is composed of extensive, expanded terminations of the Müller cells (often called **footplates**) covered by a basement membrane. The inner or vitreal surface is smooth. The connection between this membrane and the vitreous still is under investigation and may actually occur at a biochemical level (see Chapter 6); only in the periphery are vitreal fibers incorporated into the internal limiting membrane.[47]

Anteriorly, the membrane is continuous with the internal limiting membrane of the ciliary body. It is present over the macula but undergoes modification at the optic disc, where processes from astrocytes replace those of the Müller cells.[52]

✍ CLINICAL COMMENTS: FUNDUS VIEW OF THE INTERNAL LIMITING MEMBRANE
Reflections from the internal limiting membrane produce the retinal sheen seen with the ophthalmoscope. In the young, this membrane gives off many reflections and appears glistening; the sheen is less evident in older individuals.

RETINAL FUNCTION

It is obvious by now that light passes through most of the retinal layers before reaching and stimulating the photoreceptor outer segment discs. The neural flow then proceeds back through the retinal elements in the opposite direction of the incident light. The efficient and accurate performance of the retina is not hampered by this seemingly reversed situation.

Scotopic and Photopic Vision

The visual system is highly specialized for the detection and analysis of patterns of light and, by visual adaptation, can modify its capacity to respond to light at both high and low levels of illumination. Rods are extremely sensitive in poorly lit conditions (**scotopic vision**), when cones are least responsive. In scotopic vision, the light-sensitive retina allows detection of objects at low levels of illumination, but its ability to recognize fine detail is poor and color vision is absent; objects are seen in shades of gray.[54]

Cone activity dominates in **photopic vision**, when the retina is responsive to a broader range of light wave-

Ganglion cells

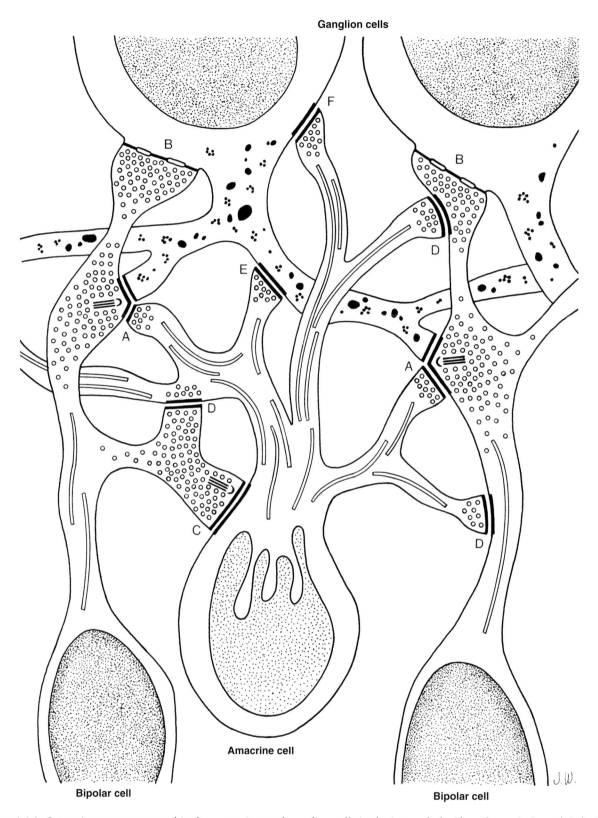

Amacrine cell

Bipolar cell   **Bipolar cell**

FIGURE 4-16. Synaptic contacts among bipolar, amacrine, and ganglion cells in the internal plexiform layer. A, B, and C depict bipolar axonal endings: (*A*) Axodendritic endings at a dyad. (*B*) Axosomatic ending on a ganglion cell. (C) A bipolar axon-amacrine soma contact. D, E, and F represent amacrine cell contacts with the other cells. (*D*) An axoaxonal contact between bipolar and amacrine cell processes. (*E*) An axodendritic contact between an amacrine and a ganglion cell. (*F*) An axosomatic contact between an amacrine cell process and the soma of a ganglion cell. (Reprinted with permission from MJ Hogan, JA Alvarado, JE Weddell. Histology of the Human Eye. Philadelphia: Saunders, 1971;476.)

FIGURE 4-17. Fundus photograph of a flame-shaped hemorrhage in the nerve fiber layer at superior nasal margin of the optic disc. (Courtesy of Dr. William Jones, Albuquerque, NM.)

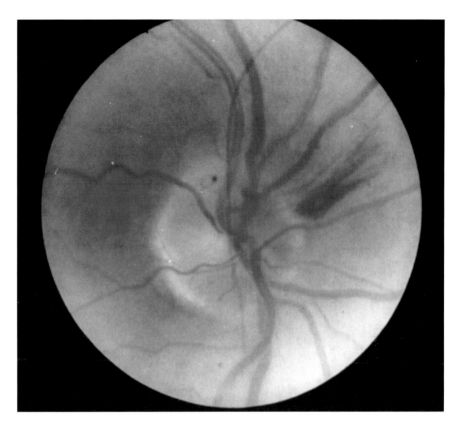

length. Bright illumination is necessary for the sharp visual acuity and color discrimination of photopic vision. Cones are designated as red, green, or blue, depending on the wavelength that they absorb.[67]

Neural Signals

The neural signal generated by the photoreceptors is modified and processed by the complex synaptic pathway through which it passes. There is a greater convergence of rods than of cones onto a ganglion cell; in some instances, there is a one-to-one ratio between ganglion and cone cells, reflecting the enormous amount of detail that the cone population can discriminate.[1] In most retinal regions, there is a high ratio of rods to ganglion cells, resulting in high sensitivity for the detection of light and motion.

Ganglion cell axons can be thought of as carrying information in processing streams, such that certain types of information are directed toward specific destinations.[6] One major target structure is the lateral geniculate body, wherein some axons terminate in the parvocellular layers, which process wavelength, shape, fine detail, and resolution of contrast. Other axons end in the magnocellular layers, which discern movements and flickering light but have poor wavelength sensitivity.[68] Visual information terminating in the midbrain is important in the autonomic control of the ciliary and iris muscles. Other centers that receive visual information can influence motor pathways that control eye, head, and neck movements.

Number and Distribution of Neural Cells

Early work by Østerberg[69] put the cell count in the retina at 110–125 million rods and 6.3–6.8 million cones. More recent research indicates that there are 80–110 million rods and 4–5 million cones.[70, 71] The density of rods is greater than that of cones except in the macular region, where cones are concentrated; rods are absent from the fovea,[13] the macular center (Figure 4-18). Rod density is greatest in an area concentric with the fovea, beginning approximately 3 mm (7 degrees) from it.[47, 54] The number of both types of photoreceptors diminishes toward the ora serrata.

There are approximately 35.68 million bipolar cells[72] and 1.12–2.22 million ganglion cells.[73] The signals from numerous photoreceptors converge at one ganglion cell, indicating integration and refinement of the initial response of the photoreceptor cells.

Retinal Synapses

There are two types of synapses in the retina, electrical and chemical. The gap junction is electrical, allowing current to pass directly between cells—that is, no chemical

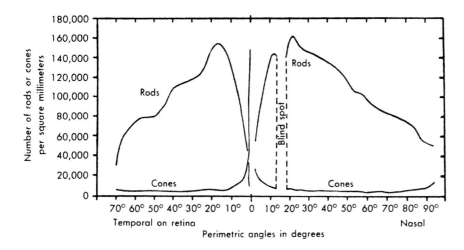

FIGURE 4-18. Distribution of rods and cones in human retina. Instead of retinal distances, Østerberg's[69] values for corresponding perimetric angles are given. Although approximate only, especially at higher angles, such values are more useful in practice than are distances on the retina. Note that the distribution of rods and cones on the nasal side in and near the fovea, not given on this graph, would be approximately the same as the distribution on the temporal side of the retina, which is seen to the left of vertical, passing through 0 degrees on the angle scale. (Reprinted from M Pirenne. Vision and the Eye. London: Pilot Press, 1948.)

mediator is necessary, which ensures a rapid rate of signal transmission. Gap junctions are found between photoreceptor, horizontal, and amacrine cells and, occasionally, between a bipolar terminal and an amacrine process.[6]

Chemical synapses contain synaptic vesicles that release a neurotransmitter from the presynaptic terminal into the synaptic cleft. The transmitter binds to specific sites on the postsynaptic membrane, eliciting a change in that neuron that may be excitatory or inhibitory. There are three types of chemical synapses in the retina—conventional, ribbon, and flat. Junctions containing a ribbonlike protein structure in the presynaptic terminal are called **ribbon junctions**. Triads are ribbon junctions that have three postsynaptic processes, whereas dyads have two. Flat junctions are found only at the cone pedicles.[6]

The extremely complex processing of neural signals in excitatory and inhibitory circuits within the retina is beyond the scope of this book. The reader is referred to any of a number of extensive works on this subject, some of which are cited in the reference list.

REGIONS OF RETINA

The retina often is described as consisting of two regions, peripheral and central. The periphery is designated for detecting gross form and motion, whereas the central area is specialized for visual acuity. In area, the periphery makes up most of the retina, and rods dominate. The central retina is rich in cones, has more ganglion cells per area than elsewhere, and is a relatively small portion of the entire retina.

✍ CLINICAL COMMENT: PERIPHERAL VISION
When the eyes are looking straight ahead, the object of interest is imaged on the macular area in the central retina, and the rest of the field that is in view, sometimes described as that which is seen out of the corner of one's eye, is focused on more peripheral retinal regions. Detail and color of those objects in the central area of vision are evident. Even slight movement in the more peripheral areas often stimulates the retina and frequently elicits a turning of the eye or head toward the motion.

Central Cornea

Macula Lutea

The **macula lutea** appears as a darkened region in the central retina and may seem to have a yellow hue due to the pigment xanthophyll.[47] The macula lutea is approximately 5.5 mm in diameter; its center is approximately 3.5 mm lateral to the edge of the disc and approximately 1 mm inferior to the center of the disc. The pigment epithelial cells are taller and contain more pigment than do cells elsewhere in the retina, which contributes to the darkness of this area. However, the intensity of the pigment varies greatly from person to person.[52] The choroidal capillary bed also is thicker here than elsewhere.

Useful color vision occupies an area approximately 9 mm in diameter, the center of which is the macula lutea.[6] The entire macular region consists of the foveola, the fovea, and the parafoveal and perifoveal areas (the annular regions) (Figure 4-19). These areas are described and delineated on the basis of histologic findings, with consideration given to the number and rows of cells in the nuclear layers. However, they are not easily differentiated on viewing the living retina.

✍ CLINICAL COMMENT: TERMINOLOGY
The terms used to describe these areas differ between the histologist and the clinician. The histologist uses

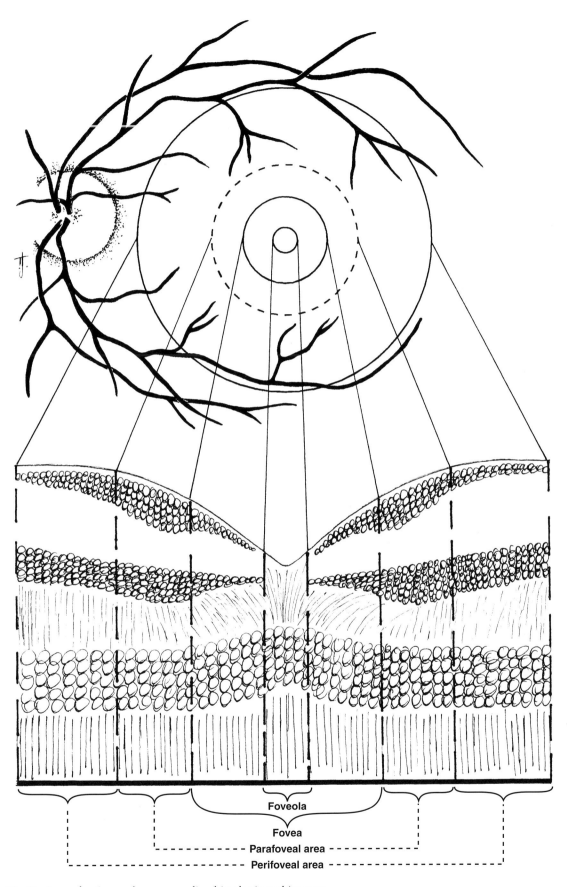

Foveola

Fovea

Parafoveal area

Perifoveal area

FIGURE 4-19. Regions of retina and corresponding histologic architecture.

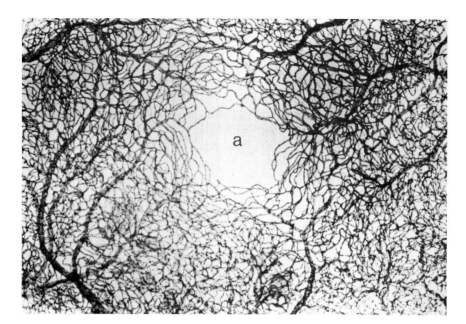

FIGURE 4-20. Capillary bed of the macular region. There is a capillary-free zone (*a*) in its center (×42.5). (Reprinted with permission from MJ Hogan, JA Alvarado, JE Weddell. Histology of the Human Eye. Philadelphia: Saunders, 1971;513.)

the word **fovea** to describe what a clinician would label **macula**, and the histologist would call the **foveola** that which a clinician would label the **fovea**. The term **macula** is purely a clinical one and usually refers to the area of darker coloration that is approximately the same size as the optic disc; the term **fovea** then refers to the very center of this area. The **posterior pole** is another term used in clinical descriptions of the fundus. There is no universal agreement regarding its definition, and its usage varies from clinician to clinician.[25]

Fovea (Centralis)

The shallow depression in the center of the macular region is the **fovea**. This depression is formed because the retinal cells are displaced, leaving only photoreceptors in the center. The fovea has a horizontal diameter of approximately 1.5 mm. The curved wall of the depression is known as the **clivus**, which gradually slopes to the floor, the foveola. The fovea has the highest concentration of cones in the retina, approximately 199,000 cones per mm[2].[71] The number falls off rapidly as one moves away from the fovea in all directions. In this area of the retina, specialized for discrimination of detail and color vision, the ratio between cone cells and ganglion cells approaches 1 to 1.[6] In more peripheral areas of the retina, which are sensitive to light detection but have poor form discrimination, there is a high ratio of rods to ganglion cells.

Within the fovea is an area that is capillary-free. This zone has a 0.40- to 0.50-mm diameter (Figure 4-20).[74] The lack of blood vessels allows light to pass unobstructed into the photoreceptor's outer segment.

The only photoreceptors located in the center of the fovea are cones. These are tightly packed, and the outer segments are elongated, appearing rodlike in shape yet containing the visual pigments of the cone population. The external limiting membrane is displaced vitreally owing to the lengthening of the outer segments. This rod-free region has a diameter of approximately 0.57 mm.[1] Most of the other retinal elements are displaced, allowing light to reach the photoreceptors directly without interference of the other retinal cells (Figure 4-21).

The cells of the INL and ganglion cell layer are displaced laterally and accumulate on the walls of the fovea. The photoreceptor axons become longer as they deviate away from the center; these fibers are called **Henle's fibers**. They must take an oblique course to reach the displaced bipolar and horizontal cells (Figure 4-22). This region of the OPL is known as **Henle's fiber layer**.[1]

Foveola

The diameter of the **foveola** is approximately 0.35 mm. At the foveola, the retina is approximately 0.13 mm thick, as compared to 0.18 mm at the equator and 0.11 mm at the ora serrata.[1] The foveola contains the densest population of cones that have the smallest cross-sectional diameters of all the photoreceptors.[6]

The layers present in the foveola are RPE, the photoreceptor layer, external limiting membrane, ONL, Henle's fiber layer, and internal limiting membrane. Moving laterally along the sides of the fovea, the other layers of the retina are increasingly represented. Müller cell processes are found throughout the macular, foveal, and foveolar areas.

FIGURE 4-21. Light micrograph of the foveal region. The foveola is included in the area between the arrows. Only the photoreceptors, glial cells, and Müller cells are present in this area. At *a*, Henle's fiber layer is seen (×85). (Reprinted with permission from MJ Hogan, JA Alvarado, JE Weddell. Histology of the Human Eye. Philadelphia: Saunders, 1971;492.)

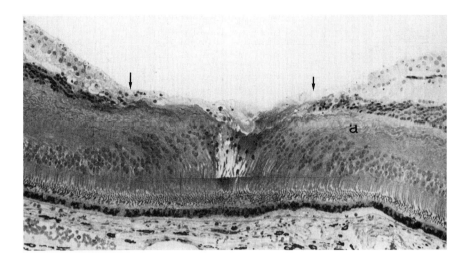

✍ CLINICAL COMMENT: CENTRAL FOVEAL REFLEX

When the ophthalmoscope light shines directly into the fovea, it reflects a pinpoint of light called the **central foveal reflex**. This pinpoint reflection is due to the parabolic shape formed by the clivus. Because the shape of the fovea is not always exactly parabolic, the reflection may vary in sharpness and regularity from person to person. The fovea is the site at which the object of interest is imaged. In the young, the sheen from the internal limiting membrane sometimes is seen as a macular reflex (Figure 4-23).

✍ CLINICAL COMMENT: METAMORPHOPSIA

The axis of the photoreceptor outer segment is oriented to accomplish capture of incident light rays. If a disruption occurs so that the outer segment is no longer oriented toward the exit pupil, vision may be altered. With macular edema, the orientation of the photoreceptors is changed, and metamorphopsia can often be elicited with an Amsler grid.[75]

Parafoveal and Perifoveal Areas

The annular zone surrounding the fovea can be divided into an inner parafoveal area and an outer perifoveal area (see Figure 4-19). The **parafoveal** zone contains the largest accumulation of retinal bipolar and ganglion cells. The INL can be 12 cells thick and the ganglion cell layer seven.[47, 52] The **perifoveal** area begins where the ganglion cell layer is four cells thick and ends where it is one cell thick. Within the perifoveal area, the fibers of Henle's fiber layer revert to the usual orientation as seen in the OPL. The width of the parafoveal area is 0.5 mm and of the perifoveal area, 1.5 mm.[1]

Peripheral Retina

Near the periphery, rods disappear and are replaced by malformed cones, and the nuclear layers merge with the

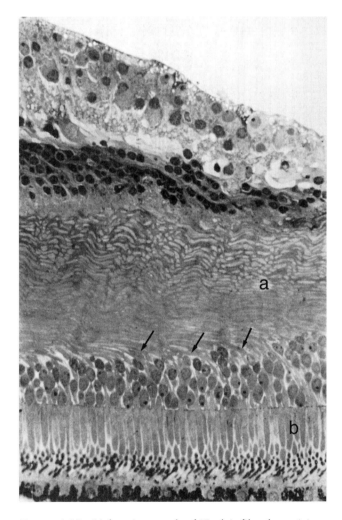

FIGURE 4-22. Light micrograph of Henle's fiber layer (*a*). The inner cone fibers (arrows) arise from the perikarya of the cells in the outer nuclear layer. At (*b*), the rodlike inner segments of the cones are seen (×425). (Reprinted with permission from MJ Hogan, JA Alvarado, JE Weddell. Histology of the Human Eye. Philadelphia: Saunders, 1971;495.)

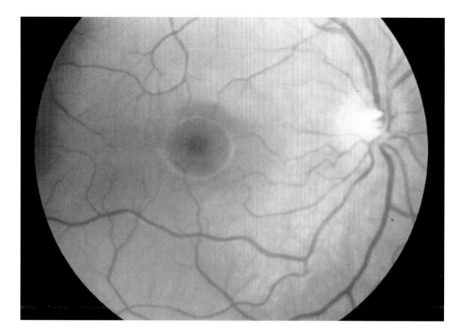

FIGURE 4-23. Normal fundus of right eye of a teenager. The sheen from the internal limiting membrane is visible as a macular reflection. (Courtesy of Pacific University Family Vision Center, Forest Grove, OR.)

plexiform layers. Finally, neural retina becomes a single layer of irregular columnar cells that continue as the nonpigmented epithelium of the ciliary body. The RPE is continuous with the outer pigmented epithelium of the ciliary body, and the internal limiting membrane continues as the internal limiting membrane of the ciliary body. There are few blood vessels in the peripheral retina.

The **ora serrata** is the peripheral termination of the retina and lies approximately 5 mm anterior to the equator of the eye.[47] Its name derives from the scalloped pattern of bays and dentate processes (see Chapter 3); the retina extends more anteriorly on the medial side of the eye. The ora serrata is approximately 2 mm wide and is the site of transition from the complex, multilayered neural retina to the single, nonpigmented layer of ciliary epithelium.[76] A firm attachment between the retina and vitreous, the vitreous base, extends several millimeters posterior to the ora serrata.

✍ CLINICAL COMMENT: PERIPHERAL
    CYSTOID DEGENERATION
Cystic spaces and atrophied areas often are found in peripheral retina, and their incidence increases with age. One cause for these changes is the poor blood supply in the extreme retinal periphery.[47, 52] A number of conditions affect the peripheral retina, some of which are normal, age-related changes and others of which might predispose the affected individual to more serious conditions; this necessitates periodic, routine, dilated fundus examinations.

Optic Disc

The **optic disc**, or **optic nerve head**, is the site where ganglion cell axons accumulate and exit the eye. It is slightly elongated vertically. The horizontal diameter of the disc is approximately 1.7 mm, and the vertical diameter is approximately 1.9 mm.[77] The number of nerve fibers appears to be positively correlated with the size of the optic nerve head—larger discs have relatively more fibers than smaller discs. Smaller discs may demonstrate optic nerve head crowding.[77, 78] Fiber number decreases with age.[73]

The disc lacks all retinal elements except the NFL and an internal limiting membrane. It is paler than the surrounding retina as there is no RPE. The pale yellow or salmon color of the optic disc is a combination of the scleral lamina cribrosa and the capillary network. In some individuals, the openings of the lamina cribrosa may be visible through the transparent nerve fibers.

Because the disc contains no photoreceptor cells, light incident on the disc does not elicit a response; hence, it represents the **physiologic blind spot**. A depression in the surface of the disc, the **physiologic cup**, varies greatly in size and depth, according to embryologic development (Figure 4-24).

Normally, the disc margins are flat and in the same plane as the retina, swelling only toward the vitreous in optic nerve head edema. Various types of crescents or rings are observed around the optic disc margin. In nearly all individuals, the disc edges are emphasized by a white rim of scleral tissue, where the sclera separates the optic nerve from the choroid. Different configurations in the anatomic arrangement at the disc border produce the pigmented crescent that often is seen outer to the scleral crescent. The RPE may not extend to the edge of the disc, and the very darkly pigmented choroid might be evident. Irregular areas of hypopigmentation and hyperpigmentation of the RPE are common near the disc.[79, 80]

FIGURE 4-24. Variability in the normal cup-to-disc ratios. (A) The cup is small and shallow. (B) The cup is large and deep. (Courtesy of Pacific University Family Vision Center, Forest Grove, OR.)

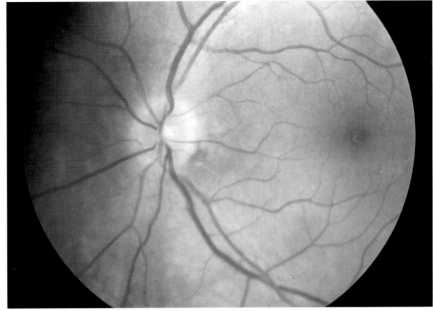

A

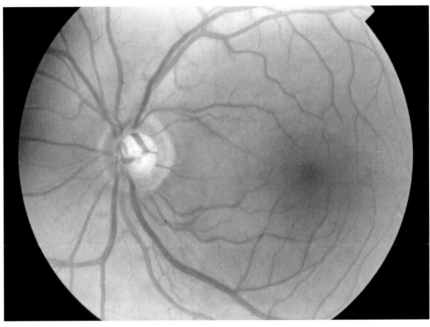

B

The optic disc serves as the site of entry for the central retinal artery and of exit for the central retinal vein.

✍ CLINICAL COMMENT: OPTIC DISC ASSESSMENT

The color of the disc, configuration and depth of the physiologic cup, the cup-to-disc ratio, and the appearance of the rim tissue and disc borders are assessed during an ocular health examination.

✍ CLINICAL COMMENT: PAPILLEDEMA

Papilledema is edema of the optic disc secondary to an increase in intracranial pressure.[81] As intracra-
nial pressure increases, pressure within the meningeal sheaths around the optic nerve slows axoplasmic flow in the ganglion fibers, causing fluid to accumulate within the fibers so that they swell.[82, 83] This accumulation of fluid is seen at the disc as an elevation of the nerve head with blurring of the disc margins (Figure 4-25). The central retinal vein may also be compromised, with hemorrhages becoming evident in the NFL in the vicinity of the disc.

Edema of the optic disc due to any other cause is referred to simply as edema of the optic disc.

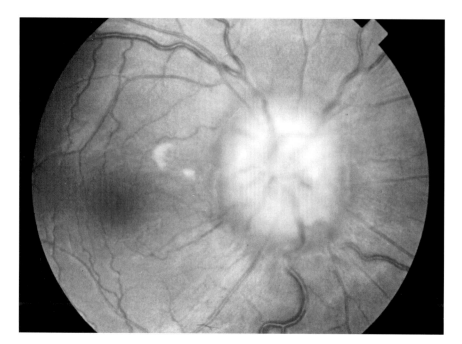

FIGURE 4-25. Papilledema of right eye. Note obvious elevation of the optic nerve head. (Courtesy of Pacific University Family Vision Center, Forest Grove, OR.)

RETINAL BLOOD SUPPLY

The outer retinal layers receive their nutrition from the choroidal capillary bed; metabolites diffuse through Bruch's membrane and the RPE into neural retina. The central retinal artery provides nutrients to the inner retinal layers. The artery enters the retina through the optic disc, usually slightly nasal of center, and branches into a superior and inferior retinal artery, each of which divides further into nasal and temporal branches, and these vessels continue to bifurcate (see Figure 4-24). The nasal branches run a relatively straight course toward the ora serrata, but the temporal vessels arch around the macular area en route to the periphery. The vessels are located in the NFL just below the transparent internal limiting membrane.

Two capillary networks are formed. The deep one lies in the INL near the OPL, and the superficial one is in the nerve fiber or ganglion cell layer.[52] The retina outer to the OPL is avascular, and the OPL is considered to receive its nutrients from both retinal and choroidal vessels. The middle limiting membrane usually is considered to be the border between the choroidal and retinal supplies.

A capillary-free zone directly surrounds the retinal vessels and, in the fovea, there is an area approximately 0.5 mm in diameter that is entirely free of all retinal vessels.[1, 25] Retinal vessels are said to be end vessels as they do not anastomose with any other system of blood vessels.[52] The vessels terminate in delicate capillary arcades approximately 1 mm from the ora serrata.[25] The retinal capillaries are made up of a single layer of unfenestrated endothelium surrounded by a basement membrane and an interrupted layer of pericytes.[25, 52, 84] Pericytes are cells with a contractile function that facilitates blood flow. The endothelial cells are one part of the blood-retinal barrier because they are joined by zonulae occludens.[1, 85]

A dense peripapillary network of capillaries, radially arranged around the optic nerve head, follows the arcuate course of the nerve fibers as they enter the disc.[86]

A cilioretinal artery is a vessel that enters the retina from the edge of the disc but has its origin in the choroidal vasculature. Such a vessel, which nourishes the macular area, is found in approximately 15–20% of the population (Figure 4-26).[87] It can maintain the viability of the macula if a blockage of the central retinal artery occurs. Smaller, less significant cilioretinal vessels can be found in 25% of the population.[87]

✐ CLINICAL COMMENT: FUNDUS VIEW OF VESSELS
The retinal blood vessels are readily visible with the ophthalmoscope and, because the vessel walls are transparent, the clinician actually is seeing the column of blood within the vessel. The lighter-colored blood is the oxygenated blood of the artery, whereas the venous deoxygenated blood is slightly darker. The artery generally lies superficial to the vein. With aging and some disease processes, such as hypertension, the arterial wall may thicken and constrict the vein; this is called **arteriovenous nicking**.

In some individuals, the pigmented choroid and its vessels are visible through the retina, and the choroidal vessels appear as flattened ribbons (see Figure 4-26).

FIGURE 4-26. Normal fundus of right eye. Note the choroidal blood vessels evident as flat, lightly colored bands and the cilioretinal artery exiting the temporal edge of the optic disc. (Courtesy of Pacific University Family Vision Center, Forest Grove, OR.)

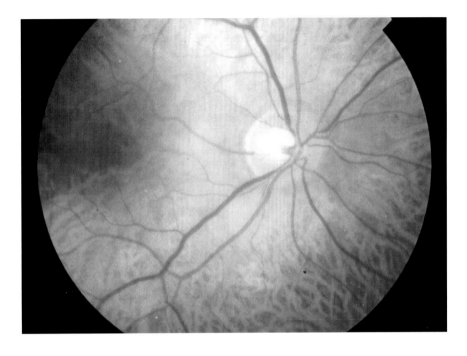

REFERENCES

1. Hogan MJ, Alvarado JA. Retina. In MJ Hogan, JA Alvarado (eds), Histology of the Human Eye. Philadelphia: Saunders, 1971;393.

2. Young RW. Pathophysiology of age-related macular degeneration. Surv Ophthalmol 1987;31:291.

3. Ko MK, Lee WR, McKechnie NM, et al. Post-traumatic hyperlipofuscinosis in the human retinal pigment epithelium. Br J Ophthalmol 1991;75(1):54.

4. Feeney-Burns L, Hildebrand ES, Eldridge S. Aging human RPE: morphometric analysis of macular, equatorial, and peripheral cells. Invest Ophthalmol Vis Sci 1984;25:195.

5. Weiter JJ, Delori FC, Wing GL, et al. Retinal pigment epithelial lipofuscin and melanin and choroidal melanin in human eyes. Invest Ophthalmol Vis Sci 1986;27:145.

6. Cohen AI. The Retina. In MJ Hart Jr (ed), Adler's Physiology of the Eye (9th ed). St. Louis: Mosby–Year Book, 1992;579.

7. Hudspeth AJ, Yee AG. The intercellular junctional complexes of retinal pigment epithelia. Invest Ophthalmol 1973;12:354.

8. Fatt I, Shantinath K. Flow conductivity of retina and its role in retinal adhesion. Exp Eye Res 1971;12:218.

9. Kita M, Marmor MF. Systemic mannitol increases the retinal adhesive force in vivo. Arch Ophthalmol 1991;109:1449.

10. Yao X-Y, Moore KT, Marmor MF. Systemic mannitol increases retinal adhesiveness measured in vitro. Arch Ophthalmol 1991;109:275.

11. Marmor FM, Abdul-Rahim AS, Cohen DS. The effect of metabolic inhibitors on retinal adhesion and subretinal fluid resorption. Invest Ophthalmol Vis Sci 1980;19:893.

12. Kita M, Marmor MF. Effects on retinal adhesive force in vivo of metabolically active agents in the subretinal space. Invest Ophthalmol Vis Sci 1992; 33:1883.

13. Foulds WS. The vitreous in retinal detachment. Trans Ophthalmol Soc U K 1975;95:412.

14. deGuillebon H, Zanberman H. Experimental retinal detachment. Biophysical aspects of retinal peeling and stretching. Arch Ophthalmol 1972;87:545.

15. Hollyfield JG, Varner HH, Rayborn ME, et al. Retinal attachment to the pigment epithelium. Retina 1989;9:59.

16. Hageman GS, Marmor MF, Yao XY, et al. The interphotoreceptor matrix mediates primate retinal adhesion. Arch Ophthalmol 1995;113(5):655.

17. Hollyfield JG, Varner HH, Rayborn ME. Regional variation within the interphotoreceptor matrix from fovea to the retinal periphery. Eye 1990;4:333.

18. Hollyfield JG, Rayborn ME, Landers RA, et al. Insoluble interphotoreceptor matrix domains surround rod photoreceptors in the human retina. Exp Eye Res 1990;51:107.

19. Marmor MF, Yao X-Y, Hageman GS. Retinal adhesiveness in surgically enucleated human eyes. Retina 1994;14(2):181.

20. Nicolaisson B, Jr. Connections between the sensory retina and the retinal pigment epithelium. Acta Ophthalmol (Copenh) 1985;63:68.

21. Lazarus HS, Hageman GS. Xyloside-induced disruption of interphotoreceptor matrix proteoglycans results in retinal detachment. Invest Ophthalmol Vis Sci 1992;33:364.

22. Sigleman J, Ozanics V. Retina. In FA Jakobiec (ed), Ocular Anatomy, Embryology, and Teratology. Philadelphia: Harper & Row, 1982;15:441.

23. Tombran-Tink J, Shivaram SM, Chader GJ, et al. Expression, secretion, and age-related regulation of pigment epithelium–derived factor, a serpin with neurotrophic activity. J Neurosci 1995;15(7,pt 1):4992.

24. Young RW. The renewal of the photoreceptor cell outer segments. J Cell Biol 1967;33:61.

25. Fine BS, Yanoff M. The Retina. In BS Fine, M Yanoff (eds), Ocular Histology (2nd ed). Hagerstown, MD: Harper & Row, 1979;59.

26. Fine BS, Zimmerman LE. Observations on the rod and cone layer of the retina. Invest Ophthalmol 1963;2:446.

27. Laties A, Liebman P, Campbell C. Photoreceptor orientation in the primate eye. Nature 1968;218:172.

28. Laties A, Enoch J. An analysis of retinal receptor orientation: I. Angular relationship of neighboring photoreceptors. Invest Ophthalmol 1971;10:69.

29. Arikawa K, Molday LL, Molday RS, et al. Localization of peripherin/rds in the disk membranes of cone and rod photoreceptors: relationship to disk membrane morphogenesis and retinal degeneration. J Cell Biol 1992;116(3):659.

30. Young RW, Bok D. Participation of the retinal pigment epithelium in the rod outer segment process. J Cell Biol 1969;42:392.

31. Young RW. The renewal of rod and cone outer segments in rhesus monkey. J Cell Biol 1971;49:303.

32. Bok D. Retinal photoreceptor-pigment epithelium interactions. Invest Ophthalmol Vis Sci 1985;26:1659.

33. Young RW. Shedding of discs from rod outer segments in the rhesus monkey. J Ultrastruct Res 1971;34:190.

34. LaVail MM. Rod outer segment disk shedding in rat retina. Science 1976;194:1071.

35. Basinger S, Hoffman R, Matthews M. Photoreceptor shedding is initiated by light in the frog retina. Science 1978;194:1074.

36. Young RW. The daily rhythm of shedding and degradation of rod and cone outer segment membranes in the chick retina. Invest Ophthalmol Vis Sci 1978;17:105.

37. Kolb H, Famiglietti EV. Rod and cone pathways in retina of cat. Invest Ophthalmol Vis Sci 1976;15:935.

38. Anderson DH, Fisher SK, Steinberg RH. Mammalian cones: disc shedding, phagocytosis, and renewal. Invest Ophthalmol Vis Sci 1978;17:117.

39. Walls GL. Human rods and cones. Arch Ophthalmol 1934;12:914

40. Young RW. A difference between rods and cones in the renewal of outer segment protein. Invest Ophthalmol 1969;8:222.

41. Eckmiller MS. Distal invaginations and the renewal of cone outer segments in anuran and monkey retinas. Cell Tissue Res 1990;260:19.

42. Hogan MJ, Wood I, Steinberg RH. Phagocytosis by pigment epithelium of human retinal cones. Nature 1974;25:305.

43. O'Day WT, Young RW. Rhythmic daily shedding of outer segment membranes by visual cells in the goldfish. J Cell Biol 1978;76:593.

44. Raviola E, Gilula NB. Intramembrane organization of specialized contacts in the outer plexiform layer of the retina: a freeze-fracture study in monkey and rabbits. J Cell Biol 1975;65:192.

45. Ayoub GS, Matthews G. Substance P modulates calcium current in retinal bipolar neurons. Vis Neurosci 1992;8(6):539.

46. Kolb H, Linberg KA, Fisher SK. Neurons of the human retina: a Golgi study. J Comp Neurol 1992;318(2):147.

47. Park SS, Sigelman J, Gragoudas ES. The Anatomy and Cell Biology of the Retina. In W Tasman, EA Jaeger (eds), Duane's Foundations of Clinical Ophthalmology (Vol 1). Philadelphia: Lippincott, 1994;1.

48. Boycott BB, Hopkins JM. Cone bipolar cells and cone synapses in the primate retina. Vis Neurosci 1991;7(1/2):19.

49. Polyak SL. The Retina. Chicago: Chicago University Press, 1941.

50. Mariani AP. Bipolar cells in the monkey retina selective for cones likely to be blue sensitive. Nature 1984;308:184.

51. Witkorsky P. Functional Anatomy of the Retina. In W Tasman, EA Jaeger (eds), Duane's Foundations of Clinical Ophthalmology (Vol 1). Philadelphia: Lippincott, 1994;1.

52. Warwick R. The Eyeball. In R Warwick (ed), Eugene Wolff's Anatomy of the Eye and Orbit (7th ed). Philadelphia: Saunders, 1976;99.

53. Kolb H, Dekorvar L. Midget ganglion cells of the parafovea of the human retina: a study by electron microscopy and serial section reconstructions. J Comp Neurol 1991;303(4):617.

54. Hart M. Visual Adaptation. In WM Hart Jr (ed), Adler's Physiology of the Eye (9th ed). St. Louis: Mosby–Year Book, 1992;523.

55. Kolb H, Ahuelt P, Fisher SK, et al. Chromatic connectivity of the three horizontal cell types in the human retina. Invest Ophthalmol Vis Sci 1989;30(Suppl):348.

56. Dowling JE, Boycott BB. Neural connections of the retina: fine structure of the inner plexiform layer. Cold Spring Harb Symp Quant Biol 1965;30:383.

57. Linberg KA, Fisher SK. Ultrastructure of the interplexiform cell of the human retina. Invest Ophthalmol Vis Sci 1983;24(Suppl):259.

58. Kuwabara T, Cogan D. Retinal glycogen. Arch Ophthalmol 1961;66:680.

59. Newman EA. Membrane physiology of retina glial (Müller) cells. J Neurosci 1985;5:2225.

60. Reichenbach A, Stolzenburg JU, Eberhardt W, et al. What do retinal Müller (glial) cells do for their neuronal "small siblings"? J Chem Neuroanat 1993;6(4): 210.

61. Bok D. The retinal epithelium: a versatile partner in vision. J Cell Sci Suppl 1993;17:189.

62. Grierson I, Hiscott P, Hogg P, et al. Development, repair and regeneration of the retinal pigment epithelium. Eye 1994;8(pt 2):255.

63. Zinn KM, Benjamin-Henkind J. Retinal Pigment Epithelium. In FA Jakobiec (ed), Ocular Anatomy, Embryology, and Teratology. Philadelphia: Harper & Row, 1982;17:533.

64. Martini B, Pandey R, Ogden TE, et al. Cultures of human retinal pigment epithelium. Modulation of extracellular matrix. Invest Ophthalmol Vis Sci 1992;33(3):516.

65. Kolb H. Organization of the outer plexiform layer of the primate retina: electron microscopy of Golgi-impregnated cells. Philos Trans R Soc Lond B Biol 1970;258:261.

66. Dowling JE, Boycott BB. Organization of the primate retina: electron microscopy. Proc R Soc Lond B Biol 1966;166:80.

67. Marks WB, Dobelle WH, MacNichol EFJ. Visual pigments of single primate cones. Science 1964; 43:1181.

68. Horton JC. The Central Visual Pathways. In WM Hart Jr (ed), Adler's Physiology of the Eye (9th ed). St. Louis: Mosby–Year Book, 1992;728.

69. Østerberg GA. Topography of the layer of rods and cones in the human retina. Acta Ophthalmol (Copenh) 1935;6:1.

70. Farber DB, Flannery JG, Lolley RN, et al. Distribution patterns of photoreceptors, protein, and cyclic nucleotides in the human retina. Invest Ophthalmol Vis Sci 1985;26:1558.

71. Curcio CA, Sloan KR, Kalina RE, et al. Human photoreceptor topography. J Comp Neurol 1990; 292:497.

72. Oppel O. Quantitative Untersuchungen Über Die Retinaganglien und Optikusfasern. In JW Rohen (ed), The Structure of the Eye (Vol 2). Stuttgart: Verlag, 1965;97.

73. Jonas JB, Gusek GC, Naumann GOH. Optic disc, cup, and neuroretinal rim size, configuration and correlations in normal eyes. Invest Ophthalmol Vis Sci 1988;29:1151.

74. Yamada E. Some structural features of the fovea centralis in the human retina. Arch Ophthalmol 1969;82:151.

75. Kanski JJ. Clinical Ophthalmology (3rd ed). London: Butterworth–Heinemann, 1994;383.

76. Pei TF, Smelser GK. Some fine structural features of the ora serrata region in primate eyes. Invest Ophthalmol Vis Sci 1968;7:672.

77. Jonas JB, Schmidt AM, Müller-Bergh JA, et al. Human optic nerve fiber count and optic disc size. Invest Ophthalmol Vis Sci 1992;33(6):2012.

78. Quigley HA, Brown AE, Morrison JD, et al. The size and shape of the optic disc in normal human eyes. Arch Ophthalmol 1990;108(1):51.

79. Hogan MJ, Alvarado JA. Histology of the Human Eye. Philadelphia: Saunders, 1971;527.

80. Fantes FE, Anderson DR. Clinical histologic correlation of human peripapillary anatomy. Ophthalmology 1989;96(1):20.

81. Alexander LJ. Diseases of the Optic Nerve. In JD Bartlett, SD Jaanus (ed), Clinical Ocular Pharmacology (2nd ed). Boston: Butterworth, 1989;690.

82. Hayreh SS. Optic disc edema in raised intracranial pressure. Arch Ophthalmol 1977;95:1566.

83. Wirtschafter JD, Rizzo FJ, Smiley BC. Optic nerve axoplasm and papilledema. Surv Ophthalmol 1977;20:157.

84. Cogan DG, Kuwabara T. The mural cell in perspective. Arch Ophthalmol 1967;78:133.

85. Shakib M, Cunha-Vaz JH. Studies on the permeability of the blood-retinal barrier: IV. Junctional complexes of the retinal vessels and their role in the permeability of the blood-retinal barrier. Exp Eye Res 1966;5:229.

86. Henkind P. Radial peripapillary capillaries of the retina. Anatomy: human and comparative. Br J Ophthalmol 1967;51:115.

87. Hayreh SS. The central artery of the retina: its role in the blood supply of the optic nerve. Br J Ophthalmol 1963;47:651.

The Crystalline Lens

Eileen C. McGill

The primary purpose of the crystalline lens is to focus images on the retina. Maintenance of lens transparency, the function of lens metabolism, is essential for performance of this vital role. The lens is composed of approximately 66% water and 33% protein. This protein concentration is double that of other bodily tissues and is responsible for the unique, refractive properties of the lens. Unlike most other tissue, the lens does not contain blood vessels or nerves.

As cells in the lens continue to divide but are not shed, the size and weight of the lens continue to increase throughout life. The oldest cells in the body are located in the lens and provide a model for investigation of the aging process. The aging process decreases the efficiency of the lens, thereby leading to loss of focusing ability (presbyopia) and loss of clarity (cataract).

This chapter introduces basic anatomy and histologic features of the lens to provide a knowledge base for effective clinical diagnosis and treatment.

OVERVIEW

The crystalline lens is an avascular, transparent, biconvex structure that functions primarily to focus images on the retina. The center of the anterior lens surface is the **anterior pole**, the center of the posterior lens surface is the **posterior pole**, and the circumferential area midway between the two poles is the lens **equator**. Attached to the lens equator are thin, threadlike zonules that suspend the lens from the ciliary body. The crystalline lens lies directly behind the iris and is the boundary that divides the globe into an aqueous chamber and a vitreous chamber (Figure 5-1).

The lens consists of long fiber cells surrounded by an acellular, elastic capsule. In the young eye, the fiber cells are soft, flexible, and easily molded by the elastic capsule. Because the lens continues to grow and produce new cells throughout life but sheds no cells in the process, the concentric formation of new, soft fiber cells inwardly displaces and compresses the older lens fibers. The crystalline lens, therefore, demonstrates a laminated onion like appearance in which the newer, softer fiber cells form the outer lens cortex and the older, compressed fiber cells form the inner lens nuclei. The lens demonstrates less intercellular space compared to other tissues because the cells are packed so tightly together.

Accommodation

A unique feature of the lens is the ability to alter its shape and thickness. The eye is able to achieve an extensive focusing range through carefully controlled changes in the shape and thickness of the lens. The lens is thinnest and flattest relative to the optical axis when the eye is focused on infinity.[1] Alteration in lens shape and thickness results in an increase in refractive power of the eye referred to as **accommodation**. Contraction of the ciliary muscle of the ciliary body releases tension on the zonules and lens capsule, allowing an increase in convexity of the anterior surface of the lens. Accommodation provides the rapid increase in refractive power necessary to image clearly on the retina objects at different distances. The maximum amount of accommodation of which an eye is capable is called the **amplitude of accommodation** and is a function of age.

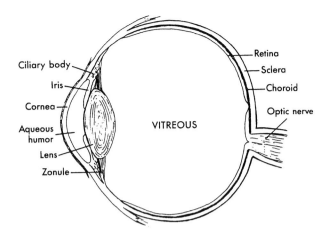

FIGURE 5-1. Sagittal section of globe shows the anterior pole of the lens facing the aqueous and the posterior pole of the lens facing the vitreous. The zonular attachment surrounds the lens at the equator. (Reprinted with permission from CA Paterson, NA Delamere. The Lens. In WM Hart Jr [ed], Adler's Physiology of the Eye [9th ed]. St. Louis: Mosby, 1992;349.)

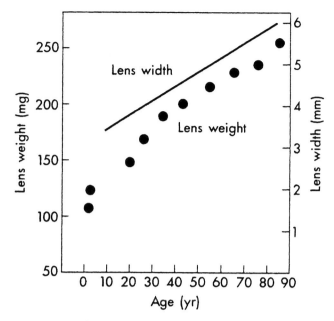

FIGURE 5-2. Changes in human lens width and weight from birth to 90 years of age. (Reprinted with permission from CA Paterson, NA Delamere. The Lens. In WM Hart Jr [ed], Adler's Physiology of the Eye [9th ed]. St. Louis: Mosby, 1992;351.)

✍ CLINICAL COMMENT: ACCOMMODATIVE AMPLITUDE

Donder's table[2] provides expected values for the amplitude of accommodation according to age. The 14-diopter (D) amplitude available at age 10 years decreases to an amplitude of approximately 2.5 D at age 50 years. The decrease in the range of accommodative amplitude with increasing age causes the nearest point that can be focused to recede gradually.

The progressive decrease in amplitude of accommodation from infancy to adulthood is attributable to the progressive increase in lens thickness and corresponding loss of flexibility of the lens fibers and lens capsule.

✍ CLINICAL COMMENT: PRESBYOPIA

Insufficient accommodative amplitude for clear near vision is called **presbyopia**. The age of onset is generally the early forties, and the patient presents with a complaint of blurry near vision. Presbyopia is treated by the addition of plus power to the optical system in the form of reading glasses, bifocals, or contact lenses, or by the removal of minus-power distance glasses from persons with myopia.

Lens Dimensions

The power of the lens is approximately 20 D,[2] and the lens increases in anteroposterior thickness by approximately 0.20 mm each year (Figure 5-2).[3,4] The equatorial lens diameter in an infant is 6.5 mm, increasing to 9 mm in an adult.[4] Values depend on the state of accommodation of the lens and on measurement techniques. In the nonaccommodated state, the anterior surface of the lens is flatter than the posterior surface. The radius of curvature anteriorly ranges from 8 to 14 mm and posteriorly from 4.5 to 7.4 mm.[3] During accommodation, the anterior lens surface curvature changes more than the posterior lens surface curvature. The average refractive index of the lens is 1.420, which progressively increases with age, particularly with cataract development.

EMBRYOLOGIC FEATURES OF THE LENS

The study of embryology and normal ocular development is essential for interpreting lens anatomy and pathologic findings in a clinical context. See Chapter 7 for more detail on the embryologic development of the lens.

A thickening of surface ectodermal cells (the lens placode) invaginates, forming a hollow sphere (the lens vesicle). As a result of the developmental process, the apical surface of the epithelial cell is oriented internally toward the lens vesicle lumen, and the basal cell surface is oriented toward the exterior. This inverted developmental plan provides a series of concentric growth layers analogous to a tree trunk in which the oldest growth layers are surrounded by progressively younger, more peripheral layers. This is in contrast to other stratified epithelia, such as that of the cornea, in which the oldest cell layers migrate toward the surface and eventually slough off. Without lens cell loss, the lens retains all cells and fibers and must maintain them physiologically to ensure transparency.

After lens vesicle formation, the anterior epithelial cells are referred to as **lens epithelium** and remain in place, whereas the posterior epithelial cells differentiate into **primary lens fibers**. Differentiation occurs as the apical surface of the posterior epithelial cell elongates anteriorly toward the anterior epithelial cell layer, ultimately obliterating the lumen of the lens vesicle (Figure 5-3).

These primary lens fibers are the first lens cells to be transformed into lens fibers and form the **embryonic lens nucleus**, which is completed at approximately 2 months' gestation.[5] All further lens growth occurs through the mitosis, elongation, and differentiation of the cells in the germinative zone anterior to the lens equator.

This process begins with an initial shape alteration from cuboidal to columnar cells with hexagonal cross-sectional profiles. The columnar epithelial cells undergo a posterior migration, rotation, and elongation to form **secondary lens fibers**. Secondary lens fibers are added in concentric layers to the lens throughout life. The **fetal nucleus** is composed of the secondary lens fiber cells laid down before birth and surrounding the embryonic nucleus (Figure 5-4). The anterior portions of the elongated fibers meet between the lens epithelium and the embryonic nucleus, whereas the posterior portions of the fibers meet between the lens capsule and the embryonic nucleus.[5]

The meeting of the ends of the elongated lens fibers produces a pattern of interconnections termed the **anterior** and **posterior lens sutures** at the anterior and posterior poles of the lens. Different layers of growth have different characteristic sutural patterns (see Figure 5-4A and B).

During lens development, a network of fine blood vessels called the **tunica vasculosa lentis** surrounds the lens and is branched from the hyaloid artery. Its function is to nourish the developing lens until the aqueous humor is available for nourishment. The tunica vasculosa lentis deteriorates by birth to allow the passage of light through the lens.

✍️ CLINICAL COMMENT: EMBRYOLOGIC REMNANTS

Remnants of the tunica vasculosa lentis are common and may be seen on slit-lamp examination. Anteriorly, epicapsular stars may be seen as small pigmented spots deposited on the anterior lens capsule. Posteriorly, a Mittendorf dot may be seen as a small gray spot on the posterior lens capsule that is attached to remnants of the hyaloid artery.

LENS EPITHELIUM

The **lens epithelium** is a single layer of cuboidal epithelium located adjacent to and beneath the anterior lens capsule. There is no corresponding lens epithelium posteriorly (see Figure 5-4C), as transformation into primary

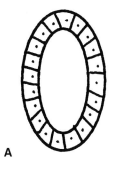

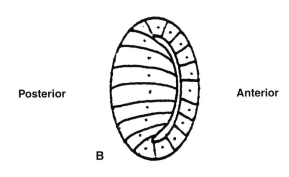

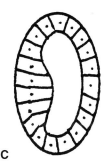

FIGURE 5-3. Development of the embryonic nucleus. (A) Hollow lens vesicle is lined with epithelium. (B) Posterior cells elongate, becoming primary lens fibers. (C) Primary lens fibers fill lumen, forming embryonic nucleus. The curved line formed by the cell nuclei is called the **lens bow**. The anterior epithelium remains in place.

lens fibers occurred with formation of the embryonic nucleus. All lens epithelial cells are nucleated, and the cytoplasm contains numerous organelles, including mitochondria, ribosomes, polysomes, Golgi bodies, and smooth and rough endoplasmic reticula.[3] A latticework organizing the cell's interior is produced by the cytoskeletal elements actin, microtubules, vimentin, and proteins (α-actinin, spectrin, and myosin). The density of cytoskeletal elements increases with age.

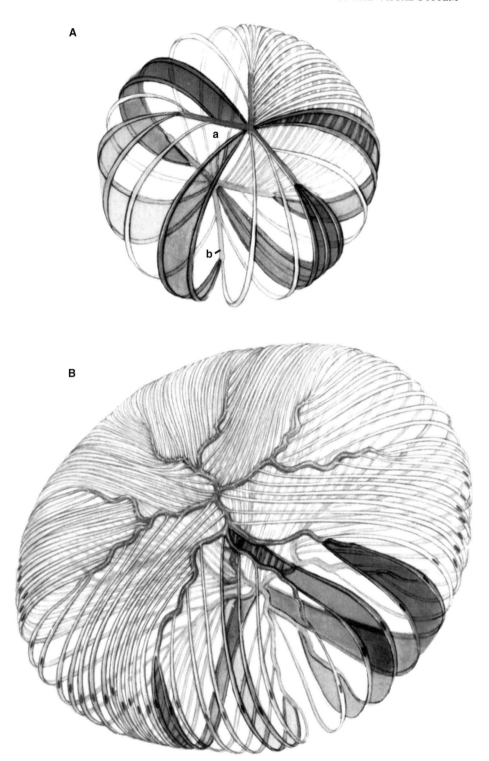

FIGURE 5-4. Fetal and adult lenses, showing the sutures and arrangement of the lens cells. (A) Fetal nucleus. The anterior Y suture is at *a* and the posterior at *b*. The lens cells are depicted as wide bands. Those cells that attach to the tips of the Y sutures at one pole of the lens attach to the fork of the Y at the opposite pole. (B) Adult lens cortex. The anterior and posterior organization of the sutures is more complex. Those lens cells that arise from the tip of a branch of the suture insert farther anteriorly or posteriorly into a fork at the opposite pole. This arrangement conserves the shape of the lens. In this drawing, for educational purposes, the suture appears to lie in a single plane, but the reader should remember that the suture extends throughout the thickness of the cortex and nucleus to the level of the Y sutures in the fetal nucleus. (C) Adult lens, showing the nuclear zones, epithelium, and capsule. The thickness of the lens capsule in various zones is shown. (Reprinted with permission from MJ Hogan, JA Alvarado, JE Weddell. Histology of the Human Eye. Philadelphia: Saunders, 1971;642.)

Functionally, the anterior lens epithelium can be divided into two regions. Located in front of and adjacent to the lens equator are the specialized cells of the **germinative zone** that undergo mitosis, elongation, and differentiation into lens cell fibers (Figure 5-5). The remaining anterior epithelial cells, in the central zone, usually do not divide. The single layer of anterior epithelial cells is responsible for the majority of metabolite and ion transport activity for the entire lens, in contrast to the metabolically less active lens fibers.[4]

Lens epithelial cells have distinct lateral, apical, and basal cell membranes. Infoldings of the lateral cell membranes enhance intercellular communication through desmosomes and an extensive network of gap junctions, which allow direct exchange of small molecules between neighboring cells.[3, 4] Because the lens is avas-

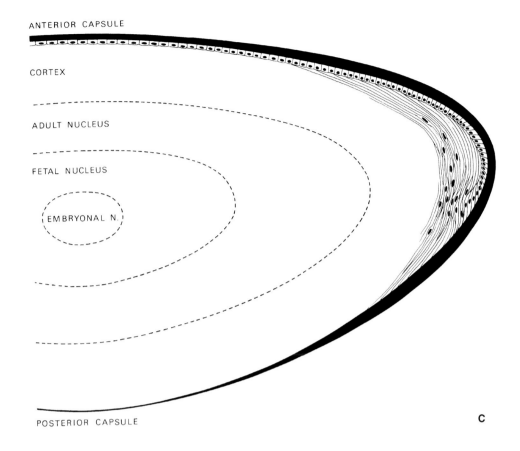

ANTERIOR CAPSULE

CORTEX

ADULT NUCLEUS

FETAL NUCLEUS

EMBRYONAL N.

POSTERIOR CAPSULE

C

cular and relies on the aqueous humor for its nutritional needs, the gap junctional network has a vital role in maintenance of lens transparency. The **epithelial-fiber interface (EFI)** is the region in which the apical membrane of the epithelial cell meets the apical membrane of the elongating fiber.[3, 4]

LENS CAPSULE

The lens **capsule** is an acellular, elastic, and transparent envelope enclosing the epithelium and fibers of the lens. Produced continuously throughout life, the lens capsule is the thickest basement membrane in the body and is composed principally of type IV collagen and 10% glycosaminoglycans.[4] It is secreted by the basal cell area of the lens epithelium anteriorly and by the basal area of the elongating fiber posteriorly. Capsule thickness varies according to age and is not consistent throughout its extent. The capsule is thicker at the anterior pole than at the posterior pole, and the anterior and posterior regions near the equatorial zone of zonular insertion are thicker than at the poles.[6]

The capsule may be divided into an inner layer and an outer, denser layer, the zonular lamella. The inner lens capsule is in contact with the anterior lens epithelium and the posterior superficial lens fibers. The outer lens capsule merges with the zonule of Zinn.

CLINICAL COMMENT: EXFOLIATION AND PSEUDOEXFOLIATION
Rare, extreme conditions, such as intense heat or trauma, can cause the two layers of the lens capsule to split, creating an exfoliation or peeling of the lens capsule. A more common finding is pseudoexfoliation of the lens, in which a material with a flaky, white, exudative appearance is deposited on the anterior lens capsule. Pseudoexfoliation is associated with glaucoma.

Zonule of Zinn

The **zonule of Zinn** suspends the lens in the visual axis (Figure 5-6). This complex network of elasticlike fibers is essential for accommodation. The fibers arise from the basement membrane of the nonpigmented epithelium of the pars plana.[7] They travel forward into the valleys between the ciliary processes. The two major sets of fibers fuse with the outer lens capsule approximately 1.5 mm anterior and posterior to the equator.[7–9] Minor fibers fuse directly to the equator.

CLINICAL COMMENT: SUBLUXATED LENS
Through trauma, disease, or congenital defects, zonular fibers may rupture or break, leading to subluxation or dislocation of the lens. In subluxa-

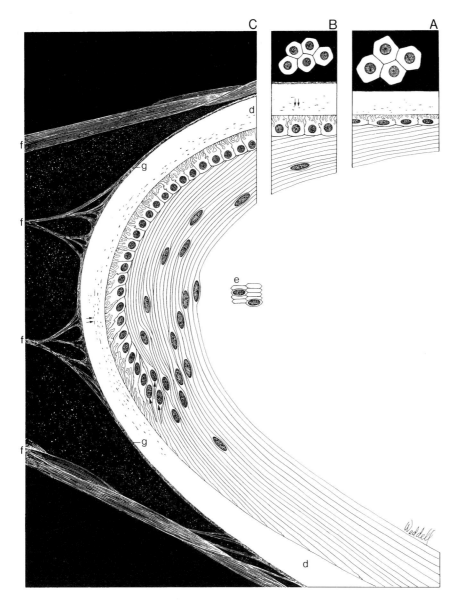

FIGURE 5-5. A composite drawing of the lens, cortex, epithelium, capsule, and zonular attachments. At (*A*) is the anterior central lens epithelium, seen in flat section and cross section. The size and shape of these cells can be compared with those of the cells in (*B*), the intermediate zone, and (*C*) the equatorial zone. At the equator, the dividing cells are elongating (arrows) to form lens cortical cells. As they elongate, they send processes anteriorly and posteriorly toward the sutures, and their nuclei migrate somewhat anterior to the equator to form the lens bow. At the same time, the nuclei become more and more displaced into the lens as new cells are formed at the equator. The lens capsule (*d*) is thicker anterior and posterior to the equator than it is at the equator itself. The anterior and equatorial capsule contains fine filamentous inclusions (double arrows); these are not present posteriorly. Lens fibers elongate into flattened hexagons (*e*) in cross section. Zonular fibers (*f*) attach to the anterior and posterior capsule and to the equatorial capsule, forming the pericapsular or zonular lamella of the lens (*g*). (Reprinted with permission from MJ Hogan, JA Alvarado, JE Weddell. Histology of the Human Eye. Philadelphia: Saunders, 1971;649.)

tion, the zonular fibers are partially disrupted, and the lens is decentered but remains in the pupillary aperture.[10] A dislocated lens involves complete disruption of zonules and is displaced out of the pupillary aperture. Couching, the intentional dislocation of an opaque lens with a needle, was the early form of cataract surgery.

Functions of the Lens Capsule

The shape of the lens is molded by the capsule in response to the tension of the zonules. Contraction of the ciliary muscle, as occurs in accommodation, creates a release of tension on the zonules and allows the capsule to mold the lens such that the anterior pole bulges forward.

In addition to its vital role in accommodation, the lens capsule functions as a selectively permeable barrier, restricting the passage of high-molecular-weight compounds while allowing low-molecular-weight compounds free passage.

LENS CELL FIBERS

New secondary lens cell fibers are formed by differentiation of equatorial epithelium from the germinative zone. The fibers elongate into flattened hexagons, and the central region remains at the equator.

The opposing ends of each fiber reach the anterior and posterior poles and form a pattern of lens sutures. Because fibers of different depths differ optically and structurally, the lens usually is described in terms of an inner nuclear and an outer cortical region. The **adult nucleus** contains the lens fibers formed from birth to sexual maturation. The **cortex** contains the secondary fiber cell layers formed after sexual maturation.[5] The difference between the age of deep cortical fibers and that of

FIGURE 5-6. Scanning electron micrograph of the anterior zonular insertion after removal of cornea and iris. Note the angle between the anterior and posterior zonules and the attachment to the lens capsule. (Reprinted with permission from BW Streeton. Zonular Apparatus. In JA Jakobiec [ed], Ocular Anatomy, Embryology, and Teratology. Hagerstown, MD: Harper & Row, 1982;341.)

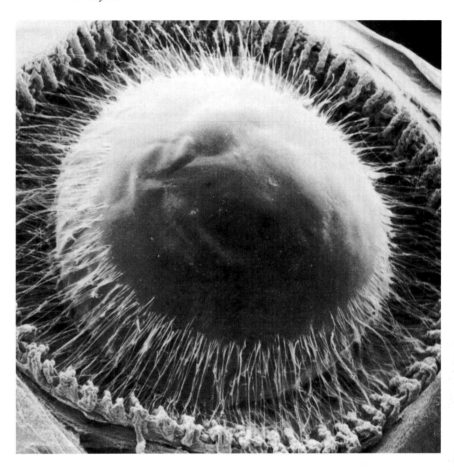

superficial cortical fibers in an elderly human eye might range to 60 years or older. Surgically defined division of the lens into nucleus and cortex differs from the distinctions made here in that the surgically defined lens nucleus includes a substantial amount of lens cortex.

Lens Sutures

The junctures between secondary lens cell fibers produce **lens sutures**. The embryonal nucleus, composed of primary fibers, does not contain lens sutures. The fetal nucleus contains an anterior, **erect Y suture**, with three suture branches positioned equidistant at 60, 180, and 300 degrees, and a posterior, **inverted Y suture** with three suture branches positioned at 0, 120, and 240 degrees (see Figure 5-4A). As a result of the curvature of the opposing ends of the lens fiber, there is an offsetting of the anterior and posterior suture branches. Symmetric and identical sutures are produced in successive secondary fiber growth layers until birth. After birth until sexual maturation, symmetric but nonidentical sutures are produced. After sexual maturation, young adult lenses demonstrate a nine-branch star suture pattern positioned equidistantly every 40 degrees.[5] Further aging and lens growth results in more complex suture formation (see Figure 5-4B).

✍ CLINICAL COMMENT: APPEARANCE OF THE LENS ON BIOMICROSCOPY

Examination of the crystalline lens is a routine part of the visual health assessment and a key indicator of a patient's age, visual acuity, and ocular and systemic health status. In contrast to the iris-covered lens equator, the central anterior and posterior areas of the lens are easily examined with the biomicroscope.

Variations in pattern of the sutural planes are responsible for the appearance of the zones of discontinuity visible on biomicroscopic examination of the lens. The zones of discontinuity appear as bright white or gray bands of convex curvature anteriorly, duplicated by zones of concave curvature posteriorly, and represent abrupt changes in the refractive index of fibers produced at various times.[11] The lens is viewed by directing a narrow optical section of light through the pupillary aperture. The beam will pass through the anterior lens capsule, anterior epithelium, anterior cortex, anterior adult nucleus, anterior fetal nucleus, embryonal nucleus, posterior fetal nucleus, posterior adult nucleus, posterior cortex, and posterior lens capsule. Table 5-1 describes the zones, and Figure 5-7 shows the biomicroscopic appearance.

TABLE 5-1. Zones of Discontinuity

Zones of discontinuity	Correlative lens morphology
Anterior capsular zone	Anterior lens capsule
Anterior subcapsular zone	Anterior lens epithelium, elongating fibers, and outermost cortical fibers
Anterior zone of disjunction	Anterior segments of cortical fibers formed after sexual maturation, complex sutures
Anterior zone of the adult nucleus	Anterior half of the adult nucleus consisting of secondary fibers formed after birth to sexual maturation
Anterior zone of the fetal nucleus	Anterior half of the fetal nucleus consisting of secondary fibers formed before birth
	Location of upright Y suture
Zone of the embryonic nucleus	Embryonic nucleus consisting of primary lens fibers formed during first 2 months of embryonic development
Posterior zone of the fetal nucleus	Posterior half of the fetal nucleus consisting of secondary fibers formed before birth
	Location of inverted Y suture
Posterior zone of the adult nucleus	Posterior half of the adult nucleus consisting of secondary fibers formed after birth to sexual maturation
Posterior subcapsular zone	Posterior segments of elongating fibers and the outermost cortical fibers, complex sutures
Posterior capsular zone	Posterior lens capsule

Source: Adapted from JR Kuszak, TA Deutsch, HG Brown. Anatomy of Aged and Senile Cataractous Lenses. In DM Albert, FA Jakobiec (eds), Principles and Practice of Ophthalmology: Basic Sciences. Philadelphia: Saunders, 1994;564.

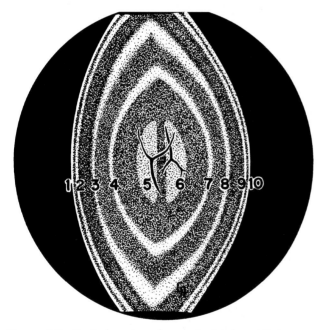

FIGURE 5-7. Optical section of normal adult lens. (1) Anterior capsule; (2) anterior line of disjunction; (3) anterior surface of adult nucleus; (4) anterior surface of fetal nucleus; (5) inner layer of anterior half of fetal nucleus, containing anterior Y suture; (6) inner layer of posterior half of fetal nucleus, containing posterior Y suture; (7) posterior surface of fetal nucleus; (8) posterior surface of adult nucleus; (9) posterior line of disjunction; and (10) posterior capsule. (Reprinted with permission from CD Phelps. Examination and Functional Evaluation of the Crystalline Lens. In TD Duane, Clinical Ophthalmology [Vol 1]. Hagerstown, MD: Harper & Row, 1978.)

The lens and the sutures are used to localize depth of an opacity. Clinically, the prominent erect anterior Y suture and inverted posterior Y suture are used as lens landmarks and demarcate the boundaries of the fetal nucleus (see Figure 5-7). Accurate lens assessment is best conducted through a dilated pupil.

Lens Cell Fiber Characteristics

Characteristics of lens cell fibers differ depending on the age of the fiber. Young fibers are uniform in shape and are most easily described as elongated hexagonal prisms with two broad sides oriented parallel to the lens surface and four narrow sides oriented at acute angles to the lens surface (Figure 5-8).[3] The uniformity and precise fiber alignment reduce large-particle scatter and contribute to lens transparency.[12]

With increasing age, fibers become less uniform in shape and demonstrate an irregular profile. Only the youngest, most superficial fibers are nucleated and contain the normal cellular organelles. As the fibers move deeper into the lens with increasing age, the nuclei and other organelles disintegrate. A characteristic pattern of nuclei called the **lens bow** or **nuclear bow** is formed as fibers move from the equator toward the center of the lens (see Figure 5-5).[6, 9]

In addition to precise alignment and organelle loss, the hexagonal fibers are packed densely. The densely packed hexagonal fibers demonstrate interdigitations along their lateral cell membranes. These numerous, fingerlike protrusions into adjacent fibers occur superficially and attain a ball-and-socket configuration (Figure 5-9).[3, 4, 12]

FIGURE 5-8. Scanning electron micrograph shows the characteristic hexagonal cross-sectional profiles of lens fiber cells. (Reprinted with permission from CA Paterson, NA Delamere. The Lens. In WM Hart Jr [ed], Adler's Physiology of the Eye [9th ed]. St. Louis: Mosby, 1992;355.)

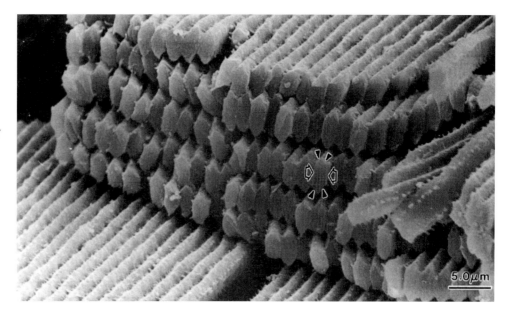

FIGURE 5-9. Fiber cells of lens cortex (transmission electron microscope, ×6,000). (Reprinted with permission from WJ Krause, JH Cutts. Concise Text of Histology. Baltimore: Williams & Wilkins, 1981;179.)

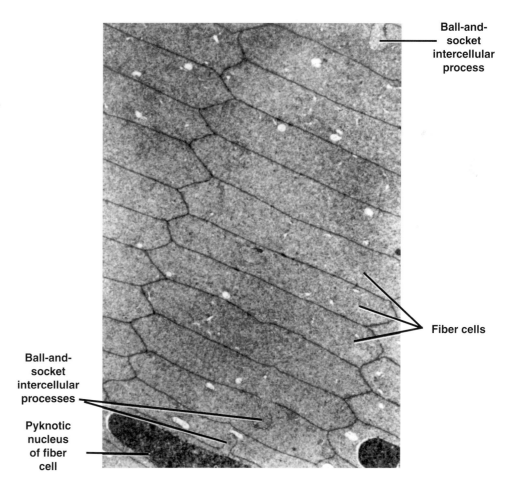

Ball-and-socket intercellular process

Fiber cells

Ball-and-socket intercellular processes

Pyknotic nucleus of fiber cell

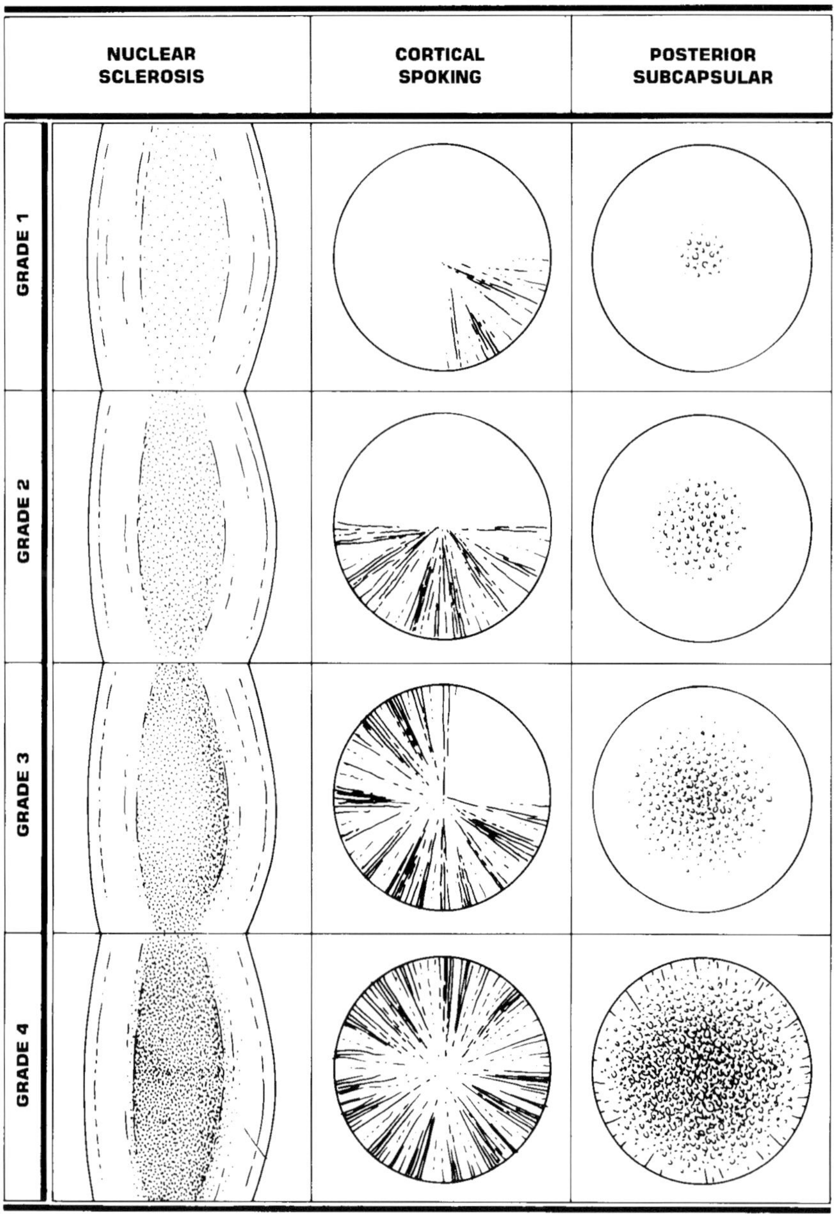

	NUCLEAR SCLEROSIS	CORTICAL SPOKING	POSTERIOR SUBCAPSULAR
GRADE 1			
GRADE 2			
GRADE 3			
GRADE 4			

FIGURE 5-10. A grading system for age-related cataracts. Nuclear sclerotic changes are shown in cross section, with the anterior surface to the left. Cortical and posterior subcapsular changes are seen in retroillumination. (Reprinted with permission from M Fingeret, L Casser, HT Woodcome. Atlas of Primary Eyecare Procedures. Norwalk, CT: Appleton & Lange, 1992;67.)

Interdigitations are most numerous in the equatorial cortical region, which demonstrates the greatest accommodative shape changes.[3] The extensive network of low-resistance gap junctions allows the lens to function as a syncytium rather than as individual cells and greatly enhances communication.

Lens Proteins

Lens proteins have the lowest turnover rate of all proteins in the body. Because most lens cells have lost their ability to synthesize new proteins, the same lens proteins must last for the life of the organism.

Lens proteins can be classified into two categories according to their solubility in water. Water-insoluble proteins are least common (10%) and include membrane and cytoskeletal proteins. Water-soluble structural proteins are called **crystallins** and are responsible for 90% of the total lens protein and, thus, the refractive indices of the lens. The abundance of the lens crystallins and their ability to be packed closely allows the lens to focus a retinal image with minimal distortion. Lens development produces layers of cells containing crystallin proteins that increase in concentration from approximately 15% in the cortex to 70% in the adult nucleus, providing a gradient of refractive index.[12] The lens crystallins are synthesized by both the anterior cuboidal epithelium and the elongated lens fiber cells.[13] The balance between soluble and insoluble proteins and the effect of these on age-related changes and lens opacities are current topics in ocular research.

CLINICAL COMMENT: CATARACTS

Technically, any opacity of the crystalline lens is termed a **cataract**. Age is the major risk factor: 95% of persons over the age of 65 years have some degree of cataract. Clinically, a cataract is considered significant when it is sufficient to alter the patient's lifestyle.

Signs and Symptoms of Cataracts

The symptoms of cataract include glare with night driving, image blur, distortion, and monocular diplopia. Some presbyopic patients report a return of "second sight" and are able to read without reading glasses owing to the refractive myopic shift of the lens nucleus. The signs of cataract include reduced visual acuity and a white or yellow-brown opacity in the lens. The red pupillary reflex may be muted or absent.

Classification of Cataracts

Cataracts generally are classified by the zones of the lens involved in the opacity. Any zone might exhibit a loss of transparency due to medications, trauma, ocular inflammations, congenital opacities, or age-related changes. Although numerous types of cataracts exist, the three most common age-related cataracts are nuclear sclerosis, cortical spokes, and posterior subcapsular cataracts (Figure 5-10).[14]

Nuclear sclerosis is a centrally located opacity initially in the embryonic nucleus and enlarging to encompass the fetal and adult nuclei. In advanced cases, it will involve the deep cortex also. Sclerosis means a hardening of the lens. Brunescence is a yellowing or browning of the nucleus.

Cortical spokes cause the least visual deficit and begin as small spokelike opacities at the lens periphery that eventually enlarge toward the center (Figure 5-11).

Posterior subcapsular cataracts begin as a spot opacity near the center of the visual axis in the posterior lens and become larger and more diffuse over time.

Treatment of Cataracts

The treatment of choice for cataract is surgical removal. To predict the potential for postoperative visual acuity, a potential acuity meter (PAM) or laser interferometer is used to bypass the cloudy lens and negate its effect on the measurement of visual acuity.

If the lens is removed and no implant is inserted, the patient is referred to as **aphakic** and requires a high plus correction in the form of spectacles or contact lenses. Today, most surgeons insert an intraocular lens (IOL) implant; this patient is

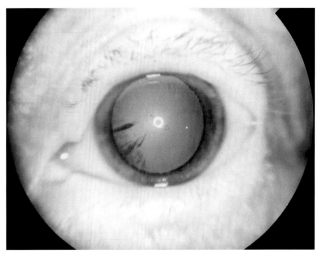

FIGURE 5-11. Spokes of a cortical cataract visible through the dilated pupil. (Courtesy of Pacific University Family Vision Center, Forest Grove, OR.)

referred to as **pseudophakic**. The IOL may be placed in the anterior chamber or, more commonly, in the posterior chamber.

The surgical procedure may be an intracapsular cataract extraction, in which the entire lens is removed, or an extracapsular cataract extraction (ECCE), in which the posterior lens capsule is left in place to support the IOL. Phacoemulsification, a variation of ECCE in which an ultrasonic probe is used to emulsify the lens nucleus, is highly successful as it allows a smaller incision and faster healing time.

REFERENCES

1. Koretz JF. Accommodation and Presbyopia. In DM Albert, FA Jakobiec (eds), Principles and Practice of Ophthalmology: Basic Sciences. Philadelphia: Saunders, 1994;270.

2. Borish IM. Clinical Refraction (3rd ed). Chicago: Professional Press, 1970;169.

3. Rafferty NS. Lens Morphology. In H Maisel (ed), The Ocular Lens: Structure, Function, and Pathology. New York: Marcel Dekker, 1985;1.

4. Paterson CA, Delamere NA. The Lens. In WM Hart Jr (ed), Adler's Physiology of the Eye (9th ed). St. Louis: Mosby, 1992;348.

5. Kuszak JR, Brown HG. Embryology and Anatomy of the Lens. In DM Albert, FA Jakobiec (eds), Principles and Practice of Ophthalmology: Basic Sciences. Philadelphia: Saunders, 1994;82.

6. Warwick R (ed). Eugene Wolff's Anatomy of the Eye and Orbit. Philadelphia: Saunders, 1976;160.

7. Kaufman PL. Accommodation and Presbyopia: Neuromuscular and Biophysical Aspects. In WM Hart Jr

(ed), Adler's Physiology of the Eye (9th ed). St. Louis: Mosby, 1992;391.

8. Streeton BW. Zonular Apparatus. In FA Jakobiec (ed), Ocular Anatomy, Embryology, and Teratology. Hagerstown, MD: Harper & Row, 1982;331.

9. Hogan MJ, Alvarado JA, Weddell JE. Histology of the Human Eye. Philadelphia: Saunders, 1971;638.

10. Cullom RD, Chang B. Wills Eye Manual: Office and Emergency Room Diagnosis and Treatment of Eye Disease. Philadelphia: Lippincott, 1994;427.

11. Kuszak JR, Deutsch TA, Brown HG. Anatomy of Aged and Senile Cataractous Lenses. In DM Albert, FA Jakobiec (eds), Principles and Practice of Ophthalmology: Basic Sciences. Philadelphia: Saunders, 1994;564.

12. Clark JI. Development and Maintenance of Lens Transparency. In DM Albert, FA Jakobiec (eds), Principles and Practice of Ophthalmology: Basic Sciences. Philadelphia: Saunders, 1994;114.

13. Hejtmancik JF, Piatigorsky J. Molecular Biology of the Lens. In DM Albert, FA Jakobiec (eds), Principles and Practice of Ophthalmology: Basic Sciences. Philadelphia: Saunders, 1994;168.

14. Fingeret M, Casser L, Woodcome HT. Atlas of Primary Eyecare Procedures. Norwalk, CT: Appleton & Lange, 1992;62.

CHAPTER

6

Aqueous and Vitreous Chambers

The eye contains three chambers—the anterior and posterior chambers, which contain aqueous humor, and the vitreous chamber, which contains the vitreous gel. The boundaries of these chambers, the contents, and the anatomic relationship with surrounding structures are discussed in this chapter.

ANTERIOR CHAMBER

The **anterior chamber** is bounded anteriorly by the corneal endothelium; peripherally by the trabecular meshwork, a portion of the ciliary body, and the iris root; and posteriorly by the anterior iris surface and the pupillary area of the anterior lens (Figure 6-1). The center of the chamber is deeper than the periphery. The **anterior chamber angle** is formed at the periphery of the chamber, where the corneoscleral and uveal coats meet. The aqueous humor exits the anterior chamber through the structures located in the angle.

Anterior Chamber Angle Structures

The structures located in the anterior chamber angle, collectively called the **filtration apparatus,** consist of the trabecular meshwork and Schlemm's canal. These structures and the scleral spur occupy the excavated area that is located at the internal corneoscleral junction and that is known as the **internal scleral sulcus.**

Scleral Spur

The **scleral spur** (described in Chapter 2) lies at the posterior edge of the internal scleral sulcus. The posterior portion of the scleral spur is the attachment site for the tendon of the longitudinal ciliary muscle fibers, whereas many of the trabecular meshwork sheets attach to the spur's anterior aspect, such that the collagen of the spur is continuous with that of the trabeculae (Figure 6-2).[1]

Trabecular Meshwork

The **trabecular meshwork** encircles the circumference of the anterior chamber. In cross-section, it has a triangular shape, its apex being at the termination of Descemet's membrane (Schwalbe's line) and its base at the scleral spur (see Figure 6-2). The inner face borders the anterior chamber, and the outer side lies against corneal stroma, sclera, and Schlemm's canal. The meshwork is composed of flattened perforated sheets, which number three to five at the apex. These sheets branch as they extend posteriorly from Schwalbe's line to the scleral spur, where they number 15–20.[2] The trabecular meshwork is an open latticework, the branches of which interlace. The intertrabecular spaces between the sheets are connected via pores, or openings within the sheets (historically called the **spaces of Fontana**).[3] The openings are of varying sizes and become smaller near Schlemm's canal. No apertures directly join the meshwork with the canal.[2]

The meshwork can be separated into two anatomic divisions. The **corneoscleral meshwork** is the outer region; its sheets attach to the scleral spur. The inner sheets, which lie inner to the spur and attach to the ciliary stroma and longitudinal muscle fibers, make up the **uveal meshwork**; some of these may attach to the iris root.[3, 4] The two portions differ slightly in structure, the corneoscleral meshwork being sheetlike and the uveal meshwork cordlike (Figure 6-3).[2] Occasional projections

91

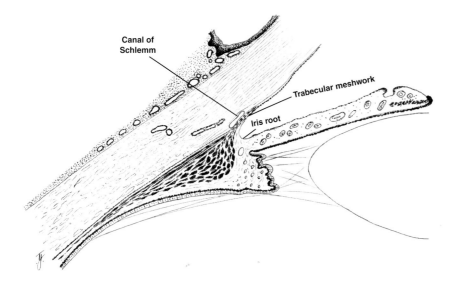

FIGURE 6-1. The periphery of the anterior segment. Structures of the anterior chamber are labeled.

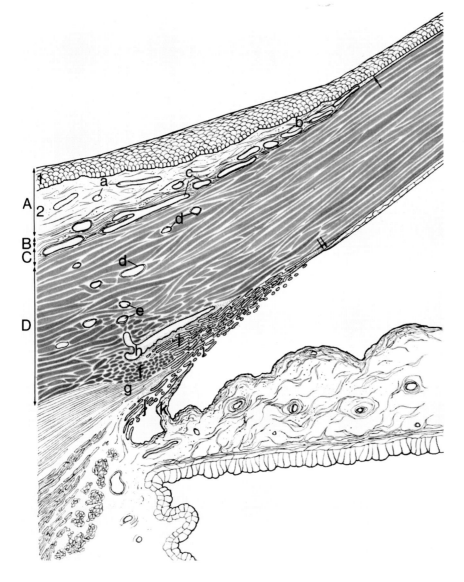

FIGURE 6-2. Drawing of the limbus. The limbal conjunctiva (A) is formed by an epithelium (1) and a loose connective tissue stroma (2). Tenon's capsule (B) forms a thin, somewhat ill-defined connective tissue layer over the episclera (C). The limbal stroma occupies the area (D) and is composed of the scleral and corneal tissues, which merge in this region. The conjunctival stromal vessels are seen at (a); they form the peripheral corneal arcades (b), which extend anteriorly to the termination of Bowman's layer (arrow). The episcleral vessels (c) are cut in different planes. Vessels forming the intrascleral (d) and deep scleral plexus (e) are shown within the limbal stroma. The scleral spur with its coarse and dense collagen fibers is shown at f. The anterior part of the longitudinal portion of the ciliary muscle (g) merges with the scleral spur and the trabecular meshwork. The lumen of Schlemm's canal (h) and the loose tissues of its wall are clearly seen. The sheets of the trabecular meshwork (i) are internal to the cords of the uveal meshwork (j). An iris process (k) arises from the iris surface and joins the trabecular meshwork at the level of the anterior portion of the scleral spur. Descemet's membrane terminates (double arrows) within the anterior portion of the triangle, outlining the aqueous outflow system. (Reprinted with permission from MJ Hogan, JA Alvarado, JE Weddell. Histology of the Human Eye. Philadelphia: Saunders, 1971;127.)

FIGURE 6-3. Drawing of the aqueous outflow apparatus and adjacent tissues. Schlemm's canal (*a*) is divided into two portions. An internal collector channel (Sondermann) (*b*) opens into the posterior part of the canal. The sheets of the corneoscleral meshwork (*c*) extend from the corneolimbus (*e*) anteriorly to the scleral spur (*d*). The ropelike components of the uveal meshwork (*f*) occupy the inner portion of the trabecular meshwork; they arise in the ciliary body (*CB*) near the angle recess and end just posterior to the termination of Descemet's membrane (*g*). An iris process (*h*) extends from the root of the iris to merge with the uveal meshwork at approximately the level of the anterior part of the scleral spur. The longitudinal ciliary muscle (*i*) is attached to the scleral spur, but a portion of it joins the corneoscleral meshwork (arrows). Descemet's membrane terminates within the deep corneolimbus. The corneal endothelium becomes continuous with the trabecular endothelium at (*j*). A broad transition zone (double-headed arrows) begins near the termination of Descemet's membrane and ends where the uveal meshwork joins the deep corneolimbus. (Reprinted with permission from MJ Hogan, JA Alvarado, JE Weddell. Histology of the Human Eye. Philadelphia: Saunders, 1971;137.)

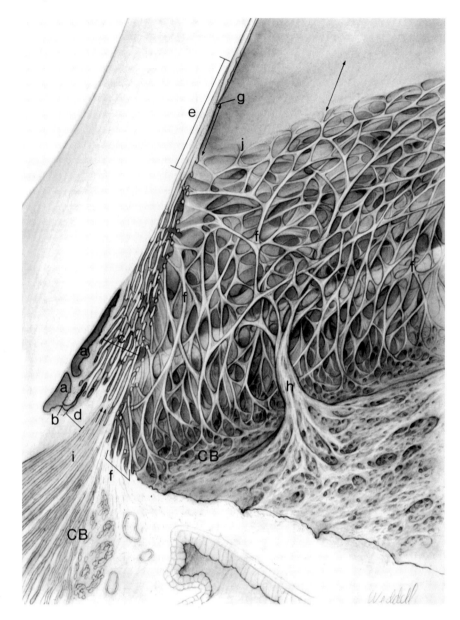

from the surface layer of the iris, known as **iris processes**, connect to the trabeculae, usually projecting no farther forward than the midpoint of the meshwork.[2]

The meshwork trabeculae consist of an inner core of collagen and elastic fibers embedded in ground substance and covered by endothelium and basement membrane (Figure 6-4). The endothelial cells are a continuation of the corneal endothelium, and the basement membrane may be a continuation of Descemet's membrane.[4, 5] The endothelial cells contain the cellular organelles for protein synthesis and apparently are capable of replacing the connective-tissue components. They also contain lysosomes, which give them the capacity for phagocytosis.[4] Gap junctions and short areas of tight junctions join the endothelial cells. No zonulae occludens are found. Cytoplasmic projections connect cells of neighboring sheets.[4, 6, 7]

At the scleral spur, the trabecular sheets lose their endothelial covering, but the collagenous and elastic fibers continue into the connective tissue of the spur and ciliary body.[2, 4] Some of the connective-tissue fibers of the ciliary muscle pass forward and merge with the inner sheets of the meshwork.

Canal of Schlemm

The Canal of Schlemm is a circular vessel and is considered to be a venous channel, although it normally contains aqueous humor rather than blood. It is located peripheral to the trabecular meshwork and anterior to the scleral spur. The external wall of the canal lies against the limbal sclera, and the internal wall lies against the trabeculae and the scleral spur (see Figure 6-2). Thin tissue septa may bridge the lumen, dividing it into two or three channels.[2, 3]

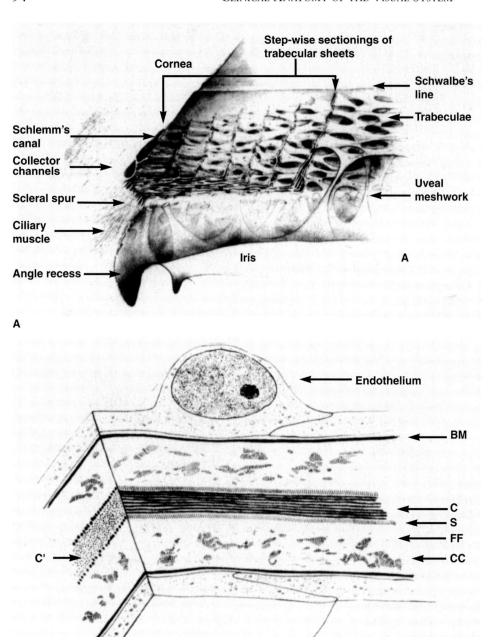

A

Schlemm's canal

Collector channels

Scleral spur

Ciliary muscle

Angle recess

Cornea

Step-wise sectionings of trabecular sheets

Schwalbe's line

Trabeculae

Uveal meshwork

Iris

A

Endothelium

BM

C

S

FF

CC

C'

B

FIGURE 6-4. (A) Trabecular area. Trabecular meshwork is cut away at progressively deeper levels to show size of openings and disposition of layer. Note large openings in uveal meshwork and progressive diminution of the size of these openings as Schlemm's canal is approached. (B) Tilted frontal and meridional representation of corneoscleral trabecular sheet. (C = central collagenous tissue; S = sheath of thick fibers; FF and CC = zone of ground substance containing irregular clumps of material and very fine fibrils; BM = basement membrane; C' = collagen fibers cut in cross section when trabeculae are sectioned in meridional plane.) (Reprinted with permission from LK Garron, ML Feeney. Electron microscopic studies of the human eye. Arch Ophthalmol 1959;62:966.)

The lumen is lined with endothelial cells, many of which are joined by zonulae occludens.[2, 7] The endothelial cells have an incomplete basement membrane.[2, 3] Pores and pinocytic vesicles in the cell membrane may be an avenue for passage of aqueous humor.[2, 3, 8, 9]

The region separating the endothelial cell lining of the canal from the trabecular meshwork is called the **cribriform layer**[4, 9, 10] or the **juxtacanalicular tissue**.[5, 11] It consists of endothelial-like cells, collagen and elasticlike fibers, and ground substance.[9, 11, 12] Schlemm's canal endothelium is anchored to the cribriform layer by a network of fibers that also is connected to the tendon of the ciliary muscle.[12]

✎ CLINICAL COMMENT: GONIOSCOPY

The condition of the anterior chamber angle structures is clinically important, as this angle is the location of exit of the aqueous humor, which must be able to flow freely from the anterior chamber. If this exit is blocked, pressure within the eye will increase, and ocular tissue damage will ensue. The width of the angle can be estimated and graded using a biomicroscope to determine whether the angle appears wide enough to provide easy access to the trabecular meshwork.

If the angle does not appear to be wide enough or if there is concern that aqueous exit is inadequate, a view of the chamber angle structures might be necessary. A direct view of the angle cannot be achieved because the limbus is opaque and light directed obliquely through the cornea into the angle does not exit, owing to total internal reflection. Therefore, a clinical procedure, **gonioscopy**, is performed that employs a special lens, a goniolens (Figure 6-5). A goniolens contains mirrors in which the examiner views the angle. The examiner sees an image as if he or she were facing the angle and sighting along the anterior surface of the iris. If all structures can be seen, they appear in the following order, beginning at the inferior aspect: the root of the iris, the ciliary body, the scleral spur, the trabecular meshwork, and Schwalbe's line (Plate 6-1). Schlemm's canal lies behind the trabecular meshwork in this view and appears as a thin red line within the meshwork if blood is backed up in the canal. Such pooling of blood occurs if the examiner exerts pressure on the lens, thereby compressing the episcleral veins and causing the episcleral venous pressure to exceed intraocular pressure (IOP).[13]

In a wide-open anterior chamber angle, the entire trabecular meshwork can be seen. As peripheral iris tissue approaches the meshwork, the angle becomes narrower, and access to the trabecular openings may be diminished. In certain conditions, cellular debris or pigment coats the meshwork, interfering with aqueous drainage; such an occurrence would be evident on gonioscopy.

Function of the Filtration Apparatus

The primary function of Schlemm's canal and the trabecular meshwork is to provide an exit for the aqueous humor. In addition, with the movement of aqueous through these structures, nutrients can diffuse into surrounding tissue, thereby supplying nutrients to the nearby deep limbal and scleral tissue.[5]

POSTERIOR CHAMBER

The **posterior chamber** is an annular area located behind the iris and bounded by the posterior iris surface, the equatorial zone of the lens, the anterior face of the vitreous, and the ciliary body. The ciliary processes that secrete the aqueous humor project into the posterior chamber. The zonule fibers arise from the internal limiting membrane of the nonpigmented epithelium of the ciliary body, pass through the posterior chamber, and insert into the lens capsule.[1] The posterior chamber contains two regions: The area occupied by the zonules is the **canal of Hannover**, and the retrozonular space, the area from the posteriormost zonules to the vitreal face, is the **canal of Petit** (Figure 6-6).[2]

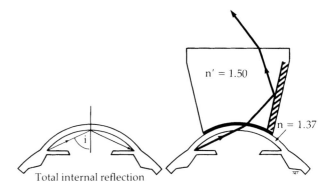

FIGURE 6-5. Optical principles of gonioscopy: (n, n' = refractive index.) (Reprinted with permission from JJ Kanski. Clinical Ophthalmology [2nd ed]. Oxford: Butterworth–Heinemann, 1989;185.)

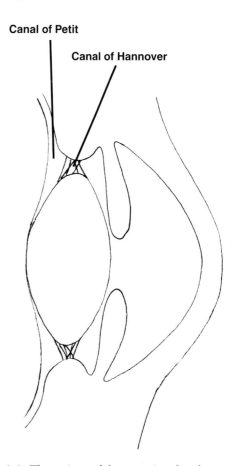

FIGURE 6-6. The regions of the posterior chamber.

AQUEOUS DYNAMICS

The aqueous humor provides necessary metabolites, primarily oxygen and glucose, to the avascular cornea and lens. It is produced by the pars plicata of the ciliary body and is secreted into the posterior chamber from the ciliary processes. It passes between the iris and lens, entering the anterior chamber through the pupil (Figure 6-7). In the anterior chamber, the aqueous circulates in con-

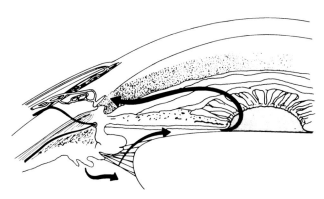

FIGURE 6-7. Normal flow of aqueous humor. Aqueous is formed in the ciliary processes, moves out around the crystalline lens and through the pupil, and flows out of the anterior chamber through the trabecular meshwork into Schlemm's canal and then to the episcleral veins. (Reprinted with permission from JD Bartlett, SD Jaanus. Clinical Ocular Pharmacology [2nd ed]. Boston: Butterworth–Heinemann, 1989;734.)

vection currents, moving down along the cooler cornea and up along the warmer iris and exiting via the periphery of the chamber.

The aqueous passes through the spaces within the uveal meshwork. A relatively small amount then passes into the connective-tissue spaces surrounding the ciliary muscle bundles.[14] The rest moves into the narrower pores of the corneoscleral meshwork and through the juxtacanalicular tissue and the endothelial lining into Schlemm's canal.[14] In histologic sections, many of the endothelial cells lining the inner wall of the canal have been found to contain giant vacuoles,[15, 16] some of which exhibit openings into the lumen.[6, 17, 18] The vacuoles apparently open and close intermittently, creating transient, transcellular, unidirectional channels that provide a means for transporting large molecules, such as proteins, across the endothelium. Flow occurs only into the canal.[8, 9, 19] As shown in Figure 6-8, an indentation forms in the basal surface of the endothelial cell, gradually enlarges, and eventually opens onto the apical surface. Then the cell cytoplasm in the basal aspect of the cell moves to occlude the opening.[19] Smaller pinocytic vesicles also provide an active transport system for substances. However, the greatest volume of aqueous humor diffuses passively into Schlemm's canal.

In the internal wall of Schlemm's canal are a number of evaginations, or blind pouches, that extend into the juxtacanalicular tissue toward the trabecular meshwork. These internal collector channels (of Sondermann)[20] can be fairly long and branching and serve to increase the surface area of the canal (Figure 6-9).[2] Their endothelium always is separated from the trabecular space by a sheet of tissue.

The endothelial cells lining the external wall of Schlemm's canal are joined by zonulae occludens and contain no vacuoles. Approximately 25–35 external collector channels branch from the outer wall of Schlemm's canal and empty into either the deep scleral or intrascleral plexus of veins,[4, 21, 22] which in turn drains into the episcleral and conjunctival veins.[2] Aqueous veins (of Ascher), which pass directly to the episcleral veins, provide another route from the canal.[23]

✍ CLINICAL COMMENT: INTRAOCULAR PRESSURE

IOP can be estimated clinically using a tonometer. IOP is maintained within a fairly small range by the complex equilibrium between production and outflow of the aqueous humor. Homeostatic mechanisms normally preserve this balance, but small variations in either the production or outflow of aqueous can cause significant changes in IOP. Production has been demonstrated to remain fairly constant. Hence, most cases of increased IOP are due to decreased aqueous outflow. Several theories have been developed to explain the decrease. Flow can be impeded at various sites along the aqueous pathway. Deposits of pigment or debris on the trabecular sheets and cords can restrict aqueous flow through the trabecular spaces. Proliferation of the juxtacanalicular tissue increases with age and has been found also to cause a decrease in outflow.[4]

✍ CLINICAL COMMENT: GLAUCOMA

Glaucoma is a complex and poorly understood disease process. One causative factor in many patients is higher-than-normal IOP. Increased IOP apparently contributes to damage of the retinal nerve fiber layer, either directly by mechanical pressure or indirectly through impeded blood flow. Treatment might consist of attempts to reduce the pressure with drugs that either decrease aqueous production

Canal of Schlemm

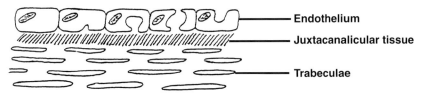

— Endothelium

— Juxtacanalicular tissue

— Trabeculae

Anterior chamber

FIGURE 6-8. The formation of giant vacuoles in the endothelial cells lining Schlemm's canal. (Redrawn from JD Bartlett, SD Jaanus. Clinical Ocular Pharmacology [2nd ed]. Boston: Butterworth–Heinemann, 1989;735.)

FIGURE 6-9. Drawing of Schlemm's canal, an internal collector channel, and adjacent tissues. The lumen of the canal (*sc*) is lined by endothelium (*e*). The endothelium of the inner wall is very irregular, with many folds and out-pouchings. Giant vacuoles (*gv*) are seen in the endothelial cells along the inner wall. The external wall of the canal (*ew*) is shown. The internal wall (*iw*) lies between the endothelium and the nearest trabecular space (*ts*). An internal collector channel (*icc*) arises near the posterior canal wall and extends into the trabecular meshwork, where it is lost. Like Schlemm's canal, it also is surrounded by a wall (*a*) that separates its lumen from the adjacent trabecular spaces. The corneoscleral trabecular sheets (*cst*) branch frequently, and their endothelial cells often form bridges between adjacent sheets. (Reprinted with permission from MJ Hogan, JA Alvarado, JE Weddell. Histology of the Human Eye. Philadelphia: Saunders, 1971;153.)

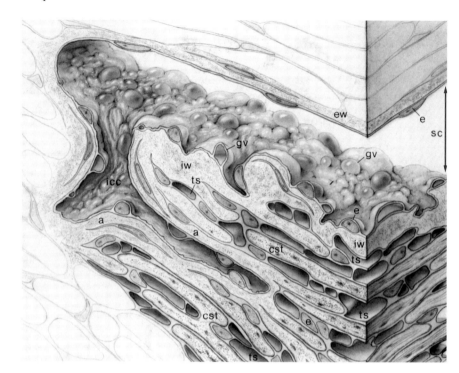

or facilitate aqueous outflow. One treatment plan includes the use of drugs that cause the iris sphincter and ciliary muscle to contract. Ciliary muscle contraction changes the configuration of the trabecular sheets, which is believed to facilitate outflow.[24, 25]

VITREOUS CHAMBER

The **vitreous chamber** is filled with the gel-like vitreous body and occupies the largest portion of the globe. It is bounded on the front by the posterior surface of the lens and the retrozonular portion of the posterior chamber. Peripherally and posteriorly, it is bounded by the pars plana of the ciliary body, the retina, and the optic disc. The center of the anterior surface contains the patellar fossa, an indentation in which the lens sits.

Vitreal Attachments

The vitreous forms several attachments to surrounding structures. The strongest of these is the vitreous base, located at the ora serrata. The other attachments (in order of decreasing strength) are to the posterior lens, to the optic disc, at the macula, and to retinal vessels.

The **vitreous base**, the most extensive adhesion, extends 1.5–2.0 mm anterior to the ora serrata, 1–3 mm posterior to it, and several millimeters into the vitreous (Figure 6-10).[2, 26] The vitreal fibers that form

the base are embedded firmly in the basement membrane of the nonpigmented epithelium of the ciliary body and the internal limiting membrane of the peripheral retina.[21, 27]

The **hyaloideocapsular ligament (of Weiger)**, or **retrolental ligament**, forms an annular attachment 1–2 mm wide and 8–9 mm in diameter between the posterior surface of the lens and the anterior face of the vitreous.[26] This is a firm attachment site in the young, but the strength of the bond diminishes with age. Within the ring formed by this ligament is a potential space, the retrolental space (of Berger), which is present because the lens and vitreous are juxtaposed but not joined.[2]

The peripapillary adhesion around the edge of the optic disc also diminishes with age. The annular ring of attachment at the macula is 3–4 mm in diameter.[2]

The attachment of the vitreous to retinal blood vessels consists of fine strands that extend through the internal limiting membrane to branch and surround the larger retinal vessels.[27, 28] These strands may account for hemorrhages that occur when there is vitreal traction on the retina. The nature of the attachment between the vitreous and the retinal internal limiting membrane remains uncertain. It is unlikely that fibrils from the posterior vitreous insert into the internal limiting membrane[29–31]; the actual interface probably is at a chemical bond level below the resolution of the electron microscope.[2, 32]

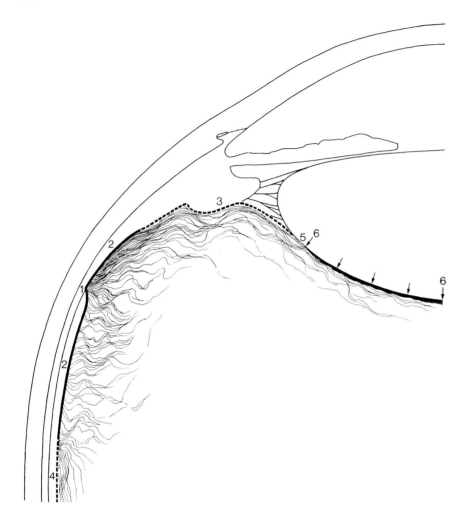

FIGURE 6-10. Vitreous relations in the anterior eye. The ora serrata (*1*) is the termination of the retina. The vitreous base (*2*) extends forward approximately 2.0 mm over the ciliary body and posteriorly approximately 4.0 mm over the peripheral retina. The collagen in this region is oriented at a right angle to the surface of the retina and ciliary body, but anteriorly over the pars plana, it is more parallel to the inner surface of the ciliary body. The posterior hyaloid (*4*) is continuous with the retina and the anterior hyaloid (*3*) with the zonules and lens. Also depicted are the hyaloideocapsular ligament (*5*) and the space of Berger (*6*). (Reprinted with permission from MJ Hogan, JA Alvarado, JE Weddell. Histology of the Human Eye. Philadelphia: Saunders, 1971;612.)

Vitreous Zones

The vitreous can be divided into zones that differ in relative density. The outermost is the cortex, the intermediate zone is inner to that, and the center is occupied by Cloquet's canal.

Vitreous Cortex

The **vitreous cortex**, also called the **hyaloid surface**, is the outer zone.[33] It is 1–3 mm wide and is composed of tightly packed collagen fibrils, some of which run parallel and some perpendicular to the retinal surface.[34, 35] The anterior cortex lies anterior to the base and is adjacent to the ciliary body, the posterior chamber, and the lens. The posterior cortex extends posterior to the base and is in contact with the retina. It contains transvitreal channels that appear as holes—the prepapillary hole, the premacular hole, and prevascular fissures. The prepapillary hole can sometimes be seen clinically when the posterior vitreous detaches from the retina.[26] The premacular hole, a weak area, may be a region of decreased density rather than an actual hole.[26, 35] The prevascular fissures provide the avenue by which fine fibers enter the retina and encircle retinal vessels.[27]

Intermediate Zone

The **intermediate zone** contains fine fibers that are continuous and unbranched and that run anteroposteriorly.[26, 34, 36] These fibers arise at the region of the vitreous base and insert into the posterior cortex.[37] The peripheral fibers parallel the cortex, whereas the more central fibers parallel Cloquet's canal. Membranelike condensations, called **vitreous tracts**, may be differentiated as areas that have differing fiber densities (Figure 6-11).[35]

Cloquet's Canal

Cloquet's canal, also called the **hyaloid channel** or the **retrolental tract**, is located in the center of the vitreous body.[2] It has an **S** shape, rotated 90 degrees with the center dip downward, and is the former site of the hyaloid artery system, which was formed during embryologic development (see Chapter 7). Cloquet's canal arises at the retrolental space. Its anterior face is approximately 4–5 mm in diameter.[2] It terminates at the area of Martegiani, a funnel-shaped space at the optic nerve head that extends forward into the vitreous to become continuous with the canal.[2, 26]

Composition

The highly transparent vitreous is a dilute solution of salts, soluble proteins, and **hyaluronic acid** (HA) contained within a meshwork of the insoluble protein collagen. It is 98.5–99.7% water.[35] Because of its high water content, study of the vitreous is difficult: Attempts at tissue fixation often have dehydrating effects that introduce artifacts.

Collagen

The collagen content of the vitreous is highest in the vitreous base, next highest in the posterior cortex, next in the anterior cortex, and lowest in the center.[26] A fine meshwork of uniform collagen fibrils, each 8–16 nm in diameter, is evident with the electron microscope and fills the vitreous body.[33, 38–41] The individual fibrils cannot be seen with the slit-lamp, but the pattern of variations in their density and regularity can. The density of this collagen fibril network differs throughout the vitreous.[33]

Hyaluronic Acid

The second major vitreal component, HA, is a long unbranched chain of molecules coiled into a twisted network.[36] This macromolecule is located in specific sites within the collagen fibril network and is believed to maintain the wide spacing between fibrils.[26] The concentration of HA is highest in the posterior cortex and decreases centrally and anteriorly.[41] The interaction between HA and collagen fibrils contributes to the viscoelastic properties of the vitreous[42, 43] and influences the physical properties (gel and liquid) of the vitreous state.[26]

Hyalocytes

Vitreous cells, or **hyalocytes**, are located in a widely spaced single layer in the cortex near the vitreal surface and parallel to it.[26, 36] Various functions have been attributed to these cells: Some investigators have determined that these cells synthesize HA.[44–46] Others have found evidence that these cells synthesize glycoproteins for the collagen fibrils.[26, 47] Still others indicate that hyalocytes have phagocytic properties.[36, 46, 48] Apparently, hyalocytes can have different appearances depending on their activity at a given time.[26] Cells located in the vitreous base are fibroblastlike anterior to the ora serrata and macrophagelike posterior to it.[29]

Fibroblasts that are present in the vitreous are located in the vitreous base near the ciliary body and near the optic disc. Although they make up less than 10% of the cell population, in the past they may have been mistaken for hyalocytes. It is believed that fibroblasts synthesize the collagen fibrils that run anteroposteriorly and are active in pathologic conditions.[26]

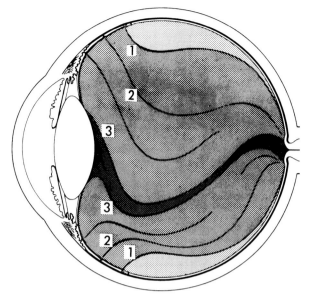

FIGURE 6-11. Eisner's interpretation of vitreous structures (according to slit-lamp examinations of eyes obtained at autopsy). The vitreous body is divided into three zones: Externally, as far as the retina extends, there is a relatively thick vitreous cortex (whitish gray). It has holes at characteristic locations: in front of the papilla, in the region of the fovea centralis, in front of vessels, and in front of anomalies of the ora serrata region (enclosed ora bays, meridional folds, zonular traction tufts). The intermediate zone (light gray) contains vitreal tracts, membranelles that form funnels packed into one another and that diverge from the region of papilla anteriorly. The central channel is space (dark gray) delimited by hyaloid tract. It is closed off anteriorly by a retrolental section of anterior vitreous membrane. It contains no typical tracts but only irregularly arranged vitreous fibers, part of which are residua of Cloquet's canal. The outermost vitreous tract, the preretinal tract (*1*), separates intermediary substance from vitreous cortex. The innermost tract, the hyaloid tract (*3*), inserts at the edge of the lens. Between them extends the median tract (*2*) to the median ligament of pars plana and the coronary tract to the coronary ligament. (Reprinted with permission from J Sebag. The Vitreous. In WM Hart Jr [ed], Adler's Physiology of the Eye [9th ed]. St. Louis: Mosby, 1992;268.)

Other cells that have been identified as macrophages and fibroblasts might originate in the nearby retinal blood vessels.[2, 35]

Vitreal Function

The vitreous body is a storage area for metabolites and catabolites for the retina and lens and provides an avenue for the movement of these substances within the eye.[23] The vitreous, because of its viscoelastic properties, acts as a shock absorber, protecting the fragile retinal tissue during rapid eye movements and strenuous physical activity.[2, 35] The vitreous transmits and refracts light, aiding in focusing the rays on the retina. Minimal light scattering occurs in the vitreous owing to its extremely low concentration of molecular substances and the wide interfibrillar spacing ensured by the HA-collagen complex. A disruption in the HA-collagen complex causes the collagen fibrils to aggregate into bundles, which may become large enough to be visible clinically, a phenomenon often referred to as **floaters**.

Age-Related Vitreal Changes

In the infant, the vitreous is a very homogeneous, gel-like body. With maturation, changes occur whereby the gel volume decreases and the liquid volume increases.[26] By age 40, the vitreous is 80% gel and 20% liquid, and by 70 or 80 years of age, it is 50% liquid,[34] with most of the liquefaction occurring in the central vitreous.[35] Conformational changes in the HA molecule and the subsequent displacement of collagen from the HA-collagen network influence the change from gel to liquid.[49] As the dissolution of the HA-collagen complex occurs, the macromolecule moves out of the collagen network, causing the fibrils to coalesce into fibers and then bands; the HA pools in areas adjacent to these bundles, forming areas of liquid vitreous.[50] The pockets of liquid formed by these changes are called **lacunae**.[51]

✎ CLINICAL COMMENT: PERIPHERAL
   RETINAL TRACTION
   With aging, the vitreous base adhesion extends further posteriorly, and the border approaches the equator.[52] These changes can increase traction on the peripheral retina and might contribute to the development of retinal tears and detachment.

✎ CLINICAL COMMENT: POSTERIOR
   VITREAL DETACHMENT
   As the HA is displaced from the collagen network and as the fibrils coalesce into bundles, the bundles can contract and apply traction to the vitreous and, consequently, to the posterior retina. One of the most common abnormalities that occur at the posterior retinal–vitreous interface is a posterior vitreal detachment caused by this traction. The vitreous usually detaches from the retinal internal limiting membrane at the peripapillary ring, forming a retrocortical space. If glial tissue is torn away with the vitreous, a circular condensation, Weiss's ring, may be visible within the vitreous.[53] If liquid vitreous seeps into the retrocortical space through the prepapillary and premacular areas, a syneresis or collapse of the vitreous can be caused by the volume displacement.[50, 54]

REFERENCES

1. Fine BS, Yanoff M. The Vitreous Body. In BS Fine, M Yanoff (eds), Ocular Histology (2nd ed). Hagerstown, MD: Harper & Row, 1979;131.

2. Hogan MJ, Alvarado JA. Histology of the Human Eye. Philadelphia: Saunders, 1971;136, 313, 493, 607.

3. Warwick R. Eugene Wolff's Anatomy of the Eye and Orbit (7th ed). Philadelphia: Saunders, 1976;52.

4. Lütjen-Drecoll E, Rohen JW. Functional Morphology of the Trabecular Meshwork. In W Tasman, EA Jaeger (eds), Duane's Foundations of Clinical Ophthalmology (Vol 1). Philadelphia: Lippincott, 1994;1.

5. Fine BS. Structure of the trabecular meshwork and Schlemm's canal. Trans Am Acad Ophthalmol Otolaryngol 1966;70:791.

6. Raviola G, Raviola E. Paracellular route of aqueous in the trabecular meshwork and canal of Schlemm. Invest Ophthalmol Vis Sci 1981;21:52.

7. Bhatt K, Gong F, Freddo TF. Freeze-fracture studies of interendothelial junctions in the angle of the human eye. Invest Ophthalmol Vis Sci 1995;36(7):1379.

8. Bill A. Scanning electron microscopic studies of the canal of Schlemm. Exp Eye Res 1970;10:214.

9. Epstein DL, Rohen JW. Morphology of the trabecular meshwork and inner wall after cationised ferritin perfusion in the monkey eye. Invest Ophthalmol Vis Sci 1991;32:160.

10. Lütjen-Drecoll E, Futa R, Rohen JW. Ultrahistochemical studies on tangential sections of the trabecular meshwork in normal and glaucomatous eyes. Invest Ophthalmol Vis Sci 1981;21:563.

11. Inomata H, Bill A, Smelser HK. Aqueous humor pathways through the trabecular meshwork and into Schlemm's canal in the cynomolgus monkey (Macaca irus). Am J Ophthalmol 1972;73:760.

12. Rohen JW, Futa R, Lütjen-Drecoll E. The fine structure of the cribriform network in normal and glaucomatous eyes seen in tangential sections. Invest Ophthalmol Vis Sci 1981;21:574.

13. Kanski JJ. Clinical Ophthalmology (3rd ed). Oxford: Butterworth–Heinemann, 1994;239.

14. Bill A. Some aspects of aqueous humour drainage. Eye 1993;7(1):14.

15. Holmberg AS. The fine structure of the inner wall of Schlemm's canal. Arch Ophthalmol 1959;62:956.

16. Speakman JS. Drainage channels in the trabecular wall of Schlemm's canal. Br J Ophthalmol 1960; 44:513.

17. Feeney ML, Wissig S. Outflow studies using an electron dense tracer. Trans Am Acad Ophthalmol Otolaryngol 1966;70:791.

18. Anderson DR. Scanning electron microscopy of primate trabecular meshwork. Am J Ophthalmol 1971; 71:90.

19. Tripathi EC. Mechanism of the aqueous outflow across the trabecular wall of Schlemm's canal. Exp Eye Res 1971;11:116.

20. Sondermann R. The formation, morphology and function of Schlemm's canal. Acta Ophthalmol 1933;11:280.

21. Theobold GD. Schlemm's canal. Its anastomosis and anatomic relations. Trans Am Ophthalmol Soc 1934;32:574.

22. Ashton N. Anatomical study of Schlemm's canal and aqueous veins by means of neoprene casts: I. Aqueous veins. Br J Ophthalmol 1951;35:291.

23. Ascher KW. Aqueous veins: preliminary notes. Am J Ophthalmol 1942;25:31.

24. Rohen JW, Unger HH. Studies on the morphology and pathology of the trabecular meshwork in the human eye. Am J Ophthalmol 1958;46:802.

25. Grierson I, Lee WR, Abraham S. Effects of pilocarpine on the morphology of human outflow apparatus. Br J Ophthalmol 1978;62:302.

26. Sebag J. The Vitreous. In WM Hart Jr (ed), Adler's Physiology of the Eye (9th ed). St. Louis: Mosby, 1992;268.

27. Mutlu F, Leopold IH. Structure of the human retinal vascular system. Arch Ophthalmol. 1964;71:93.

28. Wolter JR. Pores in the internal limiting membrane of the human retina. Arch Ophthalmol 1964;42:971.

29. Gartner J. Vitreous electron microscopic studies on the fine structure of the normal and pathologically changed vitreoretinal limiting membrane. Surv Ophthalmol 1964;9:219.

30. Matsumato B, Blanks JC, Ryan SJ. Topographic variations in rabbit and primate internal limiting membrane. Invest Ophthalmol Vis Sci 1984;25:71.

31. Malecaze F, Caratero C, Caratero A, et al. Some ultrastructural aspects of the vitreoretinal junction. Ophthalmologica 1985;191:22.

32. Russell SR, Shepherd JD, Hageman GS. Distribution of glycoconjugates in the human retinal internal limiting membrane. Invest Ophthalmol Vis Sci 1991; 32(7):1986.

33. Schwarz W. Electron microscopic observations on the human vitreous body. In GK Smelser (ed), Structure of the Eye. New York: Academic, 1961;283.

34. Balazs EA. Functional Anatomy of the Vitreous. In W Tasman, EA Jaeger (eds), Duane's Foundations of Clinical Ophthalmology (Vol 1). Philadelphia: Lippincott, 1994;1.

35. Eisner G. Clinical Anatomy of the Vitreous. In W Tasman, EA Jaeger (eds), Duane's Foundations of Clinical Ophthalmology (Vol 1). Philadelphia: Lippincott, 1994;1.

36. Balazs EA, Toth LZ, Eckle EA, et al. Studies on the structure of the vitreous body: XII. Cytological and histochemical studies on the cortical tissue. Exp Eye Res 1964;3:57.

37. Sebag J, Balazs EA. Morphology and ultrastructure of human vitreous fibers. Invest Ophthalmol Vis Sci 1989;30:1867.

38. Pirie A, Schmidt G, Waters JW. Ox vitreous humor: I. The residual protein. Br J Ophthalmol 1948;32:321.

39. Matolsy AG. A study on the structural protein of the vitreous body (vitrosin). J Gen Physiol 1952;36:29.

40. Gross J, Matoltsy AG, Cohen C. Vitrosin: a member of the collagen class. J Biophys Biochem Cytol 1955;1:215.

41. Bembridge BA, Crawford CNC, Pirie A. Phase-contrast microscopy of the animal vitreous body. Br J Ophthalmol 1952;36:131.

42. Weber H, Landwehr G. A new method for the determination of the mechanical properties of the vitreous. Ophthalmic Res 1982;14:326.

43. Weber H, Landwehr G, Kilp H, et al. The mechanical properties of the vitreous of pig and human donor eyes. Ophthalmic Res 1982;14:335.

44. Osterlin SE. The synthesis of hyaluronic acid in the vitreous: IV. Regeneration in the owl monkey. Exp Eye Res 1968;7:524.

45. Hultsch E, Balazs EA. In vitro synthesis of glycosaminoglycans and glycoproteins by cells of the vitreous. Invest Ophthalmol Vis Sci 1973;14(Suppl):43.

46. Freeman MI, Jacobson B, Balazs EA. The chemical composition of vitreous hyalocyte granules. Exp Eye Res 1979;29:479.

47. Ayad S, Weiss JB. A new look at vitreous humor collagen. Biochem J 1984;218:835.

48. Szirmai JA, Balazs EA. Studies on the structure of the vitreous body: cells in the cortical layer. Arch Ophthalmol 1958;59:34.

49. Armand G, Chakrabarti B. Conformational differences between hyaluronates of gel and liquid human vitreous—fractionation and circular dichroism studies. Curr Eye Res 1987;6:445.

50. Sebag J. Age-related differences in the human vitreoretinal interface. Arch Ophthalmol 1991;109(7):966.

51. Kishi S, Shimizu K. Posterior precortical vitreous pocket. Arch Ophthalmol 1990;108:979.

52. Teng CC, Che HH. Vitreous changes and the mechanism of retinal detachment. Am J Ophthalmol 1957;44:335.

53. Spalton DJ, Hitchings RA, Hunter PA. Atlas of Clinical Ophthalmology. Philadelphia: Lippincott, 1984; 12.4.

54. Lindner B. Acute posterior vitreous detachment and its retinal complications. Acta Ophthalmol Suppl 1966;87:1.

CHAPTER

7

Ocular Embryology

This chapter has been placed after those describing the globe and orbit because the study of embryology can be difficult if the adult structure, organization, and function are not known. Though it might seem backward to study the development of a structure *after* one has studied the structure itself, in my experience this has proved to be a useful sequence for the student. *In this chapter, the development of each structure will be described separately, but the reader must keep in mind that these events are occurring simultaneously.*

DEVELOPMENT OF OCULAR STRUCTURES

During the third week of embryonic development, the three primary germ layers—ectoderm, mesoderm, and endoderm—have formed the embryonic plate.[1] (Of these three, only ectoderm and mesoderm will take part in the developing ocular structures.) A thickening in the ectoderm forms the **neural plate** and will give rise to the central nervous system, including ocular structures. A groove forms down the center of this plate at approximately day 18 of gestation, and the ridges bordering the groove grow into **neural folds**; as the groove expands, these folds grow toward one another to form the **neural tube** along the dorsal aspect of the embryo. The neural tube is formed on or near day 22.[1]

The ectoderm now lining the tube is **neural ectoderm** and that surrounding the tube is **surface ectoderm**, which differ both in anatomic location and in differentiation potentials (Table 7-1). An area of cells on the crest of each of the neural folds separates from the ectoderm. These **neural crest cells** come to lie between the neural tube and the surface ectoderm. Cells from the middle embryonic layer, the **mesoderm**, also are located between the neural tube and the surface ectoderm. Figure 7-1 illustrates these events.

Optic Pits

The **optic pits** form as indentations on both sides of the neural tube in the forebrain region even before the tube is completely closed. On approximately day 25, after the neural tube has closed, the optic pits form lateral sac-shaped extensions, the **optic vesicles**.[2] The vesicles initially are in contact with surface ectoderm[3] but gradually are separated from it by cells of neural crest origin and mesoderm.

Neural crest cells and mesoderm collectively make up the **mesenchyme** from which the connective tissue of the globe and orbit develop. Although most orbital connective tissue is neural crest–derived, determining whether a structure is of neural crest or mesodermal origin sometimes is difficult, as mesodermal cells and neural crest cells appear similar cytologically.[4] If the origin is uncertain, mesenchyme will be cited as the germ layer.

As the optic vesicle evaginates, the tissue joining the vesicle to the neural tube constricts, forming the **optic stalk** (Figure 7-2). The cells lining the inner surface of this entire formation are ciliated, and the outer surface is covered by a thin basal lamina.[2] The cavity of the optic stalk, and that of the optic vesicle, is continuous with the space that will become the third ventricle.

While the wall of the optic vesicle is in contact with surface ectoderm, it thickens and flattens to form the retinal disc.[4] The lower wall of the optic vesicle and optic stalk begins to buckle and move inward toward the upper and posterior walls. This invagination forms

TABLE 7-1. Embryologic Derivation of Ocular Structures

Surface ectoderm gives rise to:
  Lens
  Corneal epithelium
  Conjunctival epithelium and lacrimal gland
  Epithelium of eyelids and cilia, meibomian glands, and
    glands of Zeis and Moll
  Epithelium lining nasolacrimal system

Neural ectoderm gives rise to:
  Retinal pigment epithelium
  Neural retinal fibers of optic nerve
  Neuroglia
  Epithelium of ciliary body
  Epithelium of iris, including iris sphincter and dilator
    muscles

Neural crest gives rise to:
  Corneal stroma (which gives rise to Bowman's layer)
  Corneal endothelium (which gives rise to Descemet's
    membrane)
  Most (or all) of sclera
  Trabecular structures
  Uveal pigment cells
  Uveal connective tissue
  Vascular pericytes

Source: Adapted from GR Beauchamp, PA Knepper. Role of the neural crest in anterior segment development and disease. J Pediatr Ophthalmol Strabismus 1984;21(6):209; CS Cook, V Ozanics, FA Jakobiec. Prenatal Development of the Eye and Its Adnexa. In W Tasman, EA Jaeger (eds), Duane's Foundations of Clinical Ophthalmology (Vol 1). Philadelphia: Lippincott, 1994;1; and DM Nodon. Periocular Mesenchyma: Neural Crest and Mesodermal Interactions. In W Tasman, EA Jaeger (eds), Duane's Foundations of Clinical Ophthalmology (Vol 1). Philadelphia: Lippincott, 1994;1.

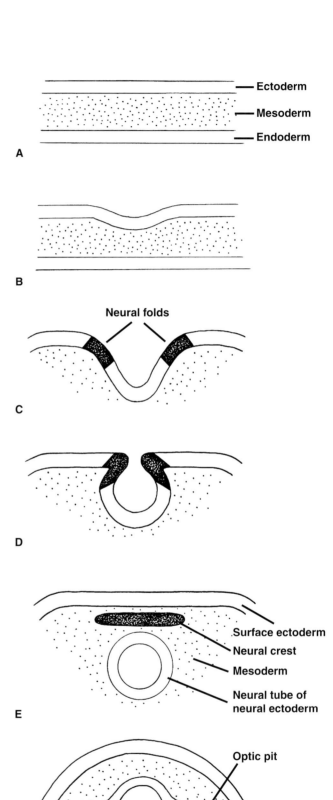

FIGURE 7-1. ▶ Formation of the neural tube. (A) Horizontal section through the three-layered embryonic disc. (B) The neural groove forms in the neural plate area of ectoderm. (C) The neural groove invaginates, and neural folds are formed. (D) The neural folds continue to grow toward each other. (E) Neural crest cells separate from the ectoderm of the neural folds as they fuse, the neural tube is formed (of neural ectoderm), and the surface ectoderm is again continuous. (F) Evaginations in the area of the forebrain form the optic pits.

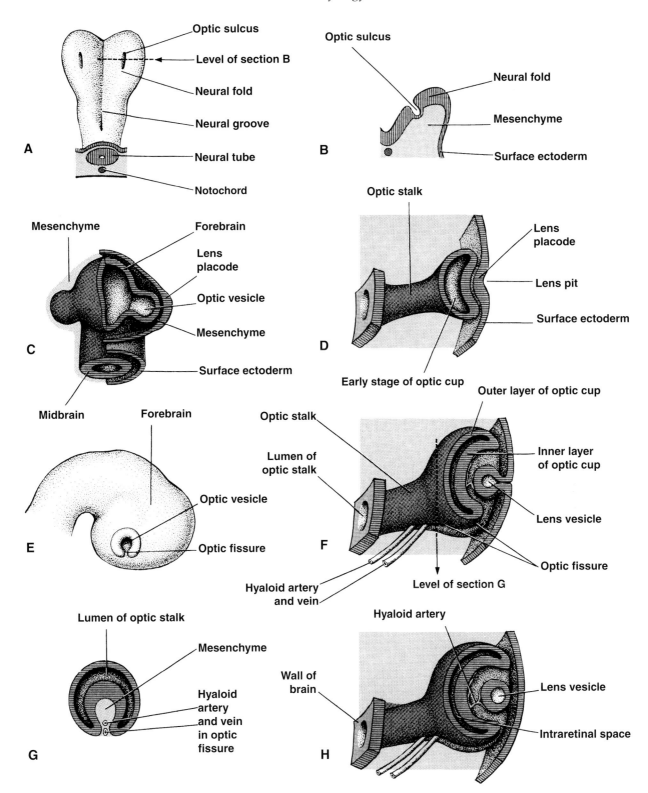

FIGURE 7-2. Early eye development. (A) Dorsal view of the cranial end of a 22-day embryo, showing the first indication of eye development. (B) Transverse section through a neural fold, showing an optic sulcus. (C) Forebrain and its covering layers of mesenchyme and surface ectoderm from an approximately 28-day-old embryo. (D, F, H) Sections of developing eye, illustrating successive stages in the development of the optic cup and the lens vesicle. (E) Lateral view of the brain of an approximately 32-day-old embryo, showing the external appearance of the optic cup. (G) Transverse section through the optic stalk, showing the optic fissure and its contents. (Reprinted with permission from KL Moore. Before We Are Born: Basic Embryology and Birth Defects [3rd ed]. Philadelphia: Saunders, 1989;270.)

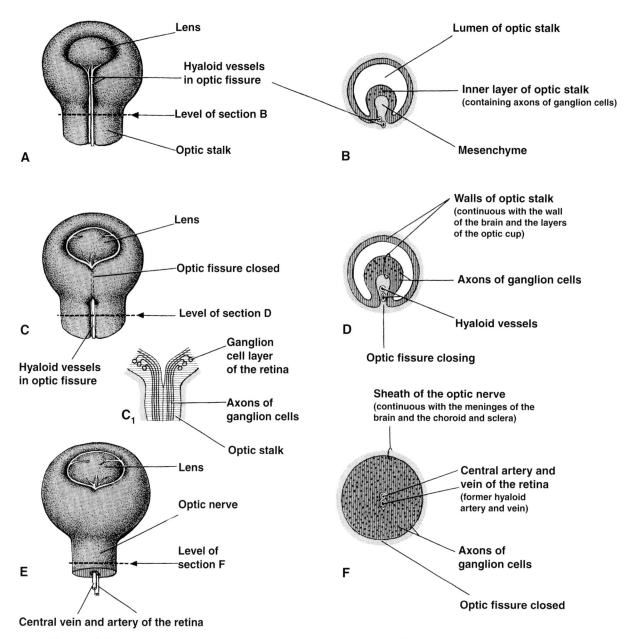

FIGURE 7-3. Closure of the optic fissure and formation of the optic nerve. (A, C, E) Views of the inferior surface of the optic cup and stalk, showing progressive stages in the closure of the optic fissure. Longitudinal section of a portion of the optic cup and optic stalk (C) shows axons of ganglion cells of the retina growing through the optic stalk to the brain. (B, D, F) Transverse sections through the optic stalk, showing successive stages in the closure of the optic fissure and in formation of the optic nerve. The optic fissure normally closes during the sixth week. Defects of closure of the optic fissure results in a defect in the iris known as **coloboma of the iris**. Note that the lumen of the optic stalk is obliterated gradually as axons of ganglion cells accumulate in the inner layer of the stalk. Formation of the optic nerve occurs between the sixth and eighth weeks. (Reprinted with permission from KL Moore. Before We Are Born: Basic Embryology and Birth Defects [3rd ed]. Philadelphia: Saunders, 1989:271.)

a cleft, variously called the **optic, embryonic,** or **fetal fissure.** (It has also been called the **choroidal fissure,** but that name will be avoided as it may imply that the choroid is involved in the fissure, which it is not.) The inferior wall continues to move inward, pulling the anterior wall of the optic vesicle with it and placing the retinal disc in the approximate location of the future retina. The edges of the fissure grow toward one another and begin to fuse at 5 weeks; fusion starts at the center and proceeds anteriorly toward the rim of the optic cup and posteriorly along the optic stalk. Closure is complete at 7 weeks, forming the two-layered optic cup (Figure 7-3).[5] Mesenchyme enters the fissure and moves into the cavity of the developing optic cup.

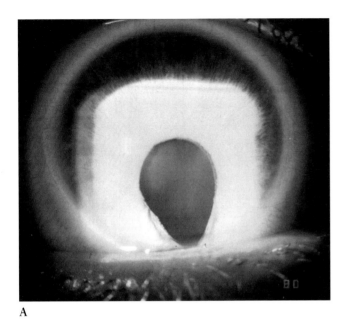

A

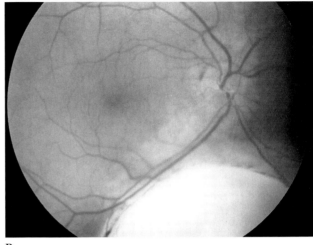

B

FIGURE 7-4. (A) Coloboma of iris gives pupil a keyhole appearance. (B) Coloboma of retina. Retinal and choroidal tissue absent; field defect results.

Optic Cup, Lens, and Related Structures

Optic Cup

The **optic cup** at this stage of development is composed of two layers of cells (both neuroectodermal in origin) that are continuous with each other at the rim of the cup. The cells of the inner and outer layers of the optic cup are positioned apex to apex and are separated by the **intraretinal space**, which, as the two layers approach each other, finally will become only a potential space. The outer layer of the optic cup will become the retinal pigment epithelium (RPE), the outer pigmented epithelium of the ciliary body, and the anterior iris epithelium. The inner layer will become the neural retina, the inner nonpigmented ciliary body epithelium, and the posterior iris epithelium.

✍ CLINICAL COMMENT: COLOBOMA

Incomplete closure of the optic fissure may affect the developing optic cup or stalk and the adult derivations of these structures, resulting in an inferior defect in the optic disc, retina, ciliary body, or iris. This defect is called a **coloboma** and can vary from a slight notch to a large wedgelike defect. A large iris coloboma produces a keyhole-shaped pupil, though the remainder of the iris develops normally.[6] Colobomas affecting the sensory retina and RPE also involve the choroid, because its differentiation depends on an intact RPE layer.[7] Bare sclera is seen in the area affected, with retinal vessels passing over the defect (Figure 7-4).

Induction

During embryologic development, formation and growth of structures depend on tissue differentiation and inter-

actions among these tissues. Some structures will not develop unless they are near another developing area at a specific time. There is some uncertainty regarding whether the two structures must actually come in contact or just be in close proximity, but substances *must* be able to pass between them.[8] This influence that one developing structure has on another is termed **induction**. It is likely that the mechanism of induction is not a single event but a series of separate steps that presumably occur on a biochemical level.[9]

Lens

Induction occurs between the developing optic cup and the developing lens, with an apparent reciprocal relationship.[10] At the time that the invagination of the optic cup begins (approximately day 27), surface ectoderm adjacent to the vesicle begins to thicken, forming the **lens plate (lens placode)**. This thickening is caused by an elongation of the ectodermal cells and by a regional increase in cell division.[4] If the area of contact between the optic vesicle and surface ectoderm is less than normal, a perfectly formed but microphthalmic eye will result.[11] Some investigators believe that transformation of the lens plate into the lens vesicle might be independent of direct contact with the optic vesicle.[12] In addition to signals from the developing optic vesicle, complete lens differentiation might also depend on factors that inhibit lens formation in the ectoderm adjacent to the lens plate.[13]

The center of the outer surface of the lens plate invaginates rapidly, forming a **lens pit**. As invagination continues, the lens vesicle is formed, which then separates from the surface ectoderm at approximately day 33.[2, 8] The **lens vesicle** is a hollow sphere composed of a

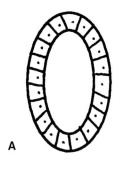

A

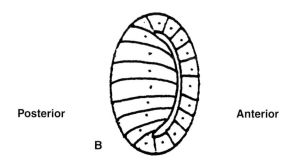

Posterior   **B**   **Anterior**

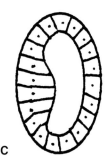

C

FIGURE 7-5. Development of the embryonic nucleus. (A) Hollow lens vesicle is lined with epithelium. (B) Posterior cells elongate, becoming primary lens fibers. (C) Primary lens fibers fill lumen, forming embryonic nucleus. The curved line formed by the cell nuclei is called the **lens bow**. The anterior epithelium remains in place.

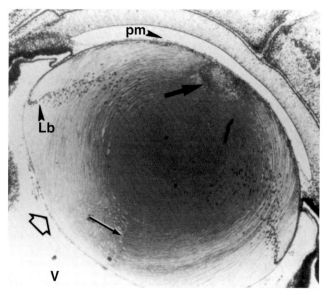

FIGURE 7-6. Lens at 65 mm (12-week fetus) in transverse section. Posterior suture (thin arrow) extends from the surface to the central, primary lens fibers (location of the embryonic nucleus). The triangular anterior suture (thick arrow) is indicated by an assembly of transversely cut fibers at the anterior pole. The posterior vascular lens capsule is indicated by a hollow arrow. The nucleated area is the location of the secondary lens fibers (×40). The lens bow (*Lb*) is formed by anteriorly migrating nuclei of newly formed lens fibers. (pm = vessels of the pupillary membrane; V = vitreous.) (Reprinted with permission from CS Cook, V Ozanics, FA Jakobiec. Prenatal Development of the Eye and Its Adnexa. In W Tasman, EA Jaeger [eds], Duane's Foundations of Clinical Ophthalmology [Vol 1]. Philadelphia: Lippincott, 1994;11.)

single layer of cells surrounded by a thin basal lamina; with the addition of more material, the basal lamina will become the lens capsule.

Once the lens vesicle is formed, the posterior epithelial cells adjacent to the future vitreous cavity elongate to fill in the lumen within the lens vesicle (Figure 7-5). The proximity of the developing retina seems to be the inducing factor for this elongation. These pos-

terior epithelial cells become the **primary lens fibers** and form the **embryonic nucleus** at the center of the lens. This nucleus has no sutures. The fact that the posterior epithelium was used to form the embryonic nucleus accounts for the lack of an epithelial layer beneath the posterior lens capsule in the fully formed lens. The anterior epithelial cells remain in place, and the cells near the equator begin to undergo mitosis. Each new cell elongates anteriorly and posteriorly, forming secondary lens fibers that are laid down around the embryonic nucleus. The first layer of **secondary fibers** is completed by week 7.[8] The ends of the secondary fibers meet in an **upright Y suture** posterior to the *anterior* epithelium and in an **inverted Y suture** anterior to the *posterior* capsule. These sutures are visible during the third month (Figure 7-6).[14] The region containing the Y sutures continues to develop until birth, forming the **fetal nucleus**. If a line were drawn to connect the cellular nuclei within the lens fibers, an arcuate shape would be revealed. This configuration is called the **lens bow** (see Figure 7-5).

FIGURE 7-7. Schema of the main features in vitreous development and regression of the hyaloid system, shown in drawings of sagittal sections. (A) At 5 weeks, the hyaloid vessels and their branches occupy much of the space between the lens and the neural ectoderm. (B) By 2 months, the vascular primary vitreous reaches its greatest extent. An avascular secondary vitreous of more finely fibrillar composition forms a narrow zone between the peripheral branches of the hyaloid system and the retina. (C) During the fourth month, the vessels of the hyaloid system atrophy progressively. Zonular fibers (tertiary vitreous) begin to stretch from the growing ciliary region toward the lens capsule. Vessels through the center of the optic nerve connect with the hyaloid vessels and send small loops into the retina. (Reprinted with permission from CS Cook, V Ozanics, FA Jakobiec. Prenatal Development of the Eye and Its Adnexa. In W Tasman, EA Jaeger [eds], Duane's Foundations of Clinical Ophthalmology [Vol 1]. Philadelphia: Lippincott, 1994;75.)

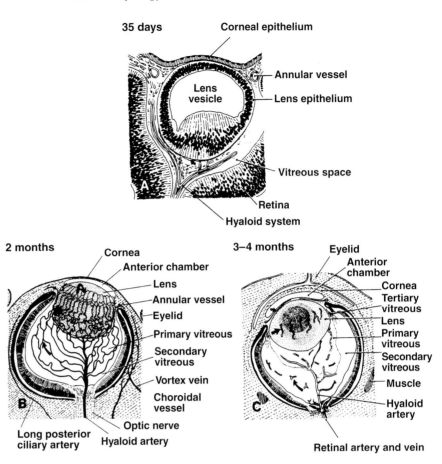

Mitosis, cell elongation, and lens fiber formation continue throughout development and throughout life. The orientation of the lens is influenced by the developing vitreous.[11, 15] The lens is initially spheric in shape but becomes more ellipsoid with additional fibers.[16] The **lens capsule** is evident at 5 weeks, evolving from the basement membrane of the invaginating surface ectoderm and from secretions of the lens epithelium.[14]

✍ CLINICAL COMMENT: CONGENITAL CATARACT

If the tissue near the developing lens fails to induce the lens fibers to elongate and pack together in an orderly way, the lens fibers will be misaligned, forming a cataract of the primary fibers. Interference with secondary lens fibers can lead to sutural cataracts.[17]

Viral infection affecting the mother during the first trimester often causes congenital malformations, one of which is a cataract. The developing lens is vulnerable to the rubella virus (German measles) between the fourth and seventh week of development, when the primary fibers are forming. After this period, the virus cannot penetrate the lens capsule and so will not affect the lens. The cataract usually is present at birth but may develop weeks to months later because the virus can persist within the lens for up to 3 years. The opacity may be dense and opaque or it may be diffuse; it can affect the nucleus only or involve most of the lens.[18]

Hyaloid Arterial System

A branch of the internal carotid artery enters the optic cup through the fetal fissure to become the **hyaloid artery**. This is a highly branching vessel that produces a network that fills the vitreous cavity and forms the **posterior tunica vasculosa lentis**, a vascular network covering the posterior lens (see Figure 7-6). Branches near the lens equator anastomose with the **annular vessel** at the margin of the optic cup. The annular vessel sends loops forward onto the anterior surface of the lens to form the **anterior tunica vasculosa lentis**.[19, 20] The tunica vasculosa lentis carries nutrients to the developing lens until production of the aqueous humor begins. These vessels drain into a network located in the region that will become the ciliary body.[2] The vessels of the hyaloid system cannot be identified as arterial or venous on the basis of their histologic makeup.[19]

Glial cells on the inner face of the optic nerve head form, around the base of the hyaloid artery, a conelike mass of tissue that proliferates, forming a glial mantle around the arterial system. The hyaloid vasculature reaches its peak development at approximately 9 weeks, begins to atrophy, and is reabsorbed during the third and fourth gestational months (Figure 7-7). By the seventh month, no blood flow is present in the hyaloid vasculature, which normally should be completely reabsorbed by birth.[2] The extent of the degeneration of the glial tissue mass defines the extent of the adult optic cup.[21]

✍ CLINICAL COMMENT: BERGMEISTER'S PAPILLA AND MITTENDORF'S DOT

Remnants of the hyaloid system often are seen clinically when a patient's ocular health is being examined. Glial tissue that persists on the nerve head is called **Bergmeister's papilla**, and a pinpoint remnant on the posterior surface of the lens is called **Mittendorf's dot**. Rarely, a remnant of the entire hyaloid artery will be seen coursing through the vitreous from its attachment at the disc to the posterior lens.

Retinal Pigment Epithelium

Apposition of the two layers of the optic cup is essential for development of the **retinal pigment epithelium**,[11] the first retinal layer to differentiate (Figure 7-8).[21] Cellular structures and melanosomes begin to appear in the outer layer of the optic cup and pigmentation of the retinal epithelium occurs at approximately week 3 or 4; this is the earliest pigmentation evident in the embryo.[2, 3, 22] After week 6, the RPE is one cell thick, the cells are cuboidal to columnar in shape, and the base of each cell is external toward the developing choroid and the apex internal toward the inner layer of the optic cup.[23, 24]

Neural Retina

By week 4 or 5, the cells of the inner layer of the optic cup, in the area that will become **neural retina**, proliferate, and two zones are evident. The cells accumulate in the outer region, the **proliferative** or **germinating zone**. The inner **marginal zone** (**of His**) is anuclear. A thin lamina—the basement membrane of the inner layer of the optic cup and the precursor of the internal limiting membrane—separates the marginal zone from the vitreal cavity.[14] At approximately week 7, cell migration occurs, forming the **inner** and **outer neuroblastic layers** between which lies the **transient fiber layer of Chievitz**, a nucleus-free area.[23, 25] The formation of these two neuroblastic layers is evident in Figure 7-8.

Ganglion cells and amacrine cells differentiate in the vitread portion of the inner neuroblastic layer.[26] The ganglion cells migrate, forming a layer close to the basement membrane, and almost immediately send out their axonal processes, which become evident by week 8.[14] Müller cells, located rather centrally in the inner neuroblastic layer, develop at the same time. The bodies of the Müller and amacrine cells remain in the inner neuroblastic layer but move slightly sclerad.[26]

Bipolar and horizontal cells migrate from the outer neuroblastic layer and settle near the Müller and amacrine

FIGURE 7-8.▶ The developing retina. The region of the posterior pole is represented in sagittal section in each diagram. (A) At 2.5 months, the transient fiber layer of Chievitz, which separated the inner from the outer neuroblastic layers of the primitive retina, is being obliterated slowly by shifting of the nuclear elements and realignment of their processes. The uppermost cells, lying vitread, are differentiating into ganglion cells. Those below the uneven transient layer of Chievitz (asterisks) are immature but are destined to differentiate into amacrine and Müller cells. The future inner plexiform layer will be located between the shifted nuclei of the Müller and amacrine cells and those of the ganglion cells. The outer neuroblastic layer contains photoreceptor, bipolar, and horizontal cell elements. (B) At midterm (4.5 months), retinal lamination essentially is complete. The ganglion cells have a multilayered arrangement. The inner plexiform layer, composed of fibers of bipolar, ganglion, and amacrine cells supported by müllerian fibers, has established sites of primitive conventional and ribbon synapses. In the inner nuclear layer, the still undifferentiated cellular components are recognizable by shape and position. In the outer nuclear layer, large cone nuclei are aligned adjacent to the pigment epithelium, and the smaller rod nuclei are positioned more vitread. The outer plexiform layer has primitive lamellar synapses between bipolar cell dendrites and cone pedicles (not indicated). Photoreceptor outer segments are not yet present. (C) At 5.5 months, the ganglion cells have thinned out to one to two layers (except in the macular area). The cellular components of the inner nuclear layer include amacrine cells with large pale nuclei in the innermost (vitread) zone of this layer and pleomorphic, dark-staining Müller cell nuclei. Both these types originally came from the inner neuroblastic layer. Also included are the smaller bipolar cells and large, pale-staining horizontal cells that are in an irregular arrangement sclerad. These two cell types, together with the photoreceptors, are derived from the outer neuroblastic layer. The outer plexiform layer has a linear arrangement of synapses between bipolar cells and rod spherules (key symbol). The outer nuclear layer consists of six to seven layers of nuclei; the outermost are cones aligned to the external limiting membrane. Growing photoreceptor outer segments projected into the space between pigment epithelium and external limiting membrane (arrowhead). Cell death is represented by the round dark-centered symbols. (D) The newborn retina has an adult configuration, with vascularization (arrowheads) reaching the outer limits of the inner nuclear layer. The outer plexiform layer is thinner than that in the adult, but the line of synapses is well established (key symbol). Rod and cone inner and outer segments are fully developed, and the tips of the outer segments contact the pigment epithelium. (Reprinted with permission from CS Cook, V Ozanics, FA Jakobiec. Prenatal Development of the Eye and Its Adnexa. In W Tasman, EA Jaeger [eds], Duane's Foundations of Clinical Ophthalmology [Vol 1]. Philadelphia: Lippincott, 1994;49.)

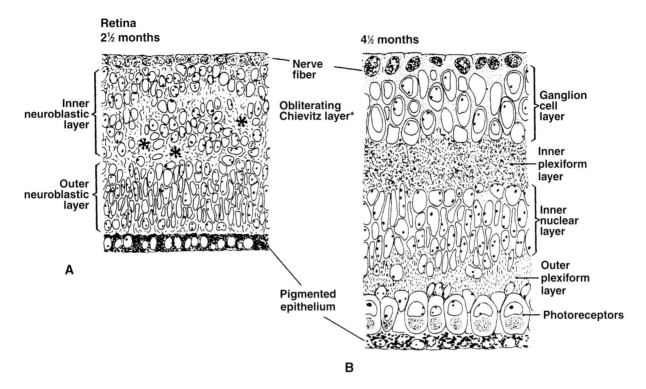

**Retina
2½ months**

Inner
neuroblastic
layer

Outer
neuroblastic
layer

A

Nerve
fiber

Obliterating
Chievitz layer*

Pigmented
epithelium

4½ months

Ganglion
cell
layer

Inner
plexiform
layer

Inner
nuclear
layer

Outer
plexiform
layer

Photoreceptors

B

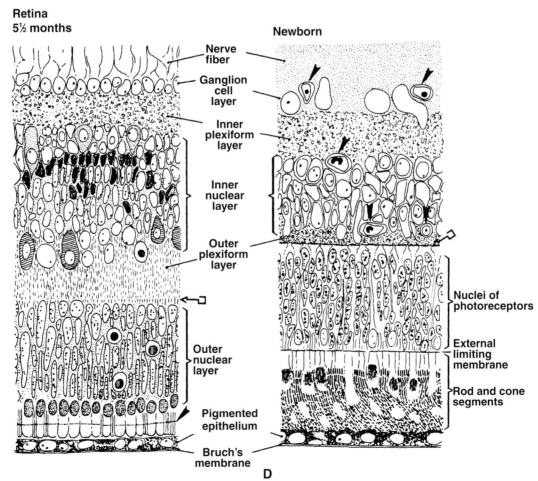

**Retina
5½ months**

Newborn

Nerve
fiber

Ganglion
cell
layer

Inner
plexiform
layer

Inner
nuclear
layer

Outer
plexiform
layer

Outer
nuclear
layer

Pigmented
epithelium

Bruch's
membrane

C

Nuclei of
photoreceptors

External
limiting
membrane

Rod and cone
segments

D

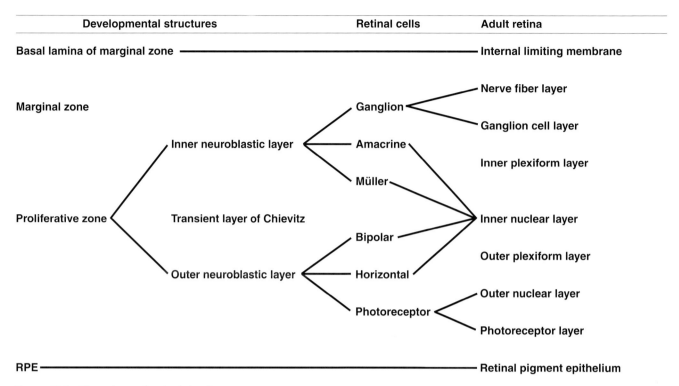

Developmental structures	Retinal cells	Adult retina

FIGURE 7-9. Flow chart of retinal development.

cells. The fiber layer of Chievitz gradually is obliterated by this move of the prospective bipolar and horizontal cells.[14] The photoreceptor cells remain in the outer neuroblastic layer. By week 12, the photoreceptors are aligned along the outer side of the inner layer of the optic cup; the horizontal, bipolar, amacrine, and Müller cells are located in the inner nuclear layer; and the ganglion cell layer is evident. In addition, the inner and outer plexiform layers are filling with cytoplasmic processes.[2] The radial fibers of the Müller cells appear and extend to the basal lamina, forming the primitive internal limiting membrane, and external processes extend between the rods and cones.[2, 23] (The developing interplexiform neuron has not yet been identified.) Figures 7-8 through 7-10 display the development of neural retina.

Synaptic complexes begin to appear at nearly the same time as the plexiform layers appear, the inner plexiform layer preceding the outer.[23, 27] Cone pedicles develop earlier than do rod spherules, and photoreceptor synapses with bipolar cells are established before the outer segments are completed.[23] The beginning of the outer segment is not evident until approximately week 23.[14]

Because retinal development is more advanced centrally than peripherally, the ganglion axons from the periphery must take an arched route above and below the macular area to reach the nerve head.[28] This line of deviation from the horizontal temporal meridian is termed the **horizontal raphe**.[2]

By 6 months of development, the dense accumulation of nuclei in the macular area makes this region thicker than the rest of the retina.[21] During the seventh month, the ganglion cells and the cells of the inner nuclear layer begin to move to the periphery of the macula. However, by birth there still is a single layer of ganglion cells and a thin inner nuclear layer across the now depressed foveal area (Figure 7-11). By 4 months postpartum, both of these layers are displaced to the sloping walls of the fovea, leaving the cones of the outer nuclear layer as the only neural cell bodies in the center of the depression.[3, 5] The cone fibers elongate and adopt an oblique orientation (forming Henle's fiber layer) so that they can synapse with the cells of the inner nuclear layer, which have been displaced to the sloping walls. The fovea, the retinal area of sharpest visual acuity, is the last to reach maturity.

Retinal Vessels

The fetal fissure along the optic stalk closes around the hyaloid artery, and those portions of the vessel within the stalk become the **central retinal artery**.[2] A branch of the primitive maxillary vein located within the optic stalk is the likely precursor of the **central retinal vein**.[22] Early in the fourth month of development, primitive retinal vessels emerge from the hyaloid artery near the optic disc and enter the developing nerve fiber layer. The vessels of the retina continue to develop but are not completed until approximately 3 months after birth, with the vessels to the nasal periphery being completed before those to the temporal periphery.[2]

✍ CLINICAL COMMENT: RETINOPATHY OF PREMATURITY

Premature infants who are exposed to a high concentration of oxygen can develop **retinopathy of prematurity** (also called **retrolental fibroplasia**). The immature retinal blood vessels respond to a high concentration of oxygen with vasoconstriction. On removal of the oxygen, vasoproliferation occurs; however, the new vessel growth is composed of "leaky" vessels with poorly formed endothelial tight junctions. Complications that can occur include neovascular invasion of the vitreous and development of vitreoretinal adhesions, which may be followed by hemorrhage and retinal detachment.[29]

Cornea

The cornea begins to develop, by induction of the lens, at about the time the lens vesicle separates from the surface ectoderm (day 33).[11, 15] One or two layers of epithelial cells from surface ectoderm become aligned and, by the fifth or sixth month, all of the cellular layers of the **corneal epithelium** are present.[30]

Corneal endothelium, formed from the first wave of mesenchyme that migrates into the space between the corneal epithelium and the lens, is one to two cells thick by week 6.[2] At 4 months, the endothelium is a single row of flattened cells with a basal lamina, the first evidence of **Descemet's membrane**.[2, 31] By the middle of the fourth month, tight junctions are apparent in the endothelium, coinciding with the beginning of aqueous formation.[32]

By week 8, a second wave of mesenchyme migrates between the developing epithelium and endothelium. It splits, with the posterior portion giving rise to the pupillary membrane. The anterior portion gives rise to the fibroblasts, collagen, and ground substance of the **stroma**.[2, 33] This mesenchyme, as well as that which gives rise to the sclera, is of neural crest origin (see Table 7-1).[2] At 3 months, all layers of the cornea are present (Figure 7-12) except **Bowman's layer**, which develops during the fifth month and is presumably formed by fibroblasts of the anterior stroma.[2] Rapid growth of the corneal stroma causes an increase in curvature relative to the rest of the globe.[4]

Sclera

The **sclera** first develops anteriorly from condensations in the mesenchyme near the limbus. Growth continues posteriorly until the sclera reaches the optic nerve and, by the end of the third month, the sclera has surrounded the developing choroid.[22] During the fourth month, connective-tissue fibers cross the scleral foramen, running through the

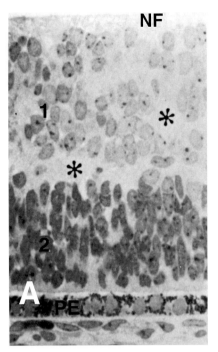

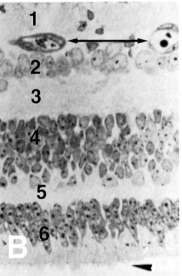

FIGURE 7-10. (A) Portion of retina of a fetus at 50–55 mm (approximately 10 weeks). The inner neuroblastic layer (*1*) is separated from the outer neuroblastic layer (*2*) by a slowly disappearing layer of Chievitz (asterisks). The pigment epithelium (*PE*) has a single layer of cells (×560). (NF = nerve fiber layer.) (B) Section through the retina of a fetus at 190 mm (estimated age, 5.5 months). (*1*) nerve fiber layer; (*2*) ganglion cell layer; (*3*) inner plexiform layer; (*4*) inner nuclear layer; (*5*) outer plexiform layer; (*6*) outer nuclear layer. The double-headed arrow indicates blood vessels in the ganglion layer. The arrowhead on the bottom points to photoreceptor inner segments protruding into the extracellular space beyond the external limiting membrane (×650). (Reprinted with permission from CS Cook, V Ozanics, FA Jakobiec. Prenatal Development of the Eye and Its Adnexa. In W Tasman, EA Jaeger [eds], Duane's Foundations of Clinical Ophthalmology. [Vol 1.] Philadelphia: Lippincott, 1994;50.)

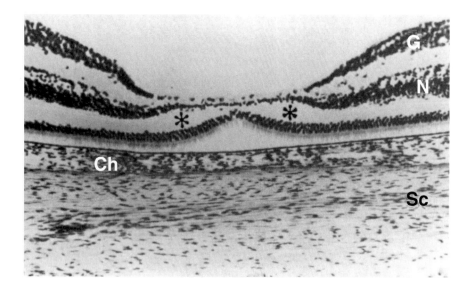

FIGURE 7-11. Fovea of *Macaca mulatta* just before birth (159 days; term at 162–165 days). One interrupted row of ganglion cells and one to two layers of bipolar cells still extend across the foveal depression. A wide and well-developed horizontal outer plexiform layer of Henle (asterisks) and elongated cone inner and outer segments are present. The parafoveal area has the large accumulation of cells in the ganglion (*G*) and inner nuclear layer (*IN*) characteristic of the mature macula (×95). (Ch = Choroid; Sc = Sclera.) (Reprinted with permission from CS Cook, V Ozanics, FA Jakobiec. Prenatal Development of the Eye and Its Adnexa. In W Tasman, EA Jaeger [eds], Duane's Foundations of Clinical Ophthalmology [Vol 1.] Philadelphia: Lippincott, 1994;75.)

optic nerve fibers and producing the first connective-tissue strands of the **lamina cribrosa**.[2] By the fifth month, the sclera (including the scleral spur) is well differentiated.[3]

Uvea

Choroid

The mesenchyme that forms the **choriocapillaris** must be in contact with the developing pigment epithelium to differentiate.[3, 5] The vessels appear during the second month, and the diaphragm-covered fenestrations are evident by week 12.[24] During the fifth month, the layers of the large and medium vessels are evident, as are the vessels that will become vortex veins.[34] The short posterior ciliary arteries also are evident and begin to anastomose to form the circle of Zinn-Haller.[2]

At midterm in fetal development, the elastic sheet of **Bruch's membrane** is present, the basement membrane of the RPE is developing, and the collagenous layers are thickening. The basement membrane of the choriocapillaris is the last component to appear.[2] By term, the choroidal stroma is pigmented.[24]

Ciliary Body

The region of the outer layer of the optic cup, which will become the outer pigmented epithelium of the ciliary body, begins to form ridges late in the third month.[35] The inner nonpigmented epithelium, from the inner optic cup layer, grows and folds with it (Figure 7-13). These folds number nearly 70 and become the **ciliary processes**. Mesenchyme differentiates into stromal elements, and the fenestrations in the capillaries are visible in week 14.[2, 35]

During the fourth month, the major arterial circle is formed, and the **ciliary muscle** begins to develop during the fifth month. However, the annular muscle (of Müller) remains incomplete at birth.[2, 3] Both epithelial layers begin to produce aqueous humor at 4–6 months.[35]

Iris

By the end of the third month, the lip of the optic cup begins to elongate and grows between the lens and the developing cornea. The proliferation of myofilaments in the basal aspect of the anterior epithelium adjoining the stroma transforms the layer into myoepithelium.[36] The group of cells that will become the **iris sphincter** breaks away from the pupillary zone of this epithelial layer during the fifth month and develops into smooth muscle within the iris stroma.[5, 36] During the sixth gestational month, the fibers of the **dilator muscle** continue to develop within the epithelial layer, and both muscles are completed by birth. That the sphincter and dilator come from neural ectoderm is unusual, as most muscle tissue is derived from mesenchyme. Pigmentation in the anterior and posterior epithelium begins to appear at approximately week 10 and is complete during the seventh month.[2]

Mesenchymal cells line up, leaving large gaps between them, to form the **anterior border layer**. A sparse distribution of collagen fibers begins to accumulate to form the **iris stroma**.[2]

Pupillary Membrane

As the lens thickens, the anterior tunica vasculosa lentis disconnects from the annular vessel, and its constituents are incorporated into the iris stroma; remnants con-

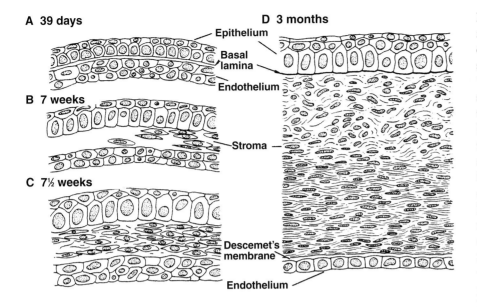

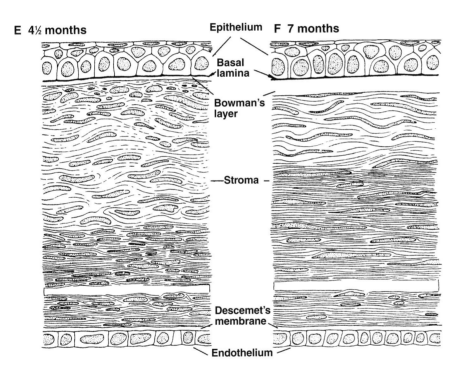

A 39 days · D 3 months · Epithelium · Basal lamina · Endothelium · B 7 weeks · Stroma · C 7½ weeks · Descemet's membrane · Endothelium · E 4½ months · Epithelium · F 7 months · Basal lamina · Bowman's layer · Stroma · Descemet's membrane · Endothelium

FIGURE 7-12. Developing cornea, central region. (A) At 39 days, the two-layered epithelium rests on a basal lamina. It is separated from a two- to three-layered "endothelium" by a narrow cellular space. (B) At 7 weeks, mesenchyme from the periphery migrates into the space between epithelium and endothelium. It is the precursor of the future corneal stroma. (C) The mesenchyme (fibroblasts) is arranged in four to five incomplete layers by 7.5 weeks, and a few collagen fibrils appear among them. (D) By 3 months, the epithelium has 2–3 layers of cells, and the stroma has approximately 25–30 layers of fibroblasts (keratoblasts), which are more regularly arranged in its posterior half. There is a thin, uneven Descemet's membrane between the posteriormost keratoblasts and the monolayered endothelium. (E) By midterm (4.5 months), some "wing cells" are forming above the basal epithelial cells, and an indefinite, acellular Bowman's layer emerges beneath the basal lamina. In nearly one-third of the anterior portion of the multilayered stroma, the keratoblasts are strewn in a disorganized formation. Descemet's membrane is well developed. (F) At 7 months, the adult structure of the cornea is established. A few mostly superficial keratoblasts still are randomly oriented with respect to the corneal surface. The collagenous lamellae in the rest of the stroma are in parallel array, and only a few spaces in the matrix lack collagen fibrils. The breaks near the bottom of (E) and (F) indicate that the central portion of the stroma is not represented. (Reprinted with permission from CS Cook, V Ozanics, FA Jakobiec. Prenatal Development of the Eye and Its Adnexa. In W Tasman, EA Jaeger [eds], Duane's Foundations of Clinical Ophthalmology [Vol 1.] Philadelphia: Lippincott, 1994;12.)

tribute to the minor circle of the iris.[2] During the third month, cells from the second wave of mesenchymal invasion migrate between the lens epithelium and the corneal epithelium to form another transitory network of vessels, the **pupillary membrane**, anterior to the lens.[37] (The pupillary membrane can be seen in Figure 7-14 just anterior to the lens.) This membrane joins with branches of the long posterior ciliary arteries and replaces the anterior tunica vasculosa lentis. It has three or four arcades

of thin-walled blood vessels separated by a thin mesodermal membrane and is complete by the end of the fifth month.[37] The vessels of the pupillary membrane cannot be identified as arterial or venous on the basis of their histologic makeup.[19]

During gestational month 6, the central vessels atrophy and become bloodless. The more peripheral vessels contribute to the lesser circle of the iris and, by 8.5 months, the central ones have fragmented and disap-

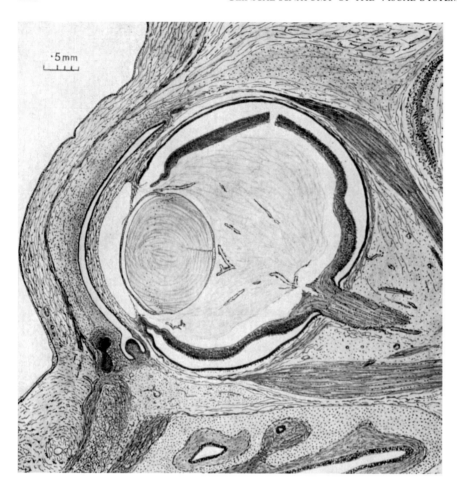

·5mm

FIGURE 7-13. Section through the eye and orbit of a 3-month-old fetus. (Reprinted with permission from I Mann. The Development of the Human Eye. New York: Grune & Stratton, 1964;95. Copyright 1964, British Medical Association.)

peared.[5, 37] As reabsorption of the central pupillary membrane occurs, the loops of the midregion form the ridge of the collarette, other components being incorporated into the anterior border layer.[2]

CLINICAL COMMENT: PERSISTENT PUPILLARY MEMBRANE

Remnants of the central portion of the pupillary membrane can be seen with a biomicroscope and appear similar to strands of a spiderweb attached to the surface of the iris. A persistent pupillary membrane may have a variety of presentations, from a single strand of connective tissue anchored at one or both ends to several interconnecting strands; pigment cells also might be incorporated. A persistent pupillary membrane is present in 17–32% of the population.[37]

Anterior Chamber

A mass of mesenchyme accumulates adjacent to the ciliary body and the iris root in the anterior chamber angle area. The method whereby this mass is eliminated to expose the angle remains a matter of controversy. The mass may atrophy,[3] the structure may split between the iris and the meshwork, with some tissue contributing to each,[38] or the intercellular spaces may enlarge and the cells reorganize into the surrounding tissue.[39]

The **trabecular meshwork** is visible as a triangular mass of mesenchymal cells during the fourth month; at least part of this tissue is of neural crest origin (see Table 7-1).[40–42] The tissue progressively becomes more organized and, by 9 months, the trabecular beams and pores are well developed. **Schlemm's canal** is derived from the deep scleral plexus.[40, 42] During the fourth month, tight junctions are evident in the canal's endothelial lining.[39]

Once the anterior chamber is formed, it is lined by a continuous endothelium that covers the trabecular meshwork and the iridocorneal angle.[43] This membrane appears continuous at gestational month 7 but, by month 9, is discontinuous in the region of the meshwork.[39, 44] During the last few weeks before birth, splits occur between cells in the membrane, and the size and number of these splits increase rapidly owing to the increase in the size of the anterior structures of the eye.[44] The loss of continuity in this membrane over the trabecular meshwork is significantly correlated with an increase in the facility of aqueous outflow.[40] Persistence of the uninterrupted endothelial membrane over the meshwork (Barkan's membrane) can be a factor in congenital glaucoma.[2, 7, 44]

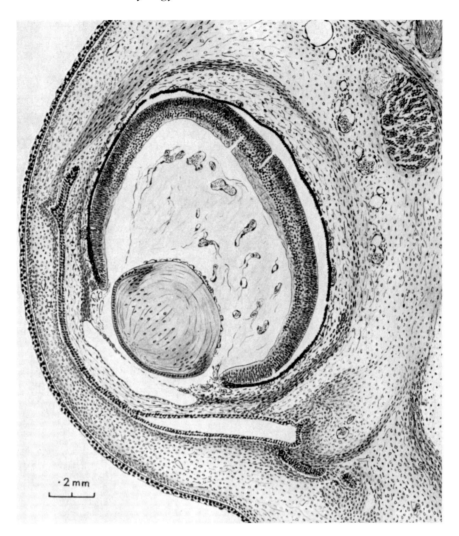

FIGURE 7-14. Section through the eye and surrounding structures in a 35-mm human embryo (approximately 8 weeks). (Reprinted with permission from I Mann. The Development of the Human Eye. New York: Grune & Stratton, 1964;170. Copyright 1964, British Medical Association.)

·2 mm

Vitreous

The presence of the developing lens is essential for normal accumulation of vitreous.[45] The **primary vitreous** fills the vitreous space early in development (see Figure 7-7) and is made up of fibrils derived from the lens, the retina, and the degenerating hyaloid system.[3]

As the **secondary vitreous** develops, it encloses the primary vitreous in the region of the atrophying hyaloid vessels, thus forming the funnel-shaped **Cloquet's canal**. This zone, with its apex at the optic disc and its base at the posterior lens, is well formed by the fourth month. It persists in the adult. The secondary vitreous contains a fibril network and primitive hyalocytes; these cells presumably are produced by the vascular primary vitreous.[2]

The zonule fibers develop from the **tertiary vitreous**, located between the lens equator and the ciliary body. Some question remains as to the precise origin of this vitreous, whether mesenchymal or epithelial.[2] Early zonule fibers appear to be a continuation of a thickening of the internal limiting membrane of the ciliary body, formed by the ciliary epithelium; they run from a zone near the ora serrata and from the valleys between the processes to the lens capsule.[4]

Optic Nerve

The optic stalk, the precursor of the optic nerve, joins the optic vesicle to the forebrain. As the optic fissure develops along the inferior stalk invagination, a two-layered optic stalk is created. The outer layer of the optic stalk becomes the neuroglial sheath that surrounds the optic nerve; it also gives rise to the glial components of the lamina cribrosa.[2] Some cells of the inner wall vacuolate, and axons from the retinal ganglion cells pass through the spaces; other cells of the inner wall become the glial cells of the optic nerve. Ganglion cell axons fill the lumen of the optic nerve (Figure 7-15) and grow toward their termination in the central nervous system. Myelination of the axons begins at the lateral geniculate body during the fifth

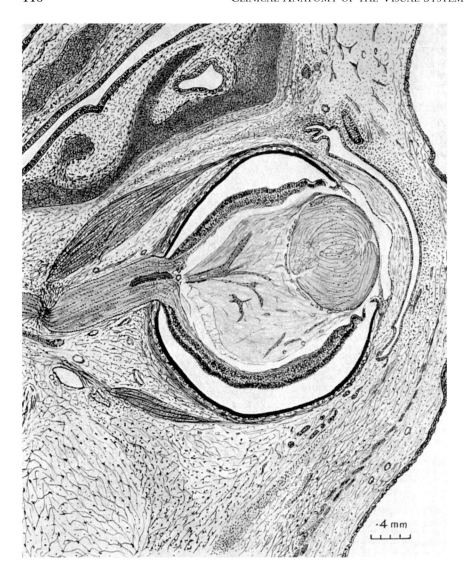

FIGURE 7-15. Section through the eye and orbit of a 48-mm human embryo (approximately 9.5 weeks). (Reprinted with permission from I Mann. The Development of the Human Eye. New York: Grune & Stratton, 1964;90. Copyright 1964, British Medical Association.)

·4 mm

month, reaches the chiasm during the sixth month, and stops at the lamina cribrosa approximately 1 month after birth.[2, 46]

DEVELOPMENT OF OCULAR ADNEXA

Eyelids

Early in the second gestational month, folds of surface ectoderm filled with mesenchyme begin to grow toward one another anterior to the developing cornea; these folds, which will become the eyelids, can be seen in Figure 7-16. The eyelid margins meet and fuse at approximately week 10 of development and remain fused until the lid structures have developed (Figure 7-17).[21] The epithelial layers of the skin and conjunctiva, the hair follicles and cilia, and the meibomian glands, Zeis glands, and glands of Moll all develop from surface ectoderm; the orbicularis oculi, levator palpebra, and tarsal mus-

cle of Müller develop from mesenchyme.[2] The fusion of the eyelids isolates the developing eye from the amniotic fluid[47] and "probably prevents the cornea and conjunctiva from keratinizing."[2] The desmosomes joining the margins break down during the fifth and sixth month, allowing the eyelids to separate; the lipid secretions of the meibomian glands may be responsible for the disjunction.[2, 4]

Orbit

Orbital fat and connective tissue are derived from neural crest cells. Most of the orbital bones ossify and fuse between the sixth and seventh months.[2] The angle between the orbits early in development is approximately 180 degrees, decreases to 105 degrees at 3 months, is 71 degrees at birth, and is 68 degrees in adulthood (Figure 7-18). The globe reaches its adult size by age 3, but the orbit is not of adult size until age 16.[2]

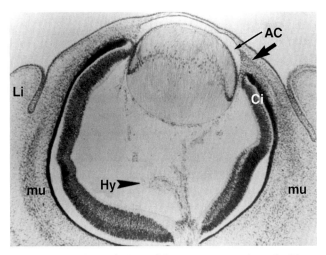

FIGURE 7-16. General view of the eye at approximately 20 mm (45 days). The ciliary portion of the neural cup (*Ci*) is relatively undifferentiated and extends to approximately the level of the lens equator. The mesenchyme around and anterior to the margin of the cup shows at least two different degrees of condensation, separated by an interface (thick arrow). The mesenchymal cells do not yet fill the center of the space between corneal epithelium and endothelium. The primordia of the extraocular muscles (*mu*) are recognizable. The upper and lower eyelids (*Li*) are undifferentiated skin folds. An anterior chamber (*AC*) is delineated by the pupillary membrane at the arrow. The major components of the hyaloid vasculature (*Hy*) are represented. (Reprinted with permission from CS Cook, V Ozanics, FA Jakobiec. Prenatal Development of the Eye and Its Adnexa. In W Tasman, EA Jaeger [eds], Duane's Foundations of Clinical Ophthalmology [Vol 1]. Philadelphia: Lippincott, 1994;37.)

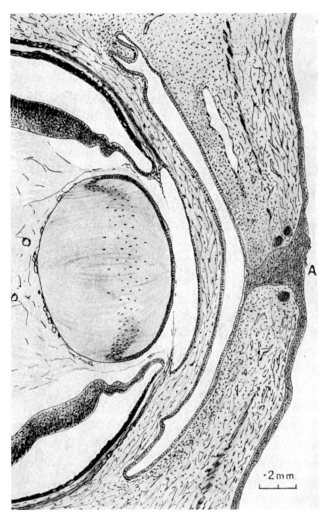

FIGURE 7-17. Section through the fused eyelids of a 48-mm human embryo (approximately 9.5 weeks). (A = area of epithelial adhesion.) (Reprinted with permission from I Mann. The Development of the Human Eye. New York: Grune & Stratton, 1964;267. Copyright 1964, British Medical Association.)

Extraocular Muscles

The extraocular muscles are of mesenchymal origin. The muscle cells are derived from mesoderm, whereas the connective-tissue components originate in neural crest. Extraocular muscles once were thought to develop in stages, first posteriorly near the orbital apex and then growing forward,[3] but recent work seems to indicate that muscle origin, belly, and insertion develop simultaneously.[48]

Nasolacrimal System

The main lacrimal gland has long been thought to develop from epithelial buds that arise from the temporal portion of the conjunctiva of the superior fornix.[2] Recently, investigators have questioned this origin and suggest a neural crest origin.[49] The lacrimal gland continues to develop after birth and is not fully developed until age 3 or 4 years.[2]

The nasolacrimal drainage system develops from a cord of surface ectodermal cells that becomes buried below the maxillary mesenchyme. This cord may fragment and form the canaliculi, the nasolacrimal duct, and the lacrimal sac, or the canaliculi might be formed from a later epithelial cord.[2]

BLOOD VESSEL PERMEABILITY AND BARRIERS

The blood-retinal and blood-aqueous barriers are recognizable early in development in the tight junctions formed in the RPE and the capillaries of the ciliary body and iris. Fenestrations that establish vessel permeability in the capillaries of the ciliary processes and the choriocapillaris also are evident early in the gestational period.

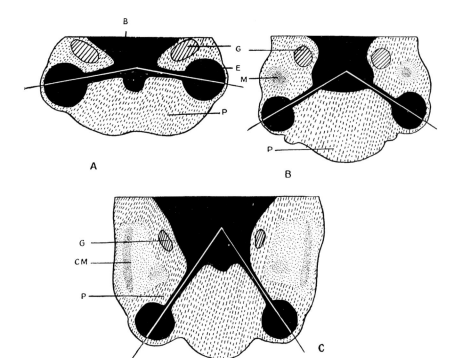

FIGURE 7-18. Sections through the developing eyes and optic stalks of human embryos of various stages. (A) Nine-millimeter embryo (approximately 37 days); 160-degree angle. (B) Sixteen-millimeter embryo; (approximately 48 days), 120-degree angle. (C) Forty-millimeter embryo (approximately 8 weeks); 72-degree angle. The decrease in the angle between the optic axes is obvious. (B = brain; E = eye; P = paraxial mesoderm; M = maxillary mesoderm; G = gasserian ganglion; CM = temporal condensation in maxillary mesoderm.) (Reprinted with permission from I Mann. The Development of the Human Eye. New York: Grune & Stratton, 1964;270. Copyright, 1964, British Medical Association.)

REFERENCES

1. Moore KL. Before We Are Born: Basic Embryology and Birth Defects (3rd ed). Philadelphia: Saunders, 1989.

2. Cook CS, Ozanics V, Jakobiec FA. Prenatal Development of the Eye and Its Adnexa. In W Tasman, EA Jaeger (eds), Duane's Foundations of Clinical Ophthalmology (Vol 1). Philadelphia: Lippincott, 1994;1.

3. Mann I. Development of the Human Eye. New York: Grune & Stratton, 1964.

4. Barishak YR. Embryology of the Eye and Its Adnexae. In W Straub (ed), Developments in Ophthalmology. New York: Karger, 1992.

5. Barber AN. Embryology of the Human Eye. St. Louis: Mosby, 1955.

6. Lovasik JV, Kothe AC. Neurophysiological correlates in a case of unilateral iris and chorioretinal coloboma. J Am Optom Assoc 1989;60:532.

7. Trachimowicz RA. Review of embryology and its relation to ocular disease in the pediatric population. Optom Vis Sci 1994;71(3):154.

8. Smelser GK. Embryology and morphology of the lens. Invest Ophthalmol 1965;4:398.

9. Matsuo T. The genes involved in the morphogenesis of the eye [abstract]. Jpn J Ophthalmol 1993; 37(3):215.

10. Harrington L, Klintworth GK, Seror TE, et al. Developmental analysis of ocular morphogenesis in alpha A-crystallin/diphtheria toxin in transgenic mice undergoing ablation of the lens. Dev Biol 1991;148(2):508.

11. Coulombre AJ. Regulation of ocular morphogenesis. Invest Ophthalmol 1969;8:25.

12. McKeehan MS. Induction of portions of the chick lens without contact with the optic cup. Anat Rec 1958;132:297.

13. Grainger RM, Henry JJ, Saha MS, et al. Recent progress on the mechanisms of embryonic lens formation. Eye 1992;6(pt 2):117.

14. O'Rahilly R. The prenatal development of the human eye. Exp Eye Res 1975;2:93.

15. Coulombre JL, Coulombre AJ. Lens development: IV. Size, shape and orientation. Invest Ophthalmol 1969;8:251.

16. Coulombre JL, Coulombre AJ. Lens development: fiber elongation and lens orientation. Science 1963;142:1489.

17. Nelson LB, Folberg R. Ocular Development Anomalies. In W Tasman, EA Jaeger (eds), Duane's Foundations of Clinical Ophthalmology (Vol 1). Philadelphia: Lippincott, 1991;1.

18. Kanski JJ. Clinical Ophthalmology (2nd ed). Oxford: Butterworth–Heinemann, 1989;238.

19. Mutlu F, Leopard IH. The structure of the fetal hyaloid system and tunica vasculosa lentis. Arch Ophthalmol 1964;71:102.

20. Jack RL. Ultrastructural aspects of hyaloid vessel development. Arch Ophthalmol 1972;87:427.

21. Warwick R. Eugene Wolff's Anatomy of the Eye and Orbit (7th ed). Philadelphia: Saunders, 1976;418.

22. Duke-Elder S, Cook C. Normal and Abnormal Development. In S Duke-Elder (ed), Embryology (Vol 3). System of Ophthalmology. St. Louis: Mosby, 1963;1.

23. Hollenberg MJ, Spira AW. Early development of the human retina. Can J Ophthalmol 1972;7:472.

24. Mund ML, Rodrigues MM, Fine BS. Light and electron microscopic observations on the pigmented layers of the developing human eye. Am J Ophthalmol 1972;73:167.

25. Smelser GK, Ozanics V, Rayborn M, et al. The fine structure of the retinal transient layer of Chiewitz. Invest Ophthalmol 1973;12:504.

26. Uga S, Smelser GK. Electron microscopic study of the development of retinal Müllerian cells. Invest Ophthalmol 1973;12:295.

27. Smelser GK, Ozanics V, Rayborn M, et al. Retinal synaptogenesis in the primate. Invest Ophthalmol 1974;13:340.

28. Vrabec F. The temporal raphé of the human retina. Am J Ophthalmol 1966;62:926.

29. Patz A, Payne JW. Retrolental Fibroplasia. In TD Duane, EA Jaeger (eds), Clinical Ophthalmology (Vol 3). Philadelphia: Harper & Row, 1982;1.

30. Zinn KM, Mockel-Pohl S. Fine structure of the developing cornea. Int Ophthalmol Clin 1975;15(1):19.

31. Wulle KG. Electron microscopy of the fetal development of the corneal endothelium and Descemet's membrane of the human eye. Invest Ophthalmol 1972;11:897.

32. Wulle KG, Ruprecht KW, Windrath LC. Electron microscopy of the development of the cell junctions in the embryonic and fetal human corneal endothelium. Invest Ophthalmol. 1974;13:923.

33. Ozanics C, Rayborn M, Sagun D. Some aspects of corneal and scleral differentiation of the primate. Exp Eye Res 1976;22:305.

34. Heinmann K. The development of the choroid in man. Choroidal vascular system. Ophthal Res 1971;3:257.

35. Wulle KG. The development of the productive and drainage system of the aqueous humor in the human eye. Adv Ophthalmol 1972;26:296.

36. Tamura T, Smelser GK. Development of the sphincter and dilator muscles of the iris. Arch Ophthalmol 1973;89:332.

37. Matsuo N, Smelser GK. Electron microscopic studies on the pupillary membrane. The fine structure of the white strands of the disappearing stage of the membrane. Invest Ophthalmol 1971;10:107.

38. Burian HM, Braley AE, Allen L. A new concept of the development of the anterior chamber angle of the human eye. Arch Ophthalmol 1956;53:439.

39. Smelser GK, Ozanics V. The development of the trabecular meshwork in primate eyes. Am J Ophthalmol 1971;71:366.

40. Rodrigues MM, Katz SI, Foidart J-M. Collagen factor VIII antigen and immunoglobulins in the human aqueous drainage channels. Ophthalmology 1980;87:337.

41. Tripathi BJ, Tripathi RC. Neural crest origin of human trabecular meshwork and its implications for the pathogenesis of glaucoma. Am J Ophthalmol 1989; 107:583.

42. Tripathi BJ, Tripathi RC. Embryology of the Anterior Segment of the Human Eye. In R Ritch, MB Shields, T Krupin (eds), The Glaucomas. St. Louis: Mosby, 1989;3.

43. Kupfer C, Ross K. The development of outflow facility in human eyes. Invest Ophthalmol 1971;10:513.

44. Hansson HA, Jerndal T. Scanning electron microscopic studies in the development of the iridocorneal angle in human eyes. Invest Ophthalmol 1971;10:252.

45. Coulombre AJ, Coulombre JL. Mechanisms of ocular development. Int Ophthalmol Clin 1975;15(1):7.

46. Sadun AA, Glaser JS. Anatomy of the Visual Sensory System. In W Tasman, EA Jaeger (eds), Duane's Foundations of Clinical Ophthalmology (Vol 1). Philadelphia: Lippincott, 1994;1.

47. Anderson G, Ehlers N, Matthiessen ME, et al. Histochemistry and development of the human eyelids. Acta Ophthalmol (Copenh) 1967;45:288.

48. Sevel D. Reappraisal of the origin of human extraocular muscles. Ophthalmology 1981;88:1330.

49. Tripathi BJ, Tripathi RC. Evidence of neuroectodermal origin of the human lacrimal gland. Invest Ophthalmol Vis Sci 1990;31:393.

SUGGESTED READING

Beauchamp GR, Knepper PA. Role of the neural crest in anterior segment development and disease. J Pediatr Ophthalmol Strabismus 1984;21(6):209.

Nodon DM. Periocular Mesenchyma: Neural Crest and Mesodermal Interactions. In W Tasman, EA Jaeger (eds), Duane's Foundations of Clinical Ophthalmology (Vol 1). Philadelphia: Lippincott, 1994;1.

Bones of the Skull and Orbit

A brief description of the bones of the skull will precede a more detailed presentation of the orbital bones. The reader is well advised to have a skull at hand while reading this section, particularly for distinguishing the relationships and articulations between bones.

The skull can be divided into two parts, the cranium and the face. The cranium consists of two parietal bones, the occipital bone, two temporal bones, the sphenoid bone, and the ethmoid bone. The face is made up of two maxillary bones, two nasal bones, the vomer, two inferior conchae, two lacrimal bones, two palatine bones, two zygomatic bones, and the mandible. The single frontal bone is a part of both the cranium and the face.

Generally, the bones of the skull unite at sutures that form immovable joints. The exception to this is the movable temporomandibular joint, which attaches the mandible to the temporal bones. Air-filled cavities called **sinuses** are contained within several of the bones.

BONES OF THE CRANIUM

The paired **parietal bones** form the roof and sides of the cranium (Figure 8-1). They articulate with each other at the midline in the sagittal suture, with the occipital bone posteriorly in the lambdoid suture, and with the frontal bone anteriorly at the coronal suture. The parietal bone articulates inferiorly with the temporal bone and the greater wing of the sphenoid bone.

The **occipital bone** forms the posterior aspect of the skull and the posterior floor of the cranial cavity. A prominence, the external occipital protuberance, or inion, is found on the external surface at the posterior midline (see Figure 8-1). The large foramen magnum is found in the inferior aspect of the occipital bone. The

inner surface of the bone forms the posterior cranial fossa, in which there are depressions in which the cerebellum, pons, and medulla oblongata lie. Figure 8-2 shows the inner aspect of the cranial floor. The occipital bone articulates with the temporal bones, the parietal bones, and the sphenoid bone.

✍ CLINICAL COMMENT: INION
 The inion, located just outer to the posterior pole of the occipital cortex, is a useful landmark in the placement of the electrodes used to record a visual evoked response (VER). This electrodiagnostic test records responses from the visual cortex. Clinical applications include the determination of visual acuity in a patient unable to respond to the typical eye chart and the assessment of impulse conduction in the patient in whom multiple sclerosis is suspected.

Each of the **temporal bones** is composed of two portions: a large, flat plate, the squamous portion; and a thickened, wedge-shaped area, the petrous portion. The squamous portion forms the side of the cranium and articulates with the parietal bone and the sphenoid bone. An anterior projection, the zygomatic process, articulates with the zygomatic bone (see Figure 8-1). The petrous portion extends within the cranium and houses the middle and inner ear structures. The mastoid process and styloid process project from the inferior aspect, and between these two is located the stylomastoid foramen, through which the facial nerve exits the skull. The petrous portion articulates with the occipital bone in the floor of the skull. The carotid canal runs superiorly and anteriorly through the petrous portion and provides entrance for the internal carotid artery into the cranial cavity.

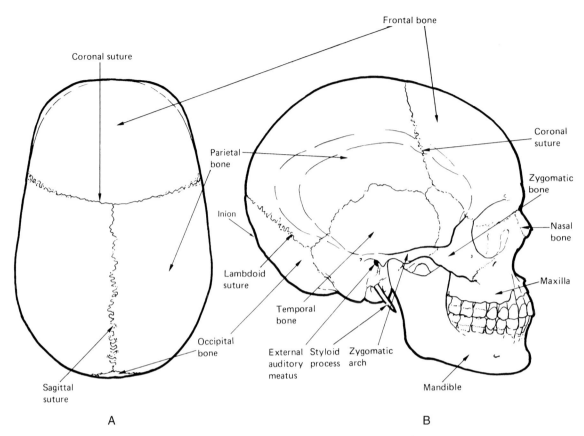

FIGURE 8-1. (A) Superior view and (B) lateral view of skull. (Reprinted with permission from N Palastanga, D Field, R Soames. Anatomy and Human Movement. Oxford: Butterworth–Heinemann, 1989;633.)

The single **frontal bone** forms the anterior portion of the cranium, the anterior floor of the cranial cavity, and the superior part of the face (see Figure 8-1). At the top of the skull, this bone articulates with the parietal bones; inferiorly it articulates with the sphenoid bone, ethmoid bone, and lacrimal bones; and inferoanteriorly it articulates with the nasal bones, maxillary bones, and zygomatic bones. The inner surface of the cranial cavity portion of the frontal bone forms the anterior cranial fossa, in which the frontal lobes of the cerebral hemispheres lie. The frontal sinuses are located within the anterior portion of the frontal bone.

The **sphenoid bone** is a single bone, the body of which lies in the midline and articulates with the occipital bone and the temporal bones to form the base of the cranium (see Figure 8-2). The sphenoid bone joins the zygomatic bones to form the lateral walls of the orbits. Anteriorly and inferiorly, the sphenoid bone articulates with the maxillary and palatine bones, superiorly with the parietal bones, and anteriorly and superiorly with the ethmoid and frontal bones. The depression on the superior cranial surface of the body of the sphenoid bone, the **hypophyseal fossa** (or the **sella turcica**), houses the pituitary gland; a portion of the body is hollow, forming the sphenoid sinus cavity.

Two pairs of wings project from the body of the sphenoid bone. The lesser wings project from the anterior aspect of the body and are more superior and smaller than the greater wings (see Figure 8-2). They are attached to the body by two small roots, and it is the gap between the two roots that forms the optic foramen or canal through which the optic nerve exits the orbit. The lesser wings articulate with the frontal and ethmoid bones.

The greater wings project from the lateral aspects of the body and articulate with the frontal bone, the parietal bones, the squamous portions of the temporal bones, and the zygomatic bones. The pterygoid process projects from the base of the greater wing and articulates with the vertical stem of the palatine bone; each contributes to a shallow depression, the pterygopalatine fossa. Three important foramina are located in the greater wing (see Figure 8-2): the **foramen rotundum**, through which the maxillary nerve passes; the **foramen ovale**, through which the mandibular nerve passes; and the **foramen spinosum**, through which the middle meningeal artery passes.

The single **ethmoid bone** resembles a rectangular box that contains a midline perpendicular plate. This plate bisects the top of the box, the horizontal cribriform plate, which is perforated for the passage of the olfactory nerves. The sides of the box parallel to the perpendicular

FIGURE 8-2. Foramina located in floor of skull.

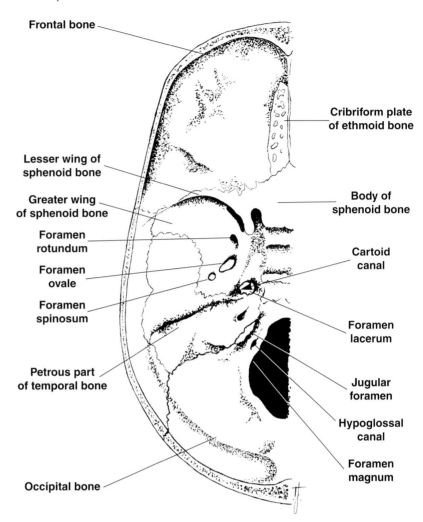

Frontal bone

Cribriform plate of ethmoid bone

Lesser wing of sphenoid bone

Greater wing of sphenoid bone

Body of sphenoid bone

Foramen rotundum

Foramen ovale

Cartoid canal

Foramen spinosum

Foramen lacerum

Jugular foramen

Petrous part of temporal bone

Hypoglossal canal

Foramen magnum

Occipital bone

plate are the orbital plates and are separated from the perpendicular plate by the ethmoid air cells. The ethmoid bone articulates with the sphenoid and frontal bones superiorly and with the vomer inferiorly; the orbital plates also articulate with the maxillary and lacrimal bones.

BONES OF THE FACE

The single **frontal bone** forms the forehead and articulates with the nasal bones, the maxillae, and the zygomatic bones in the formation of the face (Plate 8-1). The sutures joining adjacent bones of the face generally are named according to the names of the two bones that are connected (e.g., the suture between the frontal bone and the zygomatic bone is the frontozygomatic suture).

The two **maxillae**, or **maxillary bones**, form the upper jaw, the hard palate, the lateral walls of the nasal cavity, and the floor of both orbits (see Plate 8-1). Each maxillary bone articulates with the frontal, nasal, ethmoid, lacrimal, sphenoid, palatine, and zygomatic bones. That portion of the maxillary bone forming the cheek contains the maxillary sinus.

The two **nasal bones** form the bridge of the nose and articulate with each other, with the frontal bone, and with the frontal processes of the maxillary bones (see Plate 8-1). The **vomer** is a single bone that forms the posterior part of the nasal septum. It articulates with the palatine and maxillary bones inferiorly and with the ethmoid bone superiorly. The **inferior conchae** are separate bones located along the lateral walls of the nasal cavity.

The **lacrimal bone** (one in each orbit) is the smallest bone of the face and articulates with the maxillary bone, the ethmoid bone, and the frontal bone.

There are two **palatine bones**. Each is an L-shaped bone that extends from the hard palate at the back of the mouth to the orbit. The horizontal plate is found in the oral cavity; the vertical stem runs along the posterior aspect of the nasal cavity and articulates with the pterygoid process of the sphenoid bone. A small, flattened area at the top of the vertical stem is located in the orbital floor at the posterior edge of the orbital plate of the maxilla.

The paired **zygomatic bones** form the lateral part of the cheek bones and articulate with the zygomatic process of the temporal bones to form the zygomatic

Ethmoid bone

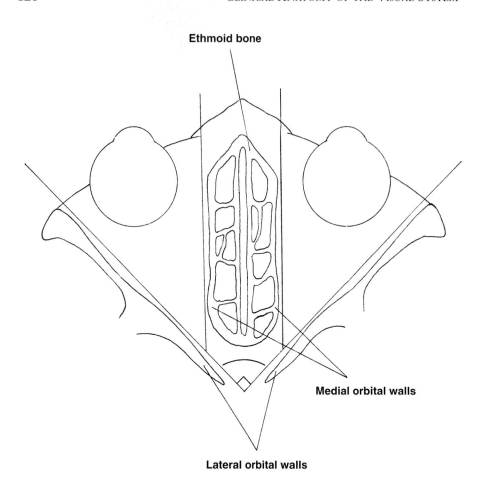

Medial orbital walls

Lateral orbital walls

FIGURE 8-3. Angular relationship of orbital walls. Medial walls are approximately parallel to each other, whereas if lines were to be extended posteriorly from the lateral walls, an approximate right angle would be formed.

arches (see Figure 8-1). They also articulate with the maxillary bones and with the greater wings of the sphenoid bone.

The **mandible** forms the movable lower jaw. It is a horseshoe-shaped bone consisting of a curved horizontal body and two perpendicular processes, the rami.

THE ORBIT

The orbits are bony cavities on either side of the midsagittal plane of the skull below the cranium. They contain the globes, the extraocular muscles, and orbital nerves, blood vessels, and connective tissue.

The orbit is shaped like a four-sided pyramid, the base of which is at the anterior orbital margin and the apex at the posterior margin within the skull. The orbital walls are referred to as **floor**, **roof**, and **medial** and **lateral walls**. As seen in Figure 8-3, the medial walls run approximately parallel to each other, whereas the two lateral walls, if extended posteriorly, would form approximately a 90-degree angle with each other.[1, 2] The orbit has also been described as pear-shaped, having its widest portion 1.5 cm inside the orbital margin.[1] The orbital floor extends to approximately two-thirds of the depth of the orbit; the other three sides extend to the apex.

Each orbit is composed of seven bones—the frontal, maxillary, zygomatic, sphenoid, ethmoid, palatine, and lacrimal bones (see Plate 8-1). The frontal, sphenoid, and ethmoid each are a single bone and take part in the formation of both orbits.

Orbital Walls

Roof

The roof is triangular and is composed primarily of the orbital plate of the **frontal bone** in front. The **lesser wing of the sphenoid** contributes a small posterior portion. The orbital plate of the frontal bone is thin in the area that separates the orbit from the anterior cranial fossa. In an elderly adult, bone in this area may resorb, leaving only the periosteal connective tissue in contact with the dural covering of the frontal lobe of the brain. The small area of the lesser wing of the sphenoid that is involved in this wall runs slightly downward, and an oval foramen, the optic canal, lies within it (see Plate 8-1). This optic foramen is located roughly at the apex of the orbit.

The frontal bone forms the ridge of the superior orbital margin. Behind the lateral aspect of this margin is an indentation in the frontal bone—the fossa for the lacrimal gland. A U-shaped piece of cartilage, the trochlea, is attached to the orbital plate of the frontal bone approximately 2 mm behind the medial aspect of the superior orbital margin. The tendon of the superior oblique muscle passes through this pulleylike structure.

Floor

The floor also is triangular and is composed of the orbital plate of the **maxillary bone** and the orbital surface of the **zygomatic bone** in front and the small orbital process of the **palatine bone** behind (see Plate 8-1). The maxillary bone makes up the largest part of the floor, and most of the remainder is provided by the zygomatic bone. The orbital process of the palatine bone is a small, flattened area at the top of the vertical arm and is located at the posteriormost edge of the orbital plate of the maxilla. Often in the adult skull, the suture between the orbital process of the palatine bone and the maxilla is indistinguishable.

The floor does not reach all the way to the apex and is separated from the lateral wall posteriorly by the inferior orbital fissure. The infraorbital groove runs across the floor from the inferior orbital fissure and anteriorly becomes a canal that runs within the maxillary bone. This canal opens on the facial surface of the maxilla below the inferior orbital margin as the infraorbital foramen (see Plate 8-1). The inferior orbital margin is composed of the maxilla and the maxillary process of the zygomatic bone.

✍ CLINICAL COMMENT: BLOW-OUT FRACTURE OF THE ORBIT

The orbital rim is strong and can withstand considerable impact. However, a blow to the orbital rim can cause compression of the orbital contents, and such a sudden increase in intraorbital pressure might cause a fracture in one of the orbital walls. In the classic blow-out fracture, the orbital rim remains intact. The floor of the orbit is particularly susceptible to such a fracture, which usually occurs in the thin region along the infraorbital canal (Figure 8-4).[2-4] Clinical signs and symptoms accompanying this damage include orbital swelling, ecchymosis, anesthesia of the area innervated by the infraorbital nerve, and diplopia caused by restriction of ocular motility (particularly noted in upward gaze).[4] Limitations in ocular motility are caused by damage to the inferior extraocular muscles, either from bruising or hematoma or from entrapment of the muscle or adjoining connective tissue within the fracture.[3, 5, 6]

Medial Wall

The medial wall is rectangular. From front to back, it is formed by the frontal process of the **maxilla**, the

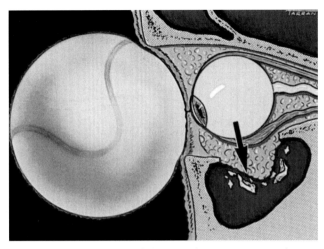

FIGURE 8-4. Mechanism of blow-out fracture; arrow indicates that the force damages the weakest orbital wall, the floor. (Reprinted with permission from JJ Kanski. Clinical Ophthalmology [3rd ed]. Oxford: Butterworth–Heinemann, 1994;52.)

lacrimal bone, the orbital plate of the **ethmoid**, and a part of the **body of the sphenoid** (Figure 8-5). A ridge on the frontal process of the maxilla that forms the inferior part of the medial orbital margin also forms the **anterior lacrimal crest**, which demarcates one border of the fossa for the lacrimal sac. The lacrimal bone, a small bone approximately the size of a thumbnail, together with the frontal process of the maxillary bone forms the wall of this fossa. The lower portion of the fossa is a groove that is continuous inferiorly with the **nasolacrimal canal**, which continues into the nasal cavity. A ridge in the lacrimal bone forms the **posterior lacrimal crest** and is continuous superiorly with the prominence of the frontal bone, forming the superior margin of the orbit (see Plate 8-1).

The ethmoid bone forms most of the medial wall. The orbital plate of the ethmoid sometimes is said to be "paper-thin" (lamina papyracea); hence, the medial wall is the thinnest of the orbital walls. The small part of the sphenoid bone present in this wall is a part of the body and is located at the posterior end adjacent to the wall of the optic canal. The floor is joined to the medial wall at the sutures connecting the bones of the two walls, and the anterior and posterior ethmoidal canals are located within the frontoethmoidal suture at the junction of the roof and medial wall.

Lateral Wall

The lateral wall is roughly triangular and is composed of the **zygomatic bone** in front and of the **greater wing of the sphenoid bone** behind (Figure 8-6). The zygomatic bone separates the orbit from the temporal fossa. One or more foramina may be present in the zygomatic bone as a conduit for nerves and vessels between the orbit and

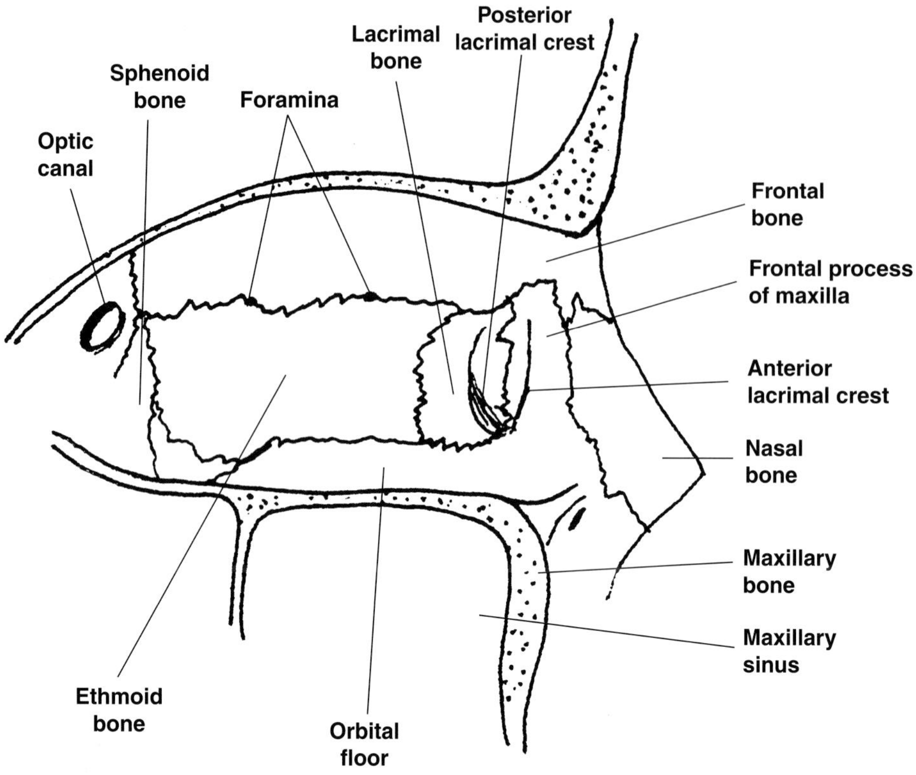

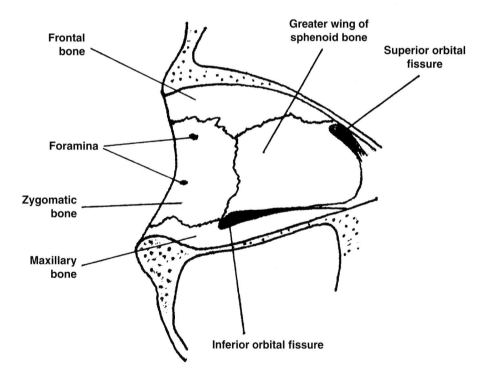

FIGURE 8-5. Structure of the medial orbital wall.

FIGURE 8-6. Structure of the lateral orbital wall.

facial areas. The **lateral** or **marginal orbital tubercle** (**Whitnall's tubercle**) is a small, bony prominence located on the orbital surface of the zygomatic bone and is the attachment site for the aponeurosis of the superior palpebral levator muscle, the lateral palpebral ligament, and the lateral check ligament.

The greater wing of the sphenoid separates the orbit from the middle cranial fossa. The roof is separated from the lateral wall in back by the superior orbital fissure and in front by the frontozygomatic and frontosphenoidal sutures. The inferior orbital fissure separates the posterior part of the floor from the lateral wall (see Figure 8-6).

Orbital Margins

Though dimensions of the orbit vary widely, the average horizontal diameter of the orbital margin is 4 cm, the average vertical diameter is 3.5 cm, and the average depth is 4.5 cm.[1, 2, 7] The frontal bone forms the superior orbital margin. The highest point of this arch is located one-third of the way along the margin from the superior medial corner of the orbit. The supraorbital notch (see Plate 8-1) is located just medial to the center of the superior orbital margin and is the conduit for the supraorbital vessels and nerves. This notch can be palpated easily. In 25% of orbits, the supraorbital notch is enclosed to form a foramen.[2, 8]

At the superior medial corner is a less well-defined groove—the supratrochlear notch—through which pass the nerve and vessels of the same name. The supratrochlear notch remains a notch or groove in the majority of orbits, becoming a foramen in just 3%.[8]

The lateral orbital margin is the orbital region most exposed to possible injury and therefore is the strongest area of the orbital margin. It is formed by the zygomatic process of the frontal bone superiorly and by the frontal process of the zygomatic bone inferiorly.

The inferior orbital margin usually is formed equally by the maxillary bone and the zygomatic bone. The zygomaticomaxillary suture can often be easily palpated through the skin along the inferior orbital edge. The infraorbital foramen (the opening from the infraorbital canal) is found in the anterior surface of the maxillary bone below the inferior orbital margin.

The frontal process of the maxillary bone articulates with the frontal bone and forms part of the medial rim of the orbital margin. Posteriorly, this process articulates with the lacrimal bone and, anteriorly, with the nasal bone. The medial margin is not continuous. Following the orbital margin around starting from the inferior nasal aspect, which is the anterior lacrimal crest, it can be seen that the margin forms a spiral (Figure 8-7). The posterior lacrimal crest completes the superior curve of the medial orbital margin.

Orbital Foramina and Fissures

A number of foramina and fissures exist between the orbit and the middle cranial fossa, the sinuses, and the face to allow the entrance and exit of vessels and nerves that supply the globe and orbital structures. The **optic foramen** or the **optic canal** (see Plate 8-1) is formed by the roots of the lesser wing of the sphenoid bone and lies just lateral to the body of the sphenoid. The canal often causes an indentation into the bone of the sphenoid sinus.[9] It provides communication between the orbital cavity and the middle cranial fossa and is separated from the medial posterior edge of the superior orbital fissure by a strip of bone. The optic

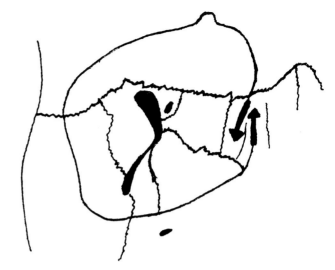

FIGURE 8-7. The orbital margin. Arrows indicate the spiral formed at the nasal margin.

nerve exits and the ophthalmic artery enters the orbit through this canal.

> ✏ CLINICAL COMMENT: OPTIC NERVE DAMAGE
> The dura mater lining the optic canal is adherent to both the dura of the optic nerve and the periosteum of the canal. This close confinement of the nerve within the bony passage predisposes the nerve to compression and damage by even very small lesions or tumors of the bony canal.[10]

The **superior orbital fissure** is the gap between the lesser wing and the greater wing of the sphenoid bone and is located between the roof and the lateral wall (see Plate 8-1). It, too, is a communication between the orbital cavity and the middle cranial fossa. The fissure usually is widest medially, becoming narrower toward the lateral portion. Approximately midway on the lower aspect is a small sharp spur (spina recti lateralis) that serves as the attachment for the lateral rectus muscle. A circular band of connective tissue, the **common tendinous ring** (or **annulus of Zinn**), is located anterior to the fissure and the optic canal. This ring is the origin for the four rectus muscles. The relationship among the superior orbital fissure, the tendinous ring, and the various nerves passing through them can be seen in Figure 8-8. The lacrimal nerve, the frontal nerve, the trochlear nerve, and the superior ophthalmic vein pass through the superior orbital fissure *above* the circular tendon. The superior and inferior divisions of the oculomotor nerve, the nasociliary nerve, and the abducens nerve pass through the fissure *and* the ring tendon. The optic nerve and the ophthalmic artery pass through the optic canal and the tendinous ring.

The **inferior orbital fissure** lies between the floor of the orbit and the lateral wall (see Figure 8-6). It allows

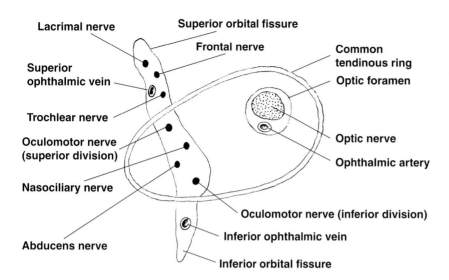

passage of vessels and nerves between the orbit and the pterygopalatine and temporal fossae. This fissure often is narrowest in its center. The foramen rotundum opens into the pterygopalatine fossa and transmits the maxillary division of the trigeminal nerve to the inferior orbital fissure. Branches of the maxillary nerve join the infraorbital nerves and vessels in passing through the inferior orbital fissure. Most of these structures continue into the infraorbital groove in the maxillary bone. The inferior ophthalmic vein exits the orbit *below* the ring tendon.

Paranasal Sinuses

The paranasal sinuses are mucosa-lined, air-filled cavities located in four of the orbital bones. These hollow spaces decrease the weight of the skull and act as a resonator for the voice. They communicate with the nasal cavity via small apertures.

The orbit is surrounded on three sides by sinuses (Figure 8-9): the frontal sinus above, the ethmoid and sphenoid sinus cavities medial to, and the maxillary sinus below the orbit. Of these, the maxillary sinus is largest. The roof of the maxillary sinus is the orbital plate of the maxilla, and this plate, which separates the sinus from the orbital contents, is only 0.5–1.0 mm thick.[1] The sphenoid sinus is within the body of the sphenoid and, in some people, continues into the lesser wing and may surround the optic canal.[1] The ethmoid sinus sometimes continues into the lacrimal bone or into the frontal process of the maxilla.[11] In a high percentage of orbits, the thin bone of both the sphenoid and ethmoid sinuses makes contact with the dural sheath of the optic nerve.[12,13] Table 8.1 shows the location of each of the sinus cavities.

✍ CLINICAL COMMENT: ORBITAL CELLULITIS
    The thin walls of the sinus cavities are poor barriers to the passage of infection from the air cavities into the orbit. If pathogens from a sinusitis pene-

trate the thin, bony barrier, a serious infection involving the orbital contents might ensue. A major infection that involves the orbital connective-tissue contents is called **orbital cellulitis,** and one of its major causes is sinusitis.[2,3,14,15] Signs and symptoms include sudden onset of pain, edema, proptosis, and a decrease in ocular motility. Orbital cellulitis is a serious medical situation because of the relatively easy access to the brain and must be treated aggressively; hospitalization may be required.[3,14] Orbital cellulitis also is a possible sequela of a blow-out fracture, which can (though rarely does) provide a pathologic avenue between the sinus cavities and the orbit that results in orbital infection.[16]

Connective Tissue of the Orbit

The connective tissue of the orbit is arranged in a complex network that serves to line, cover, and compartmentalize orbital structures, to anchor soft-tissue structures to bone, and to compartmentalize areas. Though this network is continuous, the segments will be described individually according to their position and function.

Periorbita

The **periorbita,** also called the **orbital periosteum** or **orbital fascia,** covers the bones of the orbit (Figure 8-10). This dense connective-tissue membrane serves as an attachment site for muscles, tendons, and ligaments, and is a support structure for the blood supply to the orbital bones. The periorbita is attached only loosely to the underlying bone except at the orbital margins, the sutures, and the edges of fissures and foramina. At the orbital margins, it is continuous with the periosteal covering of the bones of the face; at the edges of the superior orbital fissure, the optic canal, and the ethmoid

FIGURE 8-9. Location of the sinus cavities within the orbital walls.

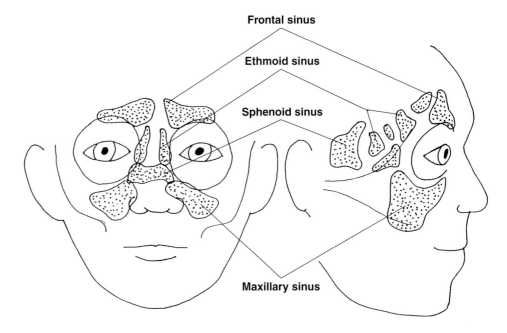

Frontal sinus

Ethmoid sinus

Sphenoid sinus

Maxillary sinus

canals, the periorbita is continuous with the periosteal layer of the dura mater. At the anterior portion of the optic canal, the periorbita splits such that a portion becomes continuous with the dura of the optic nerve and another portion reflects forward to take part in the formation of the common tendinous ring. At the inferior orbital fissure, the periorbita is continuous with the periosteum of the skull. At the lacrimal crests, a sheet of periorbita covers the lacrimal sac, and the periorbita is continuous with the tissue lining the nasolacrimal canal. Another portion of the periorbita covers the lacrimal gland.

Orbital Septum

At the orbital margins, the periorbita is continuous with a connective-tissue sheet known as the **orbital septum** (also known as the **palpebral fascia** or **septum orbitale**; see Figure 8-10). This dense connective-tissue sheet is circular and runs from the entire rim of the orbit to the tarsal plates, which are embedded in the eyelids. This strong barrier helps prevent facial infections from entering the orbit; it also maintains orbital fat in its place. In the elderly, the orbital septum often weakens, particularly in the medial inferior area, and herniation of fat and loose connective tissue might occur.

The relationship between orbital structures and these connective-tissue structures is shown in Figures 8-10 and 8-11. At the lateral margin, the orbital septum lies in front of the lateral palpebral ligament and the check ligament for the lateral rectus muscle. At the superior orbital margin, the orbital septum passes in front of the trochlea and bridges the supraorbital and supratrochlear notches. At the medial margin, the orbital sep-

TABLE 8-1. Paranasal Sinuses

Sinus	Location
Frontal	In frontal bone, on each side of midline above orbits
Ethmoid	Several air cells on both sides of perpendicular plate of ethmoid bone, medial to orbits
Sphenoid	In body of sphenoid bone, posterior and medial to orbits
Maxillary	In each maxillary bone, below orbits

tum, which attaches behind the posterior lacrimal crest, lies in front of the check ligament for the medial rectus muscle; it lies behind the medial palpebral ligament, Horner's muscle, and the lacrimal sac (see Figure 8-11), isolating the lacrimal sac (which communicates with the nasal cavity) from the orbit proper.

Tenon's Capsule

Tenon's capsule (bulbar fascia) is a sheet of dense connective tissue that encases the globe. It lies between the conjunctiva and the episclera and merges with them anteriorly in the limbal area. Tenon's capsule is pierced by the optic nerve, the vortex veins, the ciliary vessels and nerves, and the extraocular muscles. At the muscle insertions, Tenon's capsule forms sleevelike sheaths that cover the tendons.[2, 17] Posteriorly, Tenon's capsule merges with the dural sheath of the optic nerve. This dense connective-tissue capsule acts as a barrier to prevent the spread of orbital infections into the globe.

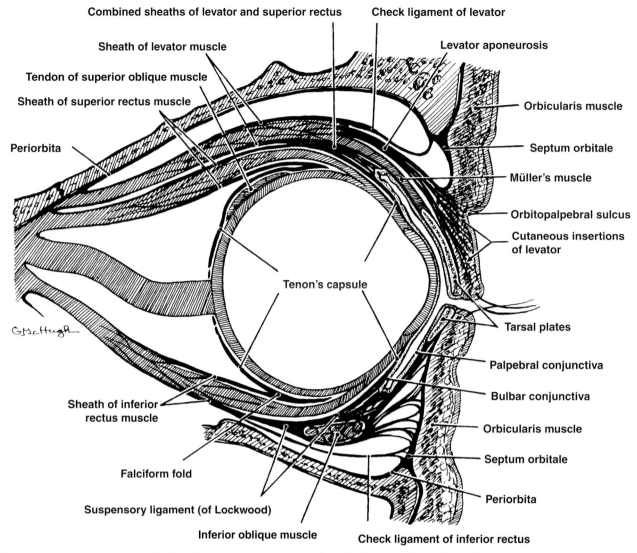

FIGURE 8-10. Fascial system of orbit, shown in vertical section through the vertical meridian of the eyeball with the latter in primary position, the eyelids being closed. (Reprinted with permission from PC Kronfeld, The Human Eye. Rochester, NY: Bausch & Lomb Press, 1943. Copyright 1943, Bausch & Lomb.)

Suspensory Ligament (of Lockwood)

The **suspensory ligament (of Lockwood)** (see Figure 8-10) is a hammocklike sheet of dense connective tissue that runs from its attachment on the lacrimal bone at the medial orbital wall to the zygomatic bone at the lateral wall. Tissue from several structures—Tenon's capsule, the sheaths of the two inferior extraocular muscles, and the inferior eyelid aponeurosis—contributes to the formation of this ligament. The suspensory ligament helps to support the globe particularly in the absence of the orbital bones of the floor.

Orbital Muscle of Müller

The **orbital muscle of Müller** is a small, smooth muscle embedded in the periorbita and covering part of the inferior orbital fissure.[6, 18] Its function in humans is unknown.

Orbital Fat

The orbital space around the globe is organized into radially arranged compartments by septa of connective tissue (Figure 8-12). The collagenous strands connect the periorbita to Tenon's capsule and intermuscular membranes. Fat pads and occasional smooth-muscle fibers are located within these spaces. This connective-tissue system anchors and supports the muscles and blood vessels within the bony orbit. The spaces not occupied by ocular structures, connective tissue, nerves, or vessels become filled with adipose tissue. Usually four adipose tissue compartments are located within the muscle cone surrounding the optic nerve and separating it from the extraocular muscles.[6] Adipose is the predominant tissue near the orbital apex.[6]

Varying degrees of connectivity occur throughout the orbit. Further description of the septa that connect

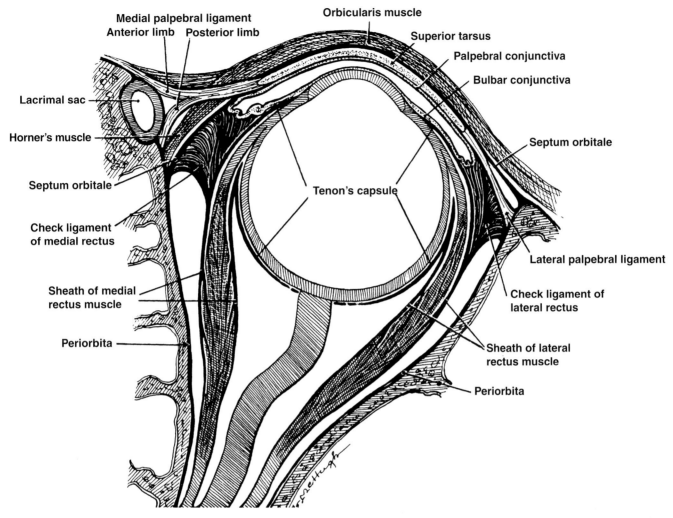

FIGURE 8-11. Fascial system of orbit, shown in horizontal section. The plane of section lies slightly above the horizontal meridian of the eyeball, which is assumed to be in primary position, the eyelids being closed. (Reprinted with permission from PC Kronfeld. The Human Eye. Rochester, NY: Bausch & Lomb Press, 1943. Copyright 1943, Bausch & Lomb.)

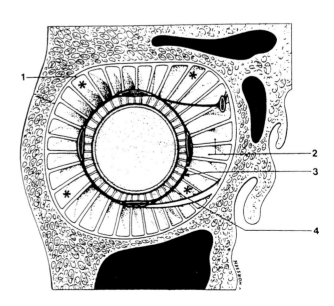

FIGURE 8-12. Anterior orbital connective tissue septa: (1) periorbita; (2) fibrous septa; (3) common muscle sheath around the eye; (4) Tenon's capsule. Asterisks indicate areas where smooth muscle tissue was found. (Reprinted with permission from L Koornneef. New insights in the human orbital connective tissue. Arch Ophthalmol 1977;95:1269. Copyright 1977, American Medical Association.)

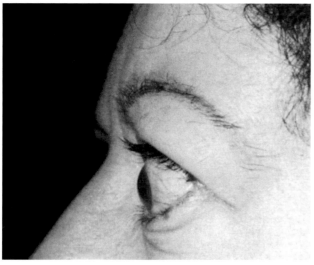

FIGURE 8-13. Fifty-year-old woman with class 3 Graves' oph-thalmopathy. Proptosis of 27 mm was measured with the Hertel exophthalmometer. (Reprinted with permission from JD Bartlett, SD Jaanus. Clinical Ocular Pharmacology [2nd ed]. Boston: Butterworth–Heinemann, 1989;707.)

extraocular muscles to one another and to other orbital structures is presented in Chapter 10. Because of the close association of the orbital contents, a space-occupying lesion will cause outward displacement of the globe.

✍ CLINICAL COMMENT: EXOPHTHALMOS

Protrusion of the globe is termed **exophthalmos** or **proptosis** (Figure 8-13) and can be caused by a number of pathologic conditions, including inflammation, edema, tumors, and injuries.[14] The most common is thyroid ophthalmopathy, which can cause hypertrophy of the extraocular muscles; in some patients, the muscles become enlarged to eight times their normal size.[3] Thyroid ophthalmopathy also causes proliferation of orbital fat and connective tissue and lymphoid infiltration.[3] Because the orbital tissue is encased in immovable bony walls, this increase in volume of the orbital contents produces protrusion of the globe and simulates eyelid retraction. At the first sign of proptosis, investigation is necessary to determine the causative factor.

REFERENCES

1. Warwick R. Eugene Wolff's Anatomy of the Eye and Orbit (7th ed). Philadelphia: Saunders, 1976;1, 8, 15, 19.

2. Doxanas MT, Anderson RL. Clinical Orbital Anatomy. Baltimore: Williams & Wilkins, 1984;20, 25, 117.

3. Kanski JJ. Clinical Ophthalmology (3rd ed). London: Butterworth–Heinemann, 1994;33, 52.

4. Forrest LA, Schuller DE, Strauss RH. Management of orbital blow-out fractures. Am J Sports Med 1989;17(2):217.

5. Taher AA. Diplopia caused by orbital floor blowout fracture. Oral Surg Oral Med Oral Pathol 1993;75(4):433.

6. Koornneef L. Orbital Connective Tissue. In FA Jakobiec (ed), Ocular Anatomy, Embryology, and Teratology. Philadelphia: Harper & Row, 1982;835.

7. Reeh MJ, Wobig JL, Wirtschafter JD. Ophthalmic Anatomy. San Francisco: American Academy of Ophthalmology 1981;11.

8. Webster RC, Gaunt JM, Hamdan US, et al. Supraorbital and supratrochlear notches and foramina: anatomical variations and surgical relevance. Laryngoscope 1986;96(3):311.

9. Goldberg RA, Hannai K, Toga AW. Microanatomy of the orbital apex. Ophthalmology 1992;99(9):1447.

10. Lang J, Kageyama I. The ophthalmic artery and its branches, measurements, and clinical importance. Surg Radiol Anat 1990;12(2):83.

11. Blaylock WK, Moore CA, Linberg JV. Anterior ethmoid anatomy facilitates dacryocystorhinostomy. Arch Ophthalmol 1990;108(12):1774.

12. Bansberg SF, Harner SG, Forbes G. Relationship of the optic nerve to the paranasal sinuses as shown by computed tomography. Otolaryngol Head Neck Surg 1987;96(4):331.

13. Cheung DK, Attia EL, Kirkpatrick DA, et al. An anatomic and CT scan study of the lateral wall of the sphenoid sinus as related to the transnasal transethmoid endoscopic approach. J Otolaryngol 1993;22(2):63.

14. Berkow R (ed). The Merck Manual (14th ed). Rahway, NJ: Merck & Co., 1982;1984.

15. Mills RP, Kartush JM. Orbital wall thickness and the spread of infection from the paranasal sinuses. Clin Otolaryngol 1985;10(4):209.

16. Silver HS, Fucci MJ, Flanagan JC, et al. Severe orbital infection as a complication of orbital fracture. Arch Otolaryngol Head Neck Surg 1992;118(8):845.

17. Eggers HM. Functional Anatomy of the Extraocular Muscles. In W Tasman, EA Jaeger (eds), Duane's Foundations of Clinical Ophthalmology (Vol 1.) Philadelphia: Lippincott, 1994;1.

18. Rodriguez-Vazquez JF, Merida-Velasco JR, Jimenez-Collado J. Orbital muscle of Müller: observations on human fetuses measuring 35–150 nm. Acta Anat (Basel) 1990;139:300.

SUGGESTED READING

Doxanas MT, Anderson RL. Osteology. In MT Doxanas, RL Anderson (eds), Clinical Orbital Anatomy. Baltimore: Williams & Wilkins, 1984;19.

Palastanga N, Field D, Soames R. Bones. The Skull. In N Palastanga, D Field, R Soames (eds), Anatomy and Human Movement. Oxford: Butterworth–Heinemann, 1989;262.

Warwick R. The Bony Orbit and Paranasal Sinuses. In R Warwick (ed), Eugene Wolff's Anatomy of the Eye and Orbit (7th ed). Philadelphia: Saunders, 1976;19.

Warwick R, Williams PL. Gray's Anatomy (35th ed). Philadelphia: Saunders, 1973;256.

Wobig JL. The Orbital Adnexae. In MJ Reeh, JL Wobig, JD Wirtschafter (eds), Ophthalmic Anatomy. San Francisco: American Academy of Ophthalmology, 1981;11.

Ocular Adnexa and Lacrimal System

The ocular adnexa includes the structures situated in proximity to the globe. Those that will be discussed in this chapter are the eyebrows, structures of the eyelids, the conjunctiva, and the structures of the medial canthus. In the discussion of the eyelids, the gross anatomy will be presented first, followed by a more detailed description of the eyelid structures. The lacrimal system consists of a secretory system, which produces the tear film, and an excretory system, which drains the tears, each of which is discussed in some detail.

EYEBROWS

The **eyebrows** consist of thick skin covered by characteristic short, prominent hairs extending across the superior orbital margin, usually arching slightly but sometimes merely running horizontally. Generally, in men the brows run along the orbital margin, whereas in women they run above the margin.[1] The first body hairs produced during embryologic development are those of the eyebrow.[2]

The muscles located in the forehead—the frontalis, procerus, corrugator superciliaris, and orbicularis oculi—produce eyebrow movements, an important element in facial expression (Figure 9-1). The **frontalis** fibers are oriented vertically and raise the eyebrow, causing a look of surprise or attention. The **corrugator** is characterized as the muscle of trouble or concentration, and its fibers are oriented obliquely; it moves the brow medially, toward the nose, creating vertical furrows between the brows. The **procerus**, the muscle of menace or aggression, extends from the medial side of the frontalis and attaches to the nasal bone; it pulls the medial portion of the eyebrow inferiorly.[2] The orbicularis oculi (described later)

lowers the entire brow. The fibers of these muscles blend with one another and are difficult to separate.[2] All are innervated by the facial nerve, cranial nerve VII.

EYELIDS

The **eyelids**, or **palpebrae**, are folds of skin and tissue that, when closed, cover the globe. The eyelids have four major functions: They (1) cover the globe for protection, (2) move the tears toward drainage at the medial canthus on closure, (3) spread the tear film over the anterior surface of the eye on opening, and (4) contain structures that produce the tear film. On closure, the upper eyelid moves down to cover the cornea, whereas the lower eyelid rises only slightly. When the eyes are closed gently, the eyelids should cover the entire globe.

✍ CLINICAL COMMENT: LAGOPHTHALMOS
Lagophthalmos refers to incomplete closure of the eyelids (Figure 9-2). Its cause may be physiologic, mechanical (such as scarring), or paralytic. Lagophthalmos is most evident during sleep, when drying of the inferior cornea may result. Scratchy, irritated eyes are evident on awakening, and punctate keratitis can occur.[3-5] Clinical assessment of the inferior cornea will show varying degrees of epithelial disruption, manifested as punctate staining with fluorescein dye.

Palpebral Fissure

The **palpebral fissure** is the area between the open eyelids. Although numerous variations exist in the positional relationship of the lid margins to the limbus, generally

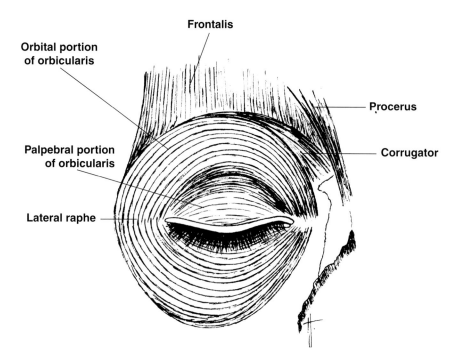

Frontalis

**Orbital portion
of orbicularis**

Procerus

**Palpebral portion
of orbicularis**

Corrugator

Lateral raphe

FIGURE 9-1. Forehead muscles that control the eyebrows.

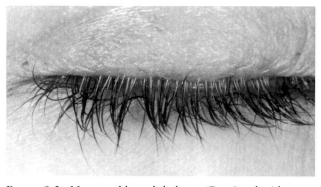

FIGURE 9-2. Nocturnal lagophthalmos. (Reprinted with permission from JD Bartlett, SD Jaanus. Clinical Ocular Pharmacology [3rd ed]. Boston: Butterworth–Heinemann, 1995;584.)

the upper lid just covers the superior limbus when one's eyes are open and looking straight ahead. The lower lid position is more variable, usually lying within 1 mm of the inferior limbus.[6–8]

The upper and lower eyelids meet at the corners of the palpebral fissure in the lateral and medial canthi. The **lateral canthus** is located approximately 5–7 mm medial to the bony orbital margin and lies directly on the globe.[8] The **medial canthus** is at the medial orbital margin but is separated from the globe by a reservoir for the pooling of tears, the **lacrimal lake**. The floor of the lacrimal lake is the plica semilunaris (Figure 9-3). This narrow, crescent-shaped fold of conjunctiva, located in the medial canthus, allows for lateral movement of the eye without stretching the bulbar conjunctiva. The caruncle is a small, pink mass of modified skin located just medial to the plica. It is covered with epithelium that contains goblet cells and fine hairs and their associated sweat and sebaceous glands.

Eyelid Topography

The upper eyelid extends to the eyebrow and is divided into the tarsal and orbital or preseptal parts. The **tarsal portion** lies closest to the lid margin, rests on the globe, and contains the tarsal plate. The skin is thin, and the underlying loose connective tissue is devoid of adipose tissue. The **orbital portion** extends from the tarsus to the eyebrow, and a furrow, the **superior palpebral sulcus**, separates the tarsal portion from the orbital portion (Figure 9-4). This sulcus separates the pretarsal skin, which is tightly adherent to the underlying tissue, from the preseptal skin, which is only loosely adherent to its underlying tissue, which contains a cushion of fat. In the eyelids of those of Eastern Asian descent, the superior orbital sulcus usually is not evident because the orbital septum inserts lower into the tarsal plate than it does in other eyelids, thus allowing more of the preseptal fat pad to encroach on the lower part of the eyelid.[2, 9, 10]

In the lower eyelid, the **inferior palpebral sulcus**, which separates the lower lid into tarsal and orbital parts, often is not very distinct. The tarsal portion rests against the globe, and the orbital portion extends from the lower border of the tarsus onto the cheek, extending just past the inferior orbital margin to the nasojugal and malar sulci (see Figure 9-4). These furrows occur at the attachment of the skin to the underlying connective tissue and become more prominent with age.

FIGURE 9-3. Structures located in the medial canthus.

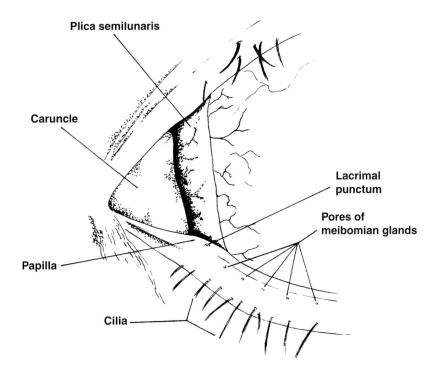

FIGURE 9-4. Surface anatomy of the eyelids.

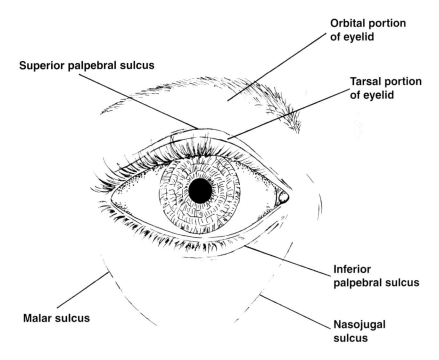

Eyelid Margin

The eyelid margin rests against the globe and contains the eyelashes and the pores of the meibomian glands. The cilia (eyelashes) are arranged at the lid margin in a double or triple row, with approximately 150 in the upper eyelid and half that many in the lower lid.[11] The lashes curl upward on the upper and downward on the lower lid. Replacement lashes will grow to full size in approximately 10 weeks, and each lash is replaced approxi-

mately every 5 months.[8] The eyelashes are richly supplied with nerves, causing them to be sensitive to even the slightest unexpected touch, which will elicit a protective response—a blink.

✍ CLINICAL COMMENT: ABNORMALITIES AFFECTING THE CILIA

Various epithelial diseases can cause madarosis (loss of eyelashes) or trichiasis (misdirected growth

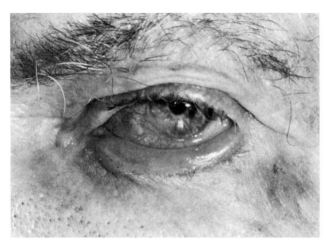

FIGURE 9-5. Tarsal ectropion with keratinized palpebral conjunctiva. (Reprinted with permission from JD Bartlett, SD Jaanus. Clinical Ocular Pharmacology [3rd ed]. Boston: Butterworth–Heinemann, 1995;585.)

of the eyelashes, in which they grow toward the palpebral fissure rather than away from it). Contact with the cornea can cause irritation and painful abrasions and can lead to ulceration.[3] The problem lashes can be removed by epilation.

The pores of the meibomian glands are located posterior to the cilia (see Figure 9-3), and the transition from skin to conjunctiva, the mucocutaneous junction, occurs just posterior to these openings.[12] A groove called the **gray line** runs along the eyelid margin between the cilia insertions and the pores of the meibomian glands. This groove is the location of a surgical plane that divides the lid into anterior and posterior portions.[2]

The eyelid margin can be divided into two parts: The medial one-sixth is the lacrimal portion, and the lateral five-sixths is the ciliary portion. The division occurs at the lacrimal papilla, a small elevation containing the lacrimal punctum, the opening that carries the tears into the nasolacrimal drainage system (see Figure 9-3). Usually, no cilia or meibomian pores are found medial to the punctum, in the lacrimal portion of the lid margin.

✍ CLINICAL COMMENT: EPICANTHUS
Epicanthus is a vertical fold of skin at the nasal canthus, arising in the medial area of the upper eyelid and terminating in the nasal canthal area. It is common in the newborn and may cause the appearance of esotropia. A concerned parent of an infant with epicanthus might be worried that the child's eyes are crossed; however, a cover test will identify a true esotropia. As the bridge of the nose develops, epicanthus gradually disappears. A form of epicanthus arising from the tarsal fold and extending into the medial canthal area is common also in those of Eastern Asian descent.[2]

Structures of the Eyelid

Orbicularis Oculi Muscle

The striated fibers of the **orbicularis oculi** muscle are located below the subcutaneous connective-tissue layer and encircle the palpebral fissure from the eyelid margin to overlap onto the orbital margin. The muscle can be divided into two regions, palpebral and orbital.

Palpebral Portion of the Muscle.   The **palpebral portion** of the orbicularis oculi muscle occupies the area of the eyelid that rests on the globe and is closest to the eyelid margin. It sometimes is divided further into pretarsal and preseptal parts. The palpebral portion is composed of semicircles of muscle fibers that run from the medial orbital margin and the medial palpebral ligament to the lateral palpebral raphe, where the superior and inferior fibers interdigitate with one another (see Figure 9-1). The lateral palpebral raphe overlies the lateral palpebral ligament.

Some fibers arise from deeper attachments on the posterior lacrimal crest. This section of the palpebral part of the orbicularis, the **muscle of Horner** or **the lacrimal part** (**pars lacrimalis**), encircles the lacrimal canaliculi.[8, 9, 13] Contraction of the orbicularis aids in moving tears through the canaliculi into the nasolacrimal drainage system. Another section of the palpebral orbicularis, called the **muscle of Riolan** or **ciliary part** (**pars ciliaris**), lies near the lid margin on both sides of the meibomian gland openings; it maintains the lid margins in close proximity to the globe.

✍ CLINICAL COMMENT: ECTROPION
AND ENTROPION
Eversion of the eyelid margin is called **ectropion** (Figure 9-5), the common cause of which is loss of muscle tone, a normal aging process. As the lid margin falls away from its position against the globe, the lacrimal punctum is no longer in position to drain the tears from the lacrimal lake. Epiphora, an overflow of tears onto the cheek, may occur, causing maceration of the delicate skin in this area.

Inversion of the lid margin is called **entropion** and may be due to spasm of the orbicularis oculi muscle that causes the lid margin to turn inward (Figure 9-6). This inward turning puts the eyelashes in contact with the globe and, unless relieved, can cause corneal abrasion. Scarring of the lid after trauma or disease also might cause entropion.

Both ectropion and entropion are more common in the lower lid and can be corrected surgically, if necessary. The anatomic relationship of the muscular and connective-tissue components is an important consideration when a repair is done.[14–16]

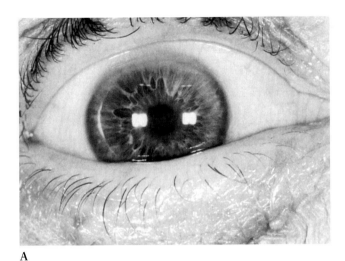

A

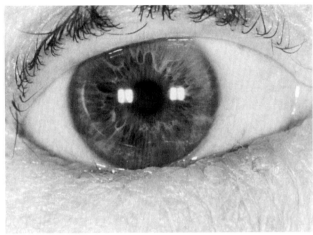

B

FIGURE 9-6. Involutional (age-related) entropion. (A) Lower eyelid margin in normal position between blinks. (B) Entropion evident immediately after tight eyelid closure. (Reprinted with permission from JD Bartlett, SD Jaanus. Clinical Ocular Pharmacology [3rd ed]. Boston: Butterworth–Heinemann, 1995;587.)

Orbital Portion of the Muscle. The **orbital portion** of the orbicularis oculi muscle is attached superiorly to the orbital margin, medial to the supraorbital notch; the fibers encircle the area outer to the palpebral portion and attach inferiorly to the orbital margin, medial to the infraorbital foramen.[2] These concentric circular fibers extend throughout the rest of the lid and over the orbital rim.

Actions of the Muscle. The orbicularis is innervated by cranial nerve VII (the facial nerve). Relaxation of the levator muscle in conjunction with contraction of the orbicularis oculi muscle causes closure of the eyelids. The palpebral portion closes the eye gently and is the muscle of action in an involuntary blink and a voluntary wink. Spontaneous involuntary blinking renews the precorneal tear film. A reflex blink is protective and may be elicited by a number of stimuli—a loud noise; corneal, conjunctival, or cilial touch; or the sudden approach of an object. When the orbital portion of the orbicularis contracts, the eye is closed tightly, and the areas surrounding the lids—the forehead, temple, and cheek—are involved in the contraction. Such eyelid closure often occurs as a protective mechanism when there is ocular pain or after an injury and is called **reflex blepharospasm**. If the lids are closed tightly in a strong contraction, forces compressing the orbital contents can significantly increase the intraocular pressure.[17]

The antagonist to the palpebral portion of the orbicularis is the levator muscle. The antagonist to the orbital portion is the frontalis muscle.

Superior Palpebral Levator Muscle

The **superior palpebral levator muscle**, the retractor of the upper eyelid, is located within the orbit above the globe and extends into the upper lid. It originates on the lesser wing of the sphenoid bone above and in front of the optic foramen, and its sheath blends with the sheath of the superior rectus muscle. As the levator approaches the eyelid from its posterior origin at the orbital apex, a ligament, the **superior transverse ligament (Whitnall's ligament)** acts as a fulcrum to change the anteroposterior direction of the levator to a superoinferior direction (Figure 9-7).[10, 18–21]

Levator Aponeurosis. As it enters the eyelid, the levator becomes a fan-shaped tendinous expansion, the **levator aponeurosis**. Unlike a typical tendon, the aponeurosis spreads out into an extensive sheet posterior to the orbital septum. The fibers of the aponeurosis penetrate the orbital septum and extend into the upper lid, fanning out across its entire width. These tendinous fibers pass through the submuscular connective tissue, the posterior fibers inserting into the lower anterior surface of the tarsal plate and the anterior fibers running between the muscle bundles of the orbicularis to insert primarily into the skin of the eyelid, though some insert into the intermuscular septa of the orbicularis (see Figure 9-7).[8, 9, 18–21] It is this attachment of the fibers from the levator aponeurosis that anchors the skin to the underlying tissues in the pretarsal area of the eyelid and that creates the palpebral sulcus. In those of Eastern Asian descent, the orbital septum attaches to the tarsal plate more inferiorly, and the aponeurotic fibers do not attach as extensively to the cutaneous tissue.[2, 9]

Two side extensions of the aponeurosis are referred to as **horns**. The lateral horn helps to support the lacrimal gland by holding it against the orbital roof and divides the gland into orbital and palpebral lobes (Figure 9-8). The lateral horn then attaches to the lateral palpebral ligament and to the lateral orbital tubercle. The

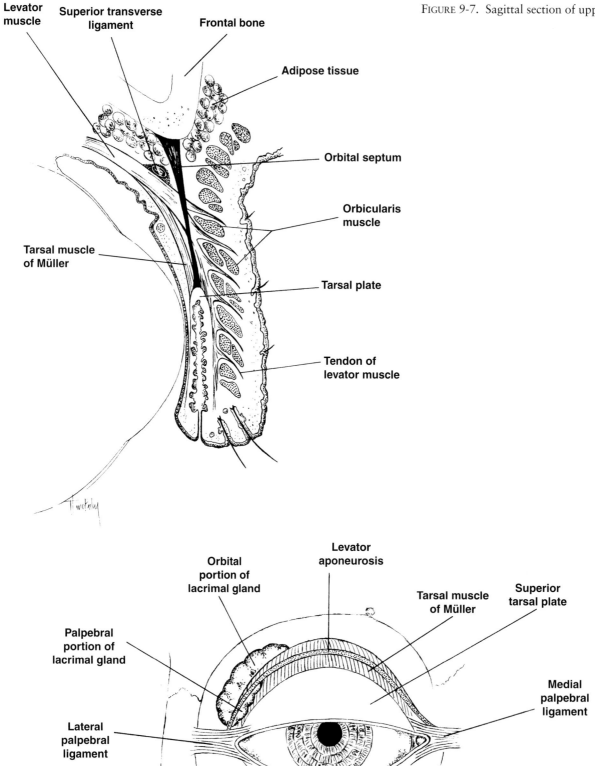

FIGURE 9-7. Sagittal section of upper eyelid.

Levator muscle

Superior transverse ligament

Frontal bone

Adipose tissue

Orbital septum

Orbicularis muscle

Tarsal muscle of Müller

Tarsal plate

Tendon of levator muscle

Orbital portion of lacrimal gland

Levator aponeurosis

Tarsal muscle of Müller

Superior tarsal plate

Palpebral portion of lacrimal gland

Lateral palpebral ligament

Medial palpebral ligament

Inferior tarsal plate

FIGURE 9-8. Orbital area viewed from in front, with skin, subcutaneous tissue, and orbital septum removed.

medial horn is attached to the medial palpebral ligament and to the medial orbital rim.

Levator Action. Contraction of the levator muscle causes elevation of the eyelid. The connection between the sheath of the levator and the sheath of the superior rectus muscle coordinates eyelid position with eye position, so that as the eye is elevated the lid is raised.[20, 21] The levator is innervated by the superior division of the oculomotor nerve, cranial nerve III.

The eyelids are closed by relaxation of the levator and contraction of the orbicularis oculi muscles. The tonic activity of the levator and the relaxation of the orbicularis holds the eyelid open. In a blink, the tonic activity of the levator is suspended and, with a burst of activity, the orbicularis rapidly lowers the lid, followed by a cessation of orbicularis activity and resumption of levator tonicity.[22]

Retractor of the Lower Eyelid

The retractor of the lower lid is the **capsulopalpebral fascia (lower eyelid aponeurosis)**.[2] The capsulopalpebral fascia, an anterior extension from the sheath of the inferior rectus muscle and the suspensory ligament, inserts into the inferior edge of the tarsal plate.[9, 20, 21] This insertion coordinates lid position with globe movement: On globe depression, the lower eyelid is depressed and, on upward movement of the globe, the lower eyelid elevates slightly.[7] The capsulopalpebral fascia also fuses with the orbital septum and sends some fibers to insert into the inferior fornix.[2, 15, 21]

Tarsal Muscle (of Müller)

The **superior tarsal muscle (muscle of Müller)** is composed of smooth muscle and originates on the posterior inferior aspect of the levator muscle. These smooth-muscle fibers begin to appear within the striated muscle at the point at which the muscle becomes aponeurotic.[2, 8, 20, 21] The superior tarsal muscle inserts on the superior edge of the tarsal plate (see Figures 9-7 and 9-8).

A similar smooth muscle, the **inferior tarsal muscle**, is found in the lower eyelid. It arises from the inferior rectus muscle sheath and inserts into the lower conjunctiva and lower border of the tarsal plate.[2, 8, 17] Investigators disagree about whether the inferior tarsal muscle actually inserts into the tarsal plate[2, 8, 20] or inserts into the tissue below the tarsal plate.[23] Both tarsal muscles are innervated by sympathetic fibers that widen the palpebral fissure when activated (as in situations associated with fear or surprise).[8, 21]

✍ CLINICAL COMMENT: PTOSIS
  Ptosis is a condition in which the upper eyelid droops or sags. It can be caused by weakness or paralysis of the levator or Müller's muscle. If Müller's muscle alone is affected, a less noticeable form of ptosis occurs than when the levator is involved.[24] An individual with ptosis might attempt to raise the lid by using the frontalis muscle, which results in elevation of the eyebrow.

Tarsal Plate

Each eyelid contains a **tarsal plate (tarsus)** that gives the lid rigidity and structure and shapes it to the curvature of the globe. The tarsal plate in the upper lid is approximately 11 mm high, and the inferior tarsal plate is approximately 5 mm high.[8] The anterior surface is adjacent to the submuscular connective tissue. The posterior surface is adherent to the palpebral conjunctiva. The orbital border of the tarsus is attached to the orbital septum, whereas the marginal border lies at the lid margin. The sides of the tarsal plates are attached to the bony orbital margin by the palpebral or tarsal ligaments (see Figure 9-8).

✍ CLINICAL COMMENT: EYELID EVERSION
  When attempting to evert the upper lid, one should place the cotton-tipped applicator or fingertip above the superior edge of the tarsal plate. The novice will experience difficulty in everting the eyelid if the applicator is placed in the middle of the tarsal plate.

Palpebral Ligaments

The palpebral or tarsal ligaments are bands of dense connective tissue connecting the tarsal plates to the orbital rim and holding the tarsal plates in position against the globe during eye and lid movements. The **medial palpebral ligament** runs from the medial edge of each tarsal plate to the medial orbital rim, where it divides into two limbs. One limb attaches to the posterior lacrimal crest and the other to the anterior lacrimal crest. Both limbs lie in front of the orbital septum (see Figure 8-11).[25]

The **lateral palpebral ligament** is located posterior to the orbital septum and attaches the lateral edges of the tarsal plates to the lateral orbital margin at the lateral orbital tubercle (see Figure 9-8). Fibrous connections between the lateral palpebral ligament and the check ligament for the lateral rectus muscle allow a slight lateral displacement of the lateral canthus with extreme abduction.[26]

The upper borders of both the medial and lateral ligaments are joined to the expansion of the levator tendon, and their lower borders are joined to an expansion of the ligament of Lockwood.[8] The connective-tissue structures at the canthi have been described as a retinaculum that is made up of the palpebral ligaments, the horns of the levator aponeurosis, the suspensory ligament, the check ligaments, and the superior transverse ligament.[2]

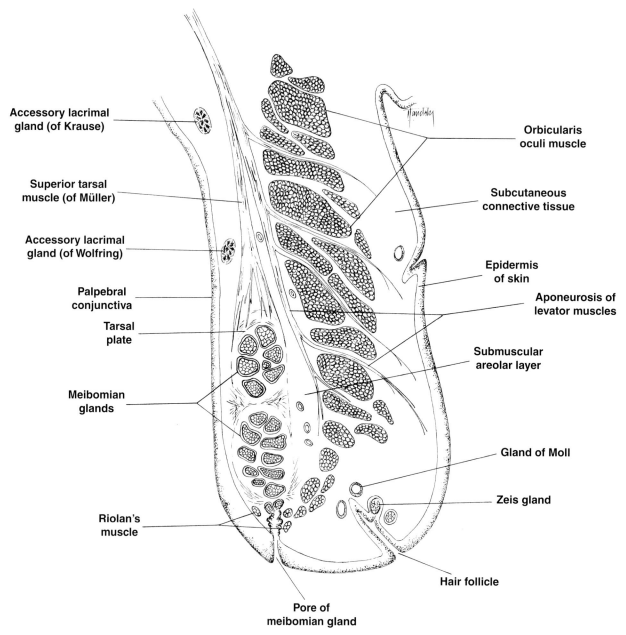

FIGURE 9-9. Sagittal section of eyelid, illustrating palpebral muscles and glands.

Glands of the Lids

The **meibomian glands (tarsal glands)** are sebaceous glands embedded in the tarsal plate. These long, multilobed glands resemble a large bunch of grapes and are arranged vertically such that their openings are located in a row along the lid margin posterior to the cilia (Figure 9-9). Approximately 30–40 meibomian glands are found in the upper lid and 20–30 in the lower lid.[11] On eyelid eversion, the vertical rows of the meibomian glands can sometimes be seen as yellow streaks through the palpebral conjunctiva. These glands' secretions provide the outer lipid layer of the tear film.

The **sebaceous glands of Zeis** secrete sebum into the hair follicle of the cilia, coating the eyelash shaft to keep it from becoming brittle.[8]

The **glands of Moll** are modified sweat glands located near the lid margin. Their ducts empty into the hair follicle, into the Zeis gland duct, or directly onto the lid margin. Similar glands found in the axillae are scent organs, but the purpose of these glands in the eyelid is not understood.[8, 11]

The **accessory lacrimal glands of Krause** are located in the stroma of the conjunctival fornix, and the **accessory lacrimal glands of Wolfring** are located along the orbital border of the tarsal plate (see Figure 9-9).[2, 8]

These glands are oval and display numerous acini. In the upper fornix, 20–40 glands of Krause are found, though only 6–8 such glands appear in the lower fornix.[2] The glands of Wolfring are less numerous. The secretion of the accessory lacrimal glands appears similar to that of the main lacrimal gland and contributes to the aqueous layer of the tear film.

Histologic Features of Eyelid Structures

Skin

The skin of the eyelid is three to four cells thick and contains many fine hairs, sebaceous glands, and sweat glands. It is the thinnest skin in the body, easily forms folds and wrinkles, and is almost transparent in the very young.[2] The epidermal layer consists of a basal germinal layer, a granular layer, and a superficial layer that is cornified. The underlying dermis is abundant in elastic fibers. A very sparse areolar connective-tissue layer, the subcutaneous tissue, lies below the dermis. This thin layer is devoid of adipose tissue in the tarsal portion. A pad of fat often is located in this region in the orbital portion that separates the orbicularis from the skin.[8]

🖎 CLINICAL COMMENT: FLUID ACCUMULATION
The loose connective-tissue layer of the eyelid can be separated from the underlying tissue easily and is the site of accumulation of blood or edema in injury or of exudates in inflammatory conditions. The thinness of the skin and the fine underlying tissue adjacent to it allows this area to be greatly distensible, as evidenced in patients with periorbital cellulitis or ecchymosis (a black eye). This skin recovers rapidly after distention because of the elasticity of the dermis. With advancing age, however, the skin loses its elasticity, and stretching will cause exaggerated skin folds.

Muscles

The **orbicularis oculi** lies deep to the subcutaneous layer. These striated muscle bundles run throughout the eyelid and, in a longitudinal section of the lid prepared for microscopic examination, are cut in cross section. Along the lid margin, small muscle bundles located on both sides of the meibomian gland represent a specific part of the orbicularis, the **pars ciliaris (Riolan's muscle)**, which holds the lid margin against the globe (see Figure 9-9).

Posterior to the orbicularis lies another layer of loose connective tissue, the **submuscular areolar layer,** which separates the muscle from the tarsal plate. Between this layer and the tarsal plate is a potential space, the pretarsal space, that contains the vessels of the palpebral arcades. The presental space is located between the orbicularis and the orbital septum; directly above it is the presental cushion of fat.[8]

Tendinous fibers of the **levator aponeurosis** run through the submuscular tissue layer between the orbicularis and the superior tarsal muscle to insert into the tarsal plate and the skin of the lid (see Figure 9-9). It is this insertion of fibers that anchors the skin so firmly in the tarsal portion of the lid. There is no such attachment of the aponeurosis in the presental area. The smooth-muscle fibers of the **superior tarsal muscle** are located above the superior tarsal plate and insert into its upper edge. Both the aponeurosis and the superior tarsal muscle are cut longitudinally in a microscope slide of a longitudinal section of the lid.

Tarsal Plates

The **tarsal plates** are composed of dense connective tissue. The collagen fibrils of this tissue are of uniform size and run both vertically and horizontally to surround the meibomian glands.

Conjunctiva

The palpebral conjunctiva is composed of two layers, a stratified epithelial layer and a connective-tissue stromal layer, the submucosa. The epithelial layer of the conjunctiva is continuous with the skin epithelium at the mucocutaneous junction of the lid margin (Figure 9-10). As the conjunctiva lines the lid, squamous cells are replaced by cuboidal and columnar cells, forming a stratified columnar mucoepithelial layer, the granular and keratinized layers having been discontinued.[11, 27] At the mucocutaneous junction, the epithelial layer is approximately five cells thick. Over much of the upper lid, the conjunctival epithelium is two to three cells thick, whereas over much of the lower lid, the epithelium is three to four cells thick.[8] This stratified columnar epithelium continues throughout the fornices into the bulbar conjunctiva, where it changes to a stratified squamous layer near the limbus, becoming continuous with the corneal epithelium.

Goblet cells, which produce the innermost mucous layer of the tear film, are scattered throughout the stratified columnar conjunctival epithelium (see Figure 9-10). These cells are most numerous in the inferior nasal aspect of the tarsal conjunctiva[28]; their number decreases with advancing age and increases in inflammatory conditions. A goblet cell produces mucin droplets that accumulate, causing the cell to swell and become goblet-shaped. The surface of the cell finally ruptures, releasing mucus. Invaginations of conjunctival epithelium, often located near the fornix, are called **crypts of Henle**. Goblet cells release their mucus into the cavity formed by these invaginations, and the mucus may become trapped if the opening to the crypt is narrow. This accumulation of

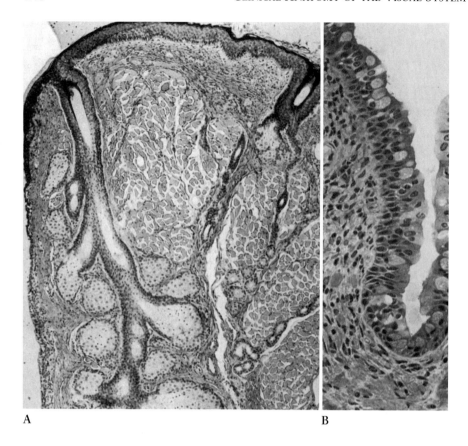

A   B

FIGURE 9-10. (A) Photomicrograph of part of an eyelid, showing conjunctiva (left), epidermis (above), and the large modified sebaceous glands (tarsal or meibomian glands). The striated muscle fibers (right) are part of the palpebral portion of orbicularis oculi muscle, and between them are parts of three glands of Moll (apocrine type sweat glands) (×25). (B) The inferior conjunctival fornix with goblet, mucus-secreting cells (pale-staining) in the epithelium (×200). (Reprinted with permission from CR Leeson, ST Leeson. Histology. Philadelphia: Saunders, 1976;567.)

mucoid material may account for the application of the misnomer "glands" of Henle to describe these structures.

✍ CLINICAL COMMENT: VITAMIN A DEFICIENCY
Vitamin A deficiency has been associated with a loss of goblet cells and keratinization of the epithelium. In dry-eye disorders showing a decrease in the number of goblet cells, treatment with vitamin A therapy can induce the reappearance of goblet cells.[29]

The **submucosa (stroma, substantia propria) of the palpebral conjunctiva** is very thin in the tarsal portion of the eyelid but becomes increasingly thick in the orbital portion. It is composed of loose, vascularized connective tissue that can be subdivided into an outer lymphoid layer and a deep fibrous layer. In addition to the normal connective-tissue components (collagen fibrils, fibroblasts, ground substance, and a few fine elastic fibers), the lymphoid layer contains macrophages, mast cells, polymorphonuclear leukocytes, eosinophils, and accumulations of lymphocytes. The immunoglobulin IgA is found in the lymphoid layer, making the conjunctiva an immunologically active tissue.[30–32]

The deep fibrous layer connects the conjunctiva to underlying structures and contains a random network of collagen fibrils and numerous fibroblasts, blood vessels, nerves, and accessory lacrimal glands. This fibrous layer merges and is continuous with the dense connective tissue of the tarsal plate. The conjunctiva is so richly supplied with blood vessels that a pale palpebral conjunctiva might signify the presence of anemia.

✍ CLINICAL COMMENT: CONJUNCTIVAL CYSTS AND CONCRETIONS
Clear conjunctival cysts, either intraepithelial or subepithelial, are filled with mucoid material and are found most commonly in the palpebral conjunctiva.[33] Conjunctival concretions are small, yellow-white nodules approximating the size of a pinhead and most often located in the tarsal conjunctiva. They are composed of finely granular material and membranous debris, products of cellular degeneration. These nodules are hard but contain no calcific deposits.[34] They are more commonly found in the elderly and can be removed if they produce a foreign-body irritation.[32]

Glands

The **meibomian glands** are large sebaceous glands occupying the length of the tarsal plate. Each consists of 10–15 lobes or acini attached to a single large central duct.[35, 36] The duct is arranged vertically such that the opening is located at the edge of the tarsal plate corresponding to the eyelid margin (see Figure 9-9).

Meibomian glands are holocrine glands; their secretion is produced by the decomposition of the entire cell. Each acinus is surrounded by a layer of myoepithelial cells and is filled with actively dividing cells. These cells become large and polyhedral and are filled with sebaceous granules. As each cell degenerates, the nucleus begins to diminish in size and the cell wall disintegrates. Cells in varying stages of decomposition pack each saccule (see Figure 9-10). Decomposed cells move down the duct to the opening, at which point the secretion forms the outermost lipid layer of the tear film.[12, 35, 36]

Histologically, the sebaceous **Zeis glands** are similar to the meibomian glands. The Zeis glands, however, are composed of just one or two acini and are associated with the eyelash follicle (Figure 9-11). Generally, two Zeis glands are present per follicle. They release sebum into the follicle, thereby preventing the cilia from becoming dry and brittle.[35]

Glands of Moll are modified sweat glands and also are located near the eyelash follicle. They consist of a spiral that begins as a large cavity, the neck of which becomes narrow as it forms a duct (see Figure 9-10). The large lumen often appears empty and is surrounded by a layer of cuboidal to columnar secretory cells.[35] Myoepithelial cells surround these cells. The Moll gland is an apocrine gland; its secretion is composed not of the whole cell but of parts of the cellular cytoplasm. The duct might empty into the duct of a Zeis gland, or it might open directly onto the lid margin between cilia.

Accessory lacrimal glands are groups of secretory cells (shaped like truncated pyramids) arranged in an oval around a central lumen.[27] The acini are surrounded, sometimes incompletely, by a row of myoepithelial cells.[2] These are merocrine glands—that is, the cell remains intact and secretes a product—and they have the same histologic makeup as the main lacrimal gland (see Figure 9-17).

✍ CLINICAL COMMENT: COMMON AFFLICTIONS OF THE EYELID

A hordeolum is an acute inflammation of an eyelid gland usually caused by staphylococci.[3] An infected Zeis or Moll gland is called an **external hordeolum** or **common stye** and usually comes to a head on the skin of the eyelid. A localized infection of a meibomian gland usually drains from the inside surface of the lid and thus is called an **internal hordeolum**. Mild cases usually resolve with hot compress treatment, but more severe cases might require medication.

A **chalazion** is a localized, sometimes painless, swelling of a meibomian gland, often caused by an obstructed duct (Figure 9-12). The gland may extrude its secretion into surrounding tissue, setting up a granulomatous inflammation. Medical or surgical therapy sometimes is necessary.[37]

Innervation of the Eyelid

The ophthalmic and maxillary divisions of the trigeminal nerve provide sensory innervation of the eyelids. The

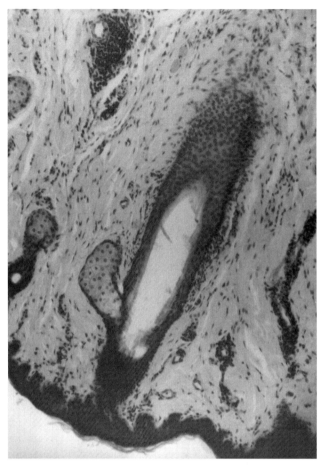

FIGURE 9-11. Photomicrograph shows Zeis gland with duct emptying into eyelash follicle (×100).

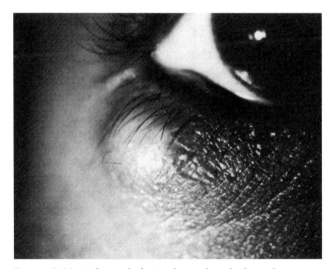

FIGURE 9-12. A large chalazion located at the lateral aspect of the lower eyelid. (Reprinted with permission from JD Bartlett, SD Jaanus. Clinical Ocular Pharmacology [3rd ed]. Boston: Butterworth–Heinemann, 1995;567.)

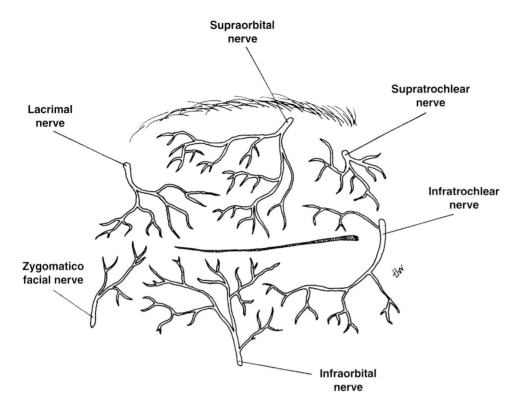

Supraorbital nerve

Supratrochlear nerve

Lacrimal nerve

Infratrochlear nerve

Zygomatico facial nerve

Infraorbital nerve

FIGURE 9-13. Palpebral innervation.

upper lid is supplied by the supraorbital, supratrochlear, infratrochlear, and lacrimal nerves, branches of the ophthalmic division. The supply to the lower lid is by the infratrochlear branch of the ophthalmic nerve and the infraorbital nerve, a branch of the maxillary division (Figure 9-13). Motor control of the orbicularis is through the temporal and zygomatic branches of the facial nerve; motor control of the levator is by the superior division of the oculomotor nerve. The tarsal smooth muscles are innervated by sympathetic fibers from the superior cervical ganglion.

Blood Supply of the Eyelid

The blood vessels are located in a series of arcades or arches in each lid. The marginal palpebral arcade lies near the lid margin, and the peripheral palpebral arcade lies near the orbital edge of the tarsal plate (Figure 9-14). The vessels forming these arcades are branches from the medial and lateral palpebral arteries. The medial and lateral palpebral arteries are branches of the ophthalmic and lacrimal arteries, respectively. Normal variations occur in the blood supply, the most common being a lack of the peripheral arcade in the lower lid.

CONJUNCTIVA

The conjunctiva is a thin, translucent mucous membrane that runs from the limbus over the anterior sclera,

forms a cul-de-sac at the superior and inferior fornices, and turns anteriorly to line the eyelids. It ensures smooth movement of the eyelids over the globe. The conjunctiva can be divided into three sections that are continuous with one another. The tissue lining the eyelids is the palpebral or tarsal conjunctiva, the bulbar conjunctiva covers the sclera, and the conjunctival fornix is the cul-de-sac connecting palpebral and bulbar sections (Figure 9-15).

At the mucocutaneous junction of the lid margin, the nonkeratinized squamous **palpebral conjunctiva** is continuous with the keratinized squamous epithelium of the epidermis of the eyelid. The conjunctiva forming the fornices is attached loosely to the fascial extensions of the levator, tarsal, and extraocular muscles, providing coordination of conjunctival movement with movement of the globe and lids. The fornices are present superiorly, inferiorly, and laterally, and ease movement of the globe without creating undue stretching of the conjunctiva. The lateral fornix is the deepest and extends posterior to the equator of the globe.

The **bulbar conjunctiva** is translucent, allowing the sclera to show through, and is colorless except when its blood vessels are engorged. Bulbar conjunctiva is loosely adherent to the underlying tissue up to within 3 mm of the cornea, where it becomes tightly adherent and merges with the underlying Tenon's capsule and sclera.

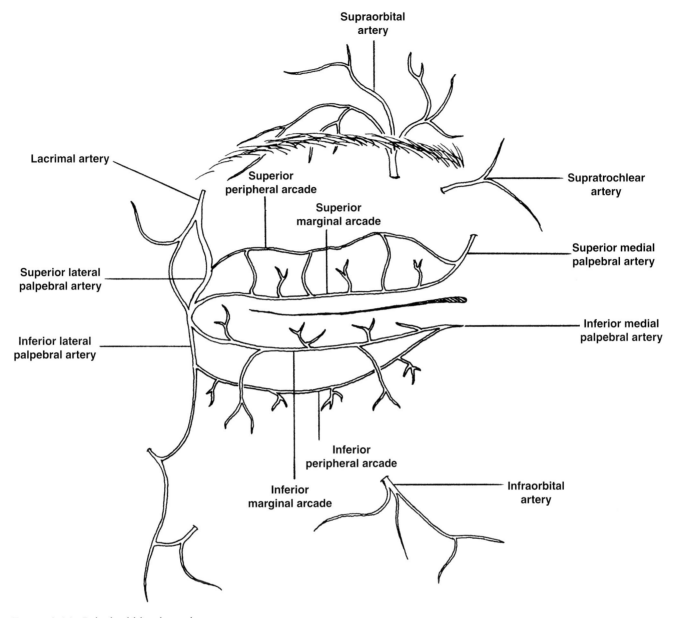

FIGURE 9-14. Palpebral blood supply.

Histologic Features of Conjunctiva

The conjunctiva is composed of two layers, a stratified epithelial layer and a connective-tissue stromal layer, the submucosa.

Conjunctival Epithelium

At the limbus, the stratified squamous conjunctival epithelium is continuous with the corneal epithelium. The superficial cells have microvilli and microplicae similar to the surface corneal cells. Melanin granules often are found in the cytoplasm of conjunctival epithelial cells, especially near the limbus; these are particularly preva-

lent in individuals with heavily pigmented skin. Goblet cells, which produce the mucus component of the tear film, also are located in the epithelium.

Subsurface vesicles, found below the outer membrane of the superficial conjunctival cell, may be an additional source of mucous material. As these vesicles fuse with the epithelial cell membrane, chains extend outward and may even form a chemical bond with the mucus layer secreted by the goblet cells. These chains increase the adherence of the tear film to the globe. These vesicle membranes may, in fact, be a source for the microvilli present on the surface epithelial cells.[38]

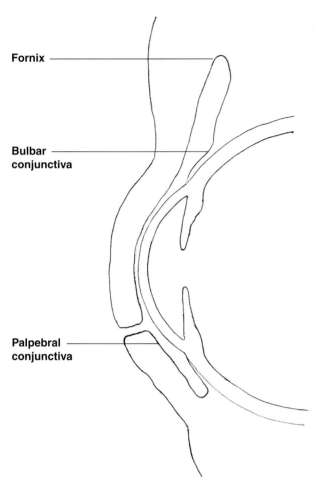

Fornix

Bulbar conjunctiva

Palpebral conjunctiva

FIGURE 9-15. The three partitions of conjunctiva.

Conjunctival Submucosa

The **submucosa** underlying the epithelium is a stromal (substantia propria) layer composed of vascularized, loose connective tissue containing the same components as are found in palpebral conjunctival stroma.

Plica Semilunaris

The **plica semilunaris** is a crescent-shaped fold of conjunctiva located at the medial canthus (see Figure 9-3). (It might be a remnant of the nictitating membrane seen in lower vertebrates.) The epithelium is 8–10 cells thick and contains numerous goblet cells, and the stroma is highly vascularized, containing smooth muscle and adipose tissue.[39] Because there is not a deep fornix at the medial side as there is at the lateral side, the evident function of the plica is to allow full lateral movement of the eye without tissue stretching.

Caruncle

The function of the **caruncle,** a mound of tissue that overlies the medial edge of the plica semilunaris (see Figure

9-3), is poorly understood. The caruncle is similar to conjunctiva in that it contains nonkeratinized epithelium and accessory lacrimal glands, but it also has skin elements—hair follicles and sebaceous and sweat glands.[39, 40] The sebaceous glands are one likely source for the occasional accumulation of matter that occurs in the medial canthus of the healthy eye.

Conjunctival Blood Vessels

The palpebral conjunctiva receives its blood supply from the palpebral arcades. Branches from the arcades anastomose on both sides of the tarsal plate; vessels from the posterior network supply the palpebral conjunctiva in both upper and lower lids.

The fornices are supplied by branches from the peripheral arcades, which then branch again and enter the bulbar conjunctiva, forming a plexus of vessels, the posterior conjunctival arteries. These anastomose with the plexus of anterior conjunctival arteries formed by branches from the anterior ciliary arteries. Conjunctival veins parallel the arteries but are more numerous. They drain into the palpebral and ophthalmic veins.

Conjunctival Lymphatics

The conjunctival lymphatic vessels are arranged in two networks within the submucosa, one superficial and one deep. These drain into the lymphatics of the eyelids, those from the lateral aspect emptying into the parotid lymph node and those from the medial aspect emptying into the submandibular lymph node (see Figure 11-11).

Conjunctival Innervation

Sensory innervation of the bulbar conjunctiva is via the long ciliary nerves. Sensory innervation of the superior palpebral conjunctiva is provided by the frontal and lacrimal branches of the ophthalmic nerve. That of the inferior palpebral conjunctiva is provided by the lacrimal nerve and the infraorbital branch of the maxillary nerve. All sensory information is carried in the trigeminal nerve.

✐ CLINICAL COMMENT: BIOMICROSCOPIC EXAMINATION

The normal bulbar conjunctiva is clear and displays a fine network of blood vessels running through it. The blood flow in an individual vessel can be seen under proper magnification. The conjunctival surface is not as smooth as the cornea, and so a small amount of fluorescein pooling might be evident in the normal eye. The palpebral conjunctiva is examined by everting the eyelids and should appear bright pink in color. The blood vessel network is evident, and arteries can be seen that run at right

FIGURE 9-16. Apex of the pterygium is encroaching onto the pupil area of the cornea. The vasculature is evident. (Courtesy of Dr. William Jones, Albuquerque, NM.)

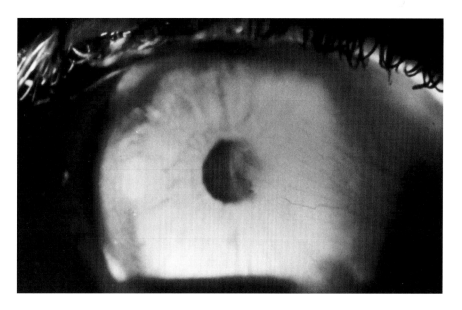

angles to the lid margins. The meibomian gland ducts, if seen, will appear as fine yellow lines.

✍ CLINICAL COMMENT: CONJUNCTIVITIS

Conjunctivitis is any inflammation of the conjunctiva and may be due to a variety of factors. Among the common causative agents are bacterial or viral invasion or an allergic reaction. In inflammatory conditions, fluids often accumulate in the loose stromal tissue; this conjunctival edema is called **chemosis**. Dilation and engorgement of the conjunctival blood vessels also occur with inflammation and irritation, and this vascular change is known as conjunctival **injection**. Both chemosis and injection are present to varying degrees in diseases and irritations of the conjunctiva. In a viral conjunctivitis, the preauricular lymph node often is prominent on the involved side.

✍ CLINICAL COMMENT: PINGUECULAE
AND PTERYGIA

A **pinguecula** consists of an opaque, slightly elevated mass of modified conjunctival tissue located in the interpalpebral area usually at the three- or nine-o'clock position. It may vary considerably in size and appearance but usually is round or oval and yellowish. Two types of histologic changes occur in the submucosal layers, whereas the epithelial layers remain unchanged. The first submucosal change is hyalinization, which occurs in a zone just below the epithelium. This zone contains degenerating collagen along with a granular material that probably results from the breakdown of connective-tissue components. The second change is in the formation of elastic fibers. Precursors of elastic fibers and abnormally immature forms of newly synthesized elastic fibers are found beneath the zone of hyalin-

ization. These fibers degenerate, and there is a marked reduction of elastic myofibrils, which prevents normal assembly of elastic fibers.[41, 42] Fibroblasts in these regions show extensive alteration.

A **pterygium** is a fibrovascular overgrowth of bulbar conjunctiva onto cornea and usually is progressive. It might be gray and is triangular, its apex (which often is called the **head**) resting on the cornea. It too occurs in the three- or nine-o'clock position of the interpalpebral area (Figure 9-16). Histologic changes have been found to be the same as those seen in pingueculae. In addition, a blood vessel network is evident within the tissue, and fibrovascular growth occurs that destroys Bowman's layer of the cornea as the pterygium grows onto the cornea.[41]

Exposure to irritants, such as wind and dust, might initiate hyperplasia and be a precursor of both of these degenerative changes. Molecular damage produced by solar radiation, particularly high-energy ultraviolet rays, can be a primary factor in pterygia.[43, 44]

Pingueculae rarely are treated unless they are inflamed. Pterygia are removed when the apex approaches the visual axis, if significant corneal astigmatism is induced, or for cosmetic concerns. Pterygia often recur after surgical removal. Patients with either condition should be advised of the relationship of these conditions to irritants and sun exposure, and ultraviolet-filtering protective lenses should be prescribed as well as artificial tears and ocular lubricants as needed.

TENON'S CAPSULE

Below the conjunctival stroma is a thin, fibrous sheet called **Tenon's capsule (fascia bulbi)**. Tenon's capsule serves as a fascial cavity within which the globe can move. It protects and supports the globe and attaches it to the orbital connective tissue.

The collagen fibrils that form Tenon's capsule are arranged in a three-dimensional network of longitudinal, horizontal, and oblique groups.[45] In young people, Tenon's capsule contains collagen fibrils of uniform shape and diameters of 70–110 nm; in older individuals, there is greater variation in fibril shape and diameters vary from 30 to 160 nm.[45, 46] Few fibroblasts and some elastic fibers are present but in a very small ratio as compared to the number of collagen fibrils.[46]

TEAR FILM

The **tear film,** which covers the anterior surface of the globe, has several functions: (1) it keeps the surface moist and serves as a lubricant between the globe and eyelids; (2) it traps debris and helps remove sloughed epithelial cells and debris; (3) it is the primary source of atmospheric oxygen for the cornea; (4) it provides a smooth refractive surface necessary for optimum optical function[47]; (5) it contains antibacterial substances (i.e., lysozyme, beta-lysin, lactoferrin, and IgA) to help protect against infection[48]; and (6) it helps to maintain corneal hydration by changes in tonicity that occur with evaporation.[49]

The tear film is composed of three layers. The outermost is a lipid layer, containing waxy esters, cholesterol, and free fatty acids, primarily produced by the meibomian glands with a small contribution from the Zeis glands. This layer retards evaporation and provides lubrication for smooth eyelid movement. The middle or aqueous layer contains inorganic salts, glucose, urea, enzymes, proteins, glycoproteins, and most of the antibacterial substances.[2] It is secreted by the main and accessory lacrimal glands. The innermost or mucous layer is adsorbed by the glycocalyx of the corneal surface and acts as an interface that facilitates adhesion of the aqueous layer of the tears to the corneal surface.[50] It is produced and secreted by the conjunctival goblet cells.

According to some sources, the tear film is 7–10 µm thick, with the aqueous layer accounting for 90% of the thickness.[8, 51] However, recent measurements using laser interferometry imply that the full thickness of the mucous layer was not recognized in the past using conventional measuring methods. The tear layer thickness may actually be in the range of 34–45 µm, and the mucous layer might be the thickest.[52, 53]

Lacrimal Secretory System

The secretory system includes the main lacrimal gland, the accessory lacrimal glands, meibomian and Zeis glands, and the conjunctival goblet cells. The main **lacrimal gland** is located in a fossa on the temporal side

of the orbital plate of the frontal bone, just posterior to the superior orbital margin.

The lacrimal gland is divided into two portions, palpebral and orbital, by the aponeurosis of the levator muscle (see Figure 9-8). The superior orbital portion is larger and almond-shaped. The superior surface lies against the periorbita of the lacrimal fossa, the inferior surface rests against the aponeurosis, the medial edge lies against the levator, and the lateral edge lies on the lateral rectus muscle. The palpebral lobe is one-third to one-half the size of the orbital lobe and is subdivided into two or three sections.[27] If the upper lid is everted, the lacrimal gland can be seen above the edge of the upper tarsal plate. Ducts from both portions of the gland exit through the palpebral lobe.

The lacrimal gland consists of lobules made up of numerous acini. Each acinus is an irregular arrangement of secretory cells around a central lumen surrounded by an incomplete layer of myoepithelial cells (Figure 9-17).[54] (Histologically, the main lacrimal gland is identical to the accessory lacrimal glands.) A network of ducts connects the acini and drains into one of the main excretory ducts. There are approximately 12 of these ducts and they empty into the conjunctival sac in the superior fornix.[31] The accessory glands are located in the subconjunctival tissue from the fornix area to near the tarsal plate. Basic secretion maintains the normal volume of aqueous, and reflex secretion increases the volume in response to a stimulus. Both main and accessory glands play a role in basic and reflex secretion.

The lacrimal gland is supplied by the lacrimal artery, a branch of the ophthalmic artery. Sensory innervation is via the lacrimal nerve, a branch of the ophthalmic division of the trigeminal nerve. The gland receives vasomotor sympathetic innervation and secretomotor parasympathetic innervation.[55] Reflex tearing occurs with stimulation of branches of the ophthalmic nerve or in response to external stimuli, such as intense light, the afferent pathway being through the trigeminal nerve and the parasympathetic pathway through the facial nerve.

Disagreement still exists regarding the relative contributions of the main and accessory lacrimal glands. One (older) view holds that the accessory glands provide basic secretion and the main lacrimal gland is primarily active during reflex or psychogenic stimulation.[55] Another, more recent view holds that all lacrimal glands produce the aqueous layer and that production is stimulus-driven, the rate of production ranging from low levels in sleep to high levels under conditions of stimulation.[56]

✍ CLINICAL COMMENT: ASSESSMENT
    OF THE TEAR FILM
    A number of clinical conditions can cause changes in the composition or stability of the tear film. A dry-eye syndrome has complex symptoms that may

be caused by a deficiency or alteration of any of the layers or by an abnormal interaction between the layers.[57] Aqueous deficiencies are common, and normal aging can cause a decrease of aqueous tear production. Patients with rheumatoid arthritis often develop Sjögren's syndrome, which includes dry-eye symptoms, caused by aqueous deficiency, and dry-mouth symptoms.[58, 59] Meibomianitis causes abnormalities of the lipid layer that result in evaporation of the tears. Conditions in which the secretion of mucus is deficient are those associated with reduced goblet-cell populations, such as chemical burns, Stevens-Johnson syndrome, and ocular pemphigoid.[60, 61] Complaints associated with dry eye include scratchy and foreign-body sensations.

Various clinical tests are used to assess the extent of tear abnormalities. The Schirmer test is a clinical measure of the adequacy of the aqueous portion of the tears. A special piece of filter paper is inserted over the inferior eyelid margin. Normally, the strip should be moistened by at least 5 mm after 5 minutes.[48, 62] This test can be done with or without topical anesthesia; if done without a topical anesthetic, the test measures both reflex and basic secretion and, if done with anesthetic, it measures merely basic secretion. The phenol red thread test, which uses a thread treated with a pH indicator, is replacing the Schirmer test in many practices.

Another clinical assessment method measures the tear film breakup time (TBUT). Fluorescein dye is instilled into the lower cul-de-sac and spreads throughout the tear film. After a blink, the thin, lipid upper layer begins to break down, and dry spots appear. The time between the completion of the blink and the first appearance of a dry spot is termed the **tear film breakup time**. Normally, the TBUT is greater than 10 seconds and usually is longer than the time between blinks.[2, 61–63] A short TBUT can occur if irregularities or disturbances in the corneal surface prevent complete tear film adherence or as a result of abnormalities in the lipid layer.[64]

Distribution of the Tear Film

The lacrimal gland fluid is secreted into the lateral part of the upper fornix and descends across the anterior surface of the globe. Each blink reforms and maintains the tear film.

At the posterior edge of both upper and lower eyelid margins, there is a meniscus of tear fluid. The meniscus at the lower lid is more easily seen. The upper tear meniscus is continuous with the lower meniscus at the lateral canthus, whereas at the medial canthus the tear menisci lead directly to the puncta and drain into them.[65] The lacrimal lake, a tear reservoir, is located in the medial

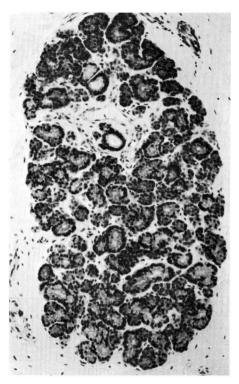

FIGURE 9-17. Photomicrograph of a lobe of the lacrimal gland, showing secretory serous acini and an intraocular duct (center) (×100). (Reprinted with permission from CR Leeson, ST Leeson. Histology. Philadelphia: Saunders, 1976;568.)

canthus. The plica semilunaris makes up the floor of the lake, and the caruncle is located at its medial side.

Nasolacrimal Drainage System

Some tear fluid is lost by evaporation and some by reabsorption through conjunctival tissue, but approximately 75% is passed through the nasolacrimal drainage system.[48] The **nasolacrimal drainage system** consists of the puncta, canaliculi, lacrimal sac, and nasolacrimal duct, which empties into the nasal cavity (Figure 9-18).

Puncta and Canaliculi

A small aperture, the **lacrimal punctum**, is located in a slight tissue elevation, the **lacrimal papilla**, at the junction of the lacrimal and ciliary portions of the eyelid margin. Both upper and lower lids have a punctum. The puncta are turned toward the globe and normally can be seen only if the eyelid edge is everted slightly. Each punctum opens into a tube, the **lacrimal canaliculus**.

The canaliculi are tubes in the upper and lower lids that join the puncta to the lacrimal sac. The walls of the canaliculi contain elastic tissue and are surrounded by fibers from the orbicularis muscle. The first portion of the canaliculus is vertical and extends approximately 2 mm; a slight dilation, the **ampulla**, is at the base of this

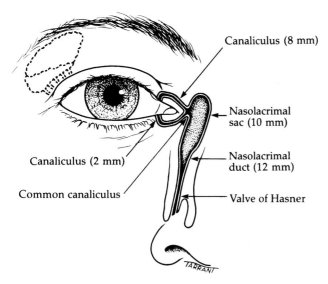

FIGURE 9-18. Anatomy of lacrimal drainage system. (Reprinted with permission from JJ Kanski. Clinical Ophthalmology [3rd ed]. Oxford: Butterworth–Heinemann, 1995;60.)

portion of the canaliculus.[8, 11, 66] The canaliculus then turns horizontally to run along the lid margin for approximately 8 mm (see Figure 9-18). The canaliculi join to form a single common canaliculus that pierces the periorbita covering the lacrimal sac and enters the lateral aspect of the sac. The angle at which the canaliculus enters the sac produces a physiologic valve that prevents reflux.[2, 66, 67]

Lacrimal Sac and Nasolacrimal Duct

The **lacrimal sac** lies within a fossa in the anterior portion of the medial orbital wall. This fossa is formed by the frontal portion of the maxillary bone and the lacrimal bone. The sac is surrounded by fascia, continuous with the periorbita, which runs from the anterior to the posterior lacrimal crest. The two limbs of the medial palpebral ligament straddle the sac to attach to the posterior and anterior crests.[68] The orbital septum and the check ligament of the medial rectus muscle lie behind the lacrimal sac (see Figure 8-11).

The lacrimal sac empties into the **nasolacrimal duct** just as it enters the nasolacrimal canal in the maxillary bone. The duct is approximately 15 mm long and terminates in the inferior meatus of the nose. At this point, the **valve of Hasner** is found. This fold of mucosal tissue prevents retrograde movement of fluid up the duct from the nasal cavity.[8, 13, 66]

Tear Drainage

During closure, the eyelids meet first at the temporal canthus; closure then moves toward the medial canthus,

where the tears pool in the lacrimal lake. The tear menisci are pushed toward the lacrimal puncta into which they drain. In the theories explaining tear drainage, the state of the lacrimal sac is variously reported to be either distended or compressed by contraction of the orbicularis. According to Jones and Marquis,[69] contraction of the ciliary part of the orbicularis compresses the canaliculi, forcing the tears into the lacrimal sac. Coincidentally, contraction of the muscle pulls on the fascial sheath attached to the lacrimal sac,[69] which causes lateral displacement of the lateral wall, expanding the sac and creating negative pressure within it—in effect, pulling tears in from the canaliculus. On relaxation of the orbicularis, the sac collapses, and the tears are driven into the nasolacrimal duct. In addition, the canaliculi open and act like siphons to pull tears in through the puncta.[69] The tears drain into the nasolacrimal duct mainly by gravity, where most are absorbed by the mucosal lining before the remainder enter the inferior meatus.[2]

Doane,[65] using high-speed photography, observed that during eye blink, the medial eyelids meet halfway through the blink, occluding the puncta. According to this theory, the canaliculi and sac are compressed, forcing all fluids into the nasolacrimal duct. As the eyelids open, compression of the canaliculi decreases, but the puncta remain occluded, creating a negative pressure in the canaliculi. When the puncta finally are opened, the negative pressure pulls the tears in immediately after the blink.[2, 67]

The primary difference in these two theories is the state of the lacrimal sac. In the first scenario, the sac is dilated, whereas in the second case the sac is compressed with orbicularis contraction. Capillary attraction plays a role in moving tears into the puncta and down into the canaliculi between blinks.[48]

REFERENCES

1. McCord CD, Doxanas MT. Browplasty and bropexy: an adjunct to blepharoplasty. Plast Reconstr Surg 1990;86(2):248.

2. Doxanas MT, Anderson RL. Clinical Orbital Anatomy. Baltimore: Williams & Wilkins, 1984;57, 89.

3. Bartlett JD, Jaanus SD. Clinical Ocular Pharmacology (3rd ed). Boston: Butterworth–Heinemann, 1995;583.

4. Katz J, Kaufman HE. Corneal exposure during sleep (nocturnal lagophthalmos). Arch Ophthalmol 1977;95:449.

5. Sturrock GD. Nocturnal lagophthalmos and recurrent erosion. Br J Ophthalmol 1976;60:97.

6. Jelks GW, Jelks EB. The influence of orbital and eyelid anatomy on the palpebral aperture. Clin Plast Surg 1991;18(1):183.

7. Fox SA. The palpebral fissure. Am J Ophthalmol 1966;62:73.

8. Warwick R. Eugene Wolff's Anatomy of the Eye and Orbit (7th ed). Philadelphia: Saunders, 1976;181.

9. Dailey RA, Wobig JL. Eyelid anatomy. J Dermatol Surg Oncol 1993;18:1023.

10. Goldberg RA, Wu JC, Jesmanwicz A, et al. Eyelid anatomy revisited. Arch Ophthalmol 1992; 110(11):1598.

11. Jakobiec FA, Iwamoto T. The Ocular Adnexa: Lids, Conjunctiva, and Orbit. In BS Fine, M Yanoff (eds), Ocular Histology (2nd ed). New York: Harper & Row, 1979;290.

12. Jester JV, Nicolaides N, Smith RE. Meibomian gland studies: histologic and ultrastructural investigations. Invest Ophthalmol Vis Sci 1981;20(4):537.

13. Fernandez-Valencia R, Pellico LG. Functional anatomy of the human saccus lacrimalis. Acta Anat (Basel) 1990;139:54.

14. Morax S, Herdan ML. The aging eyelid [abstract]. Schweiz Rundsch Med Prax 1990;9(48):1506.

15. Dryden RM, Leibsohn J, Wobig J. Senile entropion: pathogenesis and treatment. Arch Ophthalmol 1978;96:1883.

16. Fox SA. Primary congenital entropion. Arch Ophthalmol 1956;56:839.

17. Hart WM Jr. The Eyelids. In WM Hart Jr (ed), Adler's Physiology of the Eye (9th ed). St. Louis: Mosby, 1992;1.

18. Wobig JL. Surgical technique for ptosis repair. Aust N Z J Ophthalmol 1989;17(2):125.

19. Anderson RL, Beard C. The levator aponeurosis: attachments and their clinical significance. Arch Ophthalmol 1977;95:1437.

20. Kuwabara T, Cogan DG, Johnson CC. Structure of the muscles of the upper eyelid. Arch Ophthalmol 1975;93:1189.

21. Wobig JL. The Eyelids. In MJ Reeh, JL Wobig, JD Wirtschafter (eds), Ophthalmic Anatomy. San Francisco: American Academy of Ophthalmology, 1981;38.

22. Evinger C, Manning KA, Sibony PA. Eyelid movements: mechanisms and normal data. Invest Ophthalmol Vis Sci 1991;32:387.

23. Hawes MJ, Dortzbach RK. The microscopic anatomy of the lower eyelid retractors. Arch Ophthalmol 1982;100:1313.

24. Small RG, Sabates NR, Burrows D. The measurement and definition of ptosis. Ophthal Plast Reconstr Surg 1989;5(3):171.

25. Anderson RL. Medial canthal tendon branches out. Arch Ophthalmol 1977;95:2051.

26. Gioia VM, Linberg JV, McCormick SA. The anatomy of the lateral canthal tendon. Arch Ophthalmol 1987;105:529.

27. Iwamoto T, Jakobiec FA. Lacrimal Glands. In W Tasman, EA Jaeger (eds), Duane's Foundations of Clinical Ophthalmology (Vol 1). Philadelphia: Lippincott, 1994;1.

28. Kessing SV. Investigations of the conjunctival mucin. Acta Ophthalmol (Copenh) 1966;44:439.

29. Sullivan WR, McCulley JP, Dohlman CH. Return of goblet cells after vitamin A therapy in xerosis of the conjunctiva. Am J Ophthalmol 1973;75:720.

30. Hogan MJ, Alvarado JA. Histology of the Human Eye. Philadelphia: Saunders, 1971;112.

31. Allensmith MR, Greiner JV, Baird RS. Number of inflammatory cells in the normal conjunctiva. Am J Ophthalmol 1978;86:250.

32. Jakobiec FA, Iwamoto T. Ocular Adnexa: Introduction to Lids, Conjunctiva, and Orbit. In W Tasman, EA Jaeger (eds), Duane's Foundations of Clinical Ophthalmology (Vol 1). Philadelphia: Lippincott, 1994;1.

33. Srinivason BD, Jakobiec FA, Iwamoto T, et al. Epibulbar mucogenic subconjunctival cysts. Arch Ophthalmol 1978;96:857.

34. Chin GN, Chi EY, Bunt A. Ultrastructure and histochemical studies of conjunctival concretions. Arch Ophthalmol 1980;98:720.

35. Weingeist TA. The Glands of the Ocular Adnexa. In KM Zinn (ed), Ocular Structure for the Clinician. Boston: Little, Brown, 1973;13:243.

36. Sirigu P, Shen RL, Pinto-da-Silva P. Human meibomian glands: the ultrastructure of acinar cells as viewed by thin section and freeze-fracture transmission electron microscopes. Invest Ophthalmol Vis Sci 1992;33(7):2284.

37. Kanski JJ. Clinical Ophthalmology (3rd ed). London: Butterworth–Heinemann, 1994;2.

38. Dilly PN. On the nature and the role of the subsurface vesicles in the outer epithelial cells of the conjunctiva. Br J Ophthalmol 1985;69:477.

39. Fine BS, Yanoff M. Ocular Histology (2nd ed). Hagerstown, MD: Harper & Row, 1979;310.

40. Shields CL, Shields JA. Tumors of the caruncle. Int Ophthalmol Clin 1993;33(3):31.

41. Austin P, Jakobiec FA, Iwamoto T. Elastodysplasia and elastodystrophy as the pathologic bases of ocular pterygia and pinguecula. Ophthalmology 1983;90:96.

42. Li ZY, Wallace RN, Streeten BW, et al. Elastic fiber components and protease inhibitors in pinguecula. Invest Ophthalmol Vis Sci 1991;32(5):1573.

43. Mackenzie FD, Hirst LW, Battistutta D, et al. Risk analysis in the development of pterygia. Ophthalmology 1992;99(7):1056.

44. Young RW. The family of sunlight-related eye diseases. Optom Vis Sci 1994;71(2):125.

45. Shauly Y, Miller B, Lichtig C. Tenon's capsule: ultrastructure of collagen fibrils in normals and infantile esotropia. Invest Ophthalmol Vis Sci 1992;33:651.

46. Meyer E, Ludatscher RN, Miller B, et al. Connective tissue of the orbital cavity in retinal detachment: an ultrastructural study. Ophthalmic Res 1992;24:365.

47. Reiger G. The importance of the precorneal tear film for the quality of optical imaging. Br J Ophthalmol 1992;76:157.

48. Lemp MA, Wolfley DE. The Lacrimal Apparatus. In WM Hart Jr (ed), Adler's Physiology of the Eye (9th ed). St Louis: Mosby, 1992;18.

49. Mishima S, Maurice DM. The effect of normal evaporation from the eye. Exp Eye Res 1961;1:46.

50. Lemp MA, Holly FJ, Iwata S. The precorneal tear film. Arch Ophthalmol 1970;83:89.

51. Ehlers N. The thickness of the precorneal tear film. Acta Ophthalmol (Copenh) 1965;8(Suppl 81):92.

52. Prydal JI, Artal P, Woon H, et al. Study of human precorneal tear film thickness and structure using laser interferometry. Invest Ophthalmol Vis Sci 1992;33(6):2006.

53. Prydal JI, Campbell FW. Study of precorneal tear film thickness and structure by interferometry and confocal microscopy. Invest Ophthalmol Vis Sci 1992;33(6):1996.

54. Egeberg J, Jenson OA. The ultrastructure of the acini of the human lacrimal gland. Acta Ophthalmol (Copenh) 1969;47:400.

55. Jones LT. Anatomy of the tear system. Int Ophthalmol Clin 1973;13(1):3.

56. Jordan A, Baum JL. Basic tear flow, does it exist? Ophthalmology 1980;95:1.

57. Khurana AK, Chaudhary R, Ahluwalia BK, et al. Tear film profile in dry eye. Acta Ophthalmol (Copenh) 1991;69(1):79.

58. Friedlaender MH. Ocular manifestations of Sjögren's syndrome: keratoconjunctivitis sicca. Rheum Dis Clin North Am 1992;18(3):591.

59. Roberts DK. Keratoconjunctivitis sicca. J Am Optom Assoc 1991;62(3):187.

60. Ralph RA. Conjunctival goblet cell density in normal subjects and in dry eye syndromes. Invest Ophthalmol 1975;14(4):299.

61. Lemp MA, Dohlman CH, Kuwabara T, et al. Dry eye secondary to mucous deficiency. Trans Am Acad Ophthalmol Otolaryngol 1971;75:1223.

62. Cho P, Yap M. Schirmer test: a review. Optom Vis Sci 1993;70(2):152.

63. Lemp MA, Hamil JR. Factors affecting tear film breakup in normal eyes. Arch Ophthalmol 1973;89:103.

64. Mai G, Yang S. Relationship between corneal dellen and tear film breakup time [abstract]. Yen Ko Hsueh Pao 1991;7(1):43.

65. Doane MG. Blinking and the mechanics of the lacrimal drainage system. Ophthalmology 1981;88(8):844.

66. Wobig JL. The Lacrimal Apparatus. In MJ Reeh, JL Wobig, JD Wirtschafter (eds), Ophthalmic Anatomy. San Francisco: American Academy of Ophthalmology, 1981;55.

67. Doane MG. Interactions of eyelids and tears in corneal wetting and the dynamics of the normal human eyeblink. Am J Ophthalmol 1981;89:507.

68. Milder B, Demorest BH. Dacryocystography, the normal lacrimal apparatus. Arch Ophthalmol 1954;51:181.

69. Jones LT, Marquis MM. Lacrimal function. Am J Ophthalmol 1972;73:658.

Extraocular Muscles

The muscles of the globe can be divided into two groups; the involuntary intrinsic muscles and the voluntary extrinsic muscles. The intrinsic muscles—the ciliary muscle, the iris sphincter, and the iris dilator—are located within the eye; they control movement of internal structures. The extrinsic muscles—the six extraocular muscles—attach to the sclera and effect eye movement. This chapter begins with a brief review of the microscopic and macroscopic anatomy of striated muscle and follows that with a discussion of eye movements and a description of the characteristics and actions of each extraocular muscle. (The smooth intrinsic muscles are discussed in Chapter 3.)

MICROSCOPIC ANATOMY OF STRIATED MUSCLE

Striated muscle is surrounded by a connective-tissue sheath known as the **epimysium**; continuous with this sheath is a connective-tissue network, the **perimysium**, which infiltrates the muscle and divides it into bundles. The individual muscle fiber within the bundle is surrounded by a delicate connective-tissue enclosure, the **endomysium** (Figure 10-1). The individual muscle fiber is comparable to a cell; however, each is multinucleated, with the nuclei arranged in the periphery of the fiber. The plasma cell membrane surrounding each muscle fiber is called the **sarcolemma** and forms a series of invaginations into the cell. They are called the **transverse tubules (T-tubules)** and allow ions to penetrate the cell during the spread of the action potential. The cell cytoplasm is called **sarcoplasm** and contains the normal cellular structures and special muscle fibers, the myofibrils.

Histologic Features of Muscle Fibers

Myofibrils comprise two types, thick and thin. The thick myofibrils, 10 nm in diameter, are composed of hundreds of **myosin** subunits. Each subunit is a long slender filament with two globular heads attached by arms at one end. The protruding heads and arms together are called **cross-bridges**.[1] These filaments lie next to each other and form the backbone of the myofibril, with the heads projecting outward in a spiral (Figure 10-2). The thin myofibrils, 5 nm in diameter, are formed by the protein **actin** arranged in a double helical filament, with a molecular complex of **troponin** and **tropomyosin** lying within the grooves of the double helix (see Figure 10-2).

The alternating light and dark bands characteristic of striated muscle are produced by the manner in which these two types of myofibrils are arranged. The light band is the I (isotropic) band and the dark band is the A (anisotropic) band. These names describe the birefringence to polarized light exhibited by the two areas.[2]

The I band contains two sets of actin filaments connected to each other at the Z line, a dark stripe bisecting the I band. Only actin myofibrils are found in the I band. The A band contains both myosin and actin; the central lighter zone of the A band—the H zone—contains only myosin. Overlapping actin and myosin filaments form the outer darker edges of the A band (Figure 10-3).

The **sarcomere** extends from Z line to Z line and is the contractile unit of striated muscle. With muscle contraction, a change in configuration occurs; the H zone width decreases as the actin filaments slide past the myosin filaments. The sarcomere is shortened; thus, the muscle length is decreased.

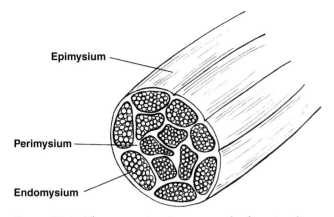

FIGURE 10-1. The connective-tissue network of a striated muscle.

Sliding Ratchet Model of Muscle Contraction

The precise biomolecular process of muscle contraction is not understood fully; however, the sliding ratchet model of muscle contraction provides a reasonable explanation.[3–5] The initiation of a muscle contraction occurs when a nerve impulse causes the release of acetylcholine into the neuromuscular junction. This action causes the sarcolemma to become more permeable to Na^+ and initiates a wave of depolarization that passes along the surface of the sarcolemma and into the T-tubule system of the muscle cell, bringing about the release of Ca^{++} from the sarcoplasmic reticulum. The Ca^{++} produces a configurational change in the troponin-tropomyosin complex, allowing an active site on the actin protein to be available

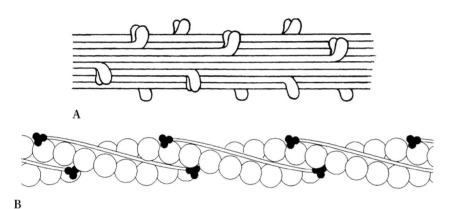

FIGURE 10-2. The myosin and actin myofibrils. (A) The myosin fibril is composed of two-headed filaments, the heads being arranged in a spiral. (B) The actin myofibril is composed of a double-helix filament to which a troponin-tropomyosin complex is attached.

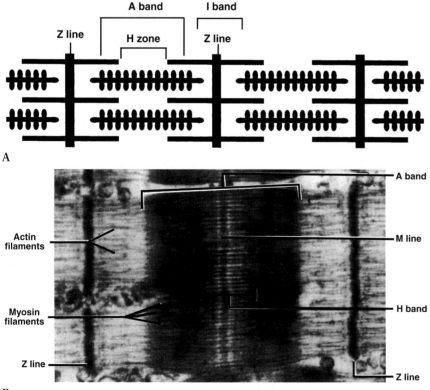

FIGURE 10-3. (A) Arrangement of the thick and thin filaments in a sarcomere. (B) Photomicrograph of striated muscle, with parts of the sarcomere indicated. For further details, see text. (Part B reprinted with permission from WJ Krause, JH Cutts. Concise Text of Histology. Baltimore: Williams & Wilkins, 1981;132.)

for binding with a myosin head. Coincidentally, adenosine triphosphate (ATP) attached to the myosin head is broken down and released, allowing the cross-bridge to bind with the active actin site. Once this bond is formed, the head tilts toward the shaft of the myosin filament, pulling the actin filament along with it (Figure 10-4).

The junction between the actin and myosin is broken by the attachment of a new ATP molecule to the myosin head. The head then rights itself, and the cross-bridge is ready to bind with the next actin site along the chain. This ratchet type of movement occurs along the length of the fiber, moving the filaments past one another with the overall effect of shortening the sarcomere and the entire muscle.

Structure of the Extraocular Muscles

The extraocular muscles have a denser blood supply, and their connective-tissue sheaths are more delicate and richer in elastic fibers than is skeletal muscle.[6] Fewer muscle fibers are included in a motor unit in extraocular muscle than are found in skeletal muscle elsewhere. Striated muscle of the leg can contain several hundred muscle fibers per motor unit[1]; in the extraocular muscles, each axon innervates 3–10 fibers.[7] Precise fine motor control and quick accurate movement of the extraocular muscles occur because of this dense innervation. Singly innervated fibers have the classic end plate (en plaque) seen in skeletal muscle; multiply innervated fibers have a neuromuscular junction resembling a bunch of grapes (en grappe).[8, 9]

The extraocular muscles have a range of fiber sizes, with the fibers closer to the surface generally having smaller diameters (5–15 μm) and those deeper within the muscle generally having larger diameters (10–40 μm).[10–13] They can be divided into five groups based on characteristics such as size, morphology, neuromuscular junction type, or various biochemical properties.[6, 11, 12, 14] The fibers range from typical twitch fibers at one end of the spectrum to typical slow fibers at the other end, with gradations between. It would seem that the fast twitch fibers should produce the quick saccadic type movements and the slow fibers should produce the slower pursuit movements and provide muscle tone. However, all fibers apparently are active at all times and share some level of involvement in all ocular movements.[11, 13, 15]

Those fibers that provide the contractility of the muscle are called **extrafusal fibers**. Other fibers found within the muscle are **intrafusal fibers** and have a proprioceptive function; these are the muscle spindles.[16] They provide a continuous feedback mechanism to regulatory centers in the central nervous system, providing information on muscle position and activity.[6, 17] Muscle spindles are sensitive to changes in muscle length; Golgi tendon organs are additional proprioceptive structures that are located in the tendon and are sensitive to changes in muscle tension.[6]

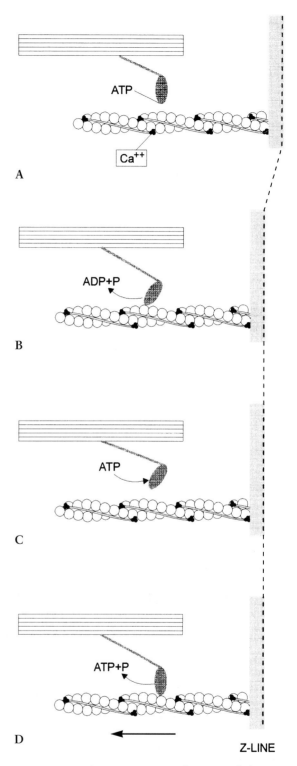

FIGURE 10-4. (A) Ca++ causes configurational change in troponin-tropomyosin complex. (B) Adenosine triphosphate (ATP) is freed from the myosin head, releasing ADP+P; a cross-bridge forms a link with the active actin site; the head tilts toward the shaft; and the actin filament is pulled along the myosin filament. (C) New ATP molecule attaches to the head, breaking the cross-bridge bond. (D) The process continues with the appearance of a cross-bridge linkage at a new site on the actin filament.

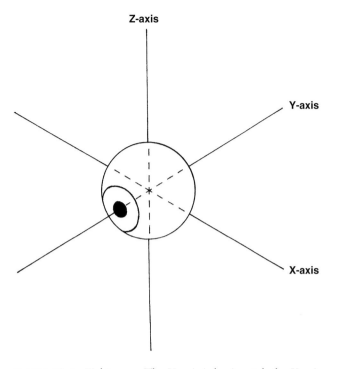

Z-axis

Y-axis

X-axis

FIGURE 10-5. Fick's axes. The X-axis is horizontal, the Y-axis is sagittal, and the Z-axis is vertical.

EYE MOVEMENTS

Fick's Axes

Before a discussion of the individual muscles and the resultant eye movements caused by their contraction, it is necessary to define certain terms. All eye movement can be described as rotations around one or more axes (**Fick's axes**). These axes divide the globe into quadrants and intersect at the approximate center of rotation, a fixed nonmoving point.[18] For convenience, it is assumed that the eye rotates around this fixed point located 13.5 mm behind the cornea; this point varies in ametropia, being slightly more posterior in myopia and slightly more anterior in hyperopia.[6] The **X-axis** is the horizontal or transverse axis and runs from nasal to temporal. The **Y-axis** is the sagittal axis running from the anterior pole to the posterior pole. The **Z-axis** is the vertical axis and runs from superior to inferior (Figure 10-5). The anterior pole of the globe is the reference point used in the description of any eye movement.

Ductions

Movements involving just one eye are called **ductions** and are shown in Figure 10-6. Rotations around the vertical Z-axis move the anterior pole of the globe medially—**adduction**—or laterally—**abduction**. Rotations around the horizontal X-axis move the anterior pole of

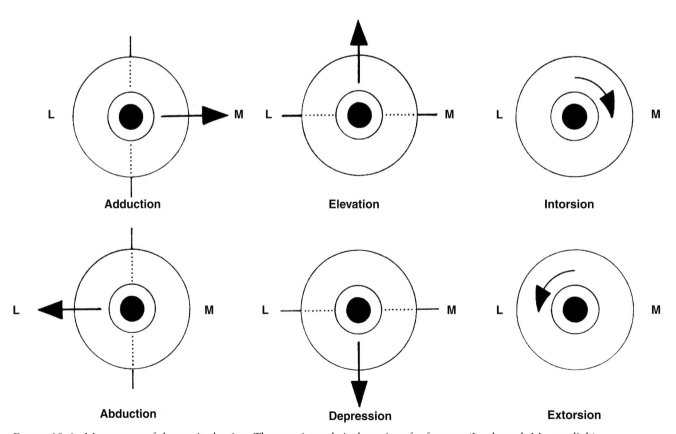

| Adduction | Elevation | Intorsion |
| Abduction | Depression | Extorsion |

FIGURE 10-6. Movements of the eye in duction. The anterior pole is the point of reference. (L = lateral; M = medial.)

TABLE 10-1. Ocular Movement Terminology

Monocular		Binocular	
Movement	Term	Movement	Term
Medial	Adduction	Right	Dextroversion
Lateral	Abduction	Left	Levoversion
Up	Elevation, supraduction, or sursumduction	Up	Supraversion or sursumversion
		Down	Infraversion or deorsumversion
Down	Depression, infraduction, or deorsumduction	Up and right	Dextroelevation
		Up and left	Levoelevation
Rotation of 12-o'clock position medially	Intorsion, incyclorotation, or incycloduction	Down and right	Dextrodepression
		Down and left	Levodepression
Rotation of 12-o'clock position laterally	Extorsion, excyclorotation, or excycloduction	Both eyes adduct	Convergence
		Both eyes abduct	Divergence
Anterior out of orbit	Protrusion or exophthalmos	Both eyes extort	Excyclovergence
Posterior into orbit	Retraction or enophthalmos	Both eyes intort	Incyclovergence
		Rotation of 12-o'clock position to right	Dextrocycloversion
		Rotation of 12 o'clock position to left	Levocycloversion

Note: For all movements, the anterior pole of the globe is the reference point unless otherwise noted.

the globe up—**elevation (supraduction)**—or down—**depression (infraduction)**.

Torsions or cyclorotations are rotations around the sagittal Y-axis and are described in relation to a point at the 12-o'clock position on the superior limbus. **Intorsion (incyclorotation)** is the rotation of that point nasally, and **extorsion (excyclorotation)** is the rotation of that point temporally. Torsional movements may occur in an attempt to keep the horizontal retinal raphe parallel to the horizon.[19] With a head tilt of 30 degrees, the ipsilateral eye is intorted approximately 7 degrees, and the contralateral eye is extorted approximately 8 degrees.[20]

Torsional movements have been questioned by some investigators who believe that true torsion occurs only in pathologic conditions.[21] Others have documented torsion in normal eye movements and with head tilt.[22–25]

Vergences and Versions

Movements involving both eyes are either vergences or versions, depending on the relative directions of movement. In vergence movements, the eyes move in opposite left-right directions; these are disjunctive movements. In **convergence**, each eye is adducted; in **divergence**, each eye is abducted. Version movements are conjugate movements and occur when the eyes move in the same direction. **Dextroversion** is right gaze, and **levoversion** is left gaze. In **supraversion**, both eyes are elevated and, in

infraversion, both eyes are depressed. Table 10.1 lists terms for monocular and binocular movement and some combination movements.

Positions of Gaze

The **primary position of gaze** is defined as the position of the eye with the head erect, the eye located at the intersection of the sagittal plane of the head and the horizontal plane passing through the centers of rotation of both eyes, and the eye focused for infinity.[15] Secondary positions of gaze are rotations around either the vertical or the horizontal axis; tertiary positions are rotations around both the vertical and horizontal axes.

MACROSCOPIC ANATOMY OF THE EXTRAOCULAR MUSCLES

The six extraocular muscles are medial rectus, lateral rectus, superior rectus, inferior rectus, superior oblique, and inferior oblique (Figure 10-7). From longest to shortest, the rectus muscles are the superior, the medial, the lateral, and the inferior.[17]

Origin of the Rectus Muscles

The four rectus muscles have their origin on the **common tendinous ring (annulus of Zinn)**. This oval band

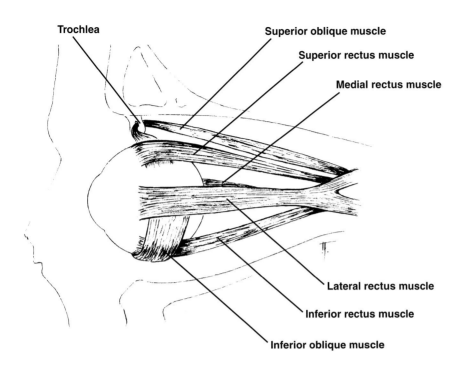

FIGURE 10-7. Globe in orbit as viewed from the lateral side.

Labels in figure:
Trochlea
Superior oblique muscle
Superior rectus muscle
Medial rectus muscle
Lateral rectus muscle
Inferior rectus muscle
Inferior oblique muscle

of connective tissue is continuous with the periorbita and is located at the apex of the orbit anterior to the optic foramen and the medial part of the superior orbital fissure. The upper and lower areas are thickened bands and sometimes are referred to as the **upper and lower tendons** or **limbs**. The medial and lateral rectus muscles take their origin from both parts of the tendinous ring. The superior rectus is attached to the upper limb, and the inferior rectus is joined to the lower. The medial rectus and the superior rectus also attach to the dural sheath of the optic nerve (Figure 10-8).[17]

CLINICAL COMMENT: RETROBULBAR OPTIC NEURITIS

Retrobulbar optic neuritis is an inflammation affecting the sheaths of the optic nerve. Generally,

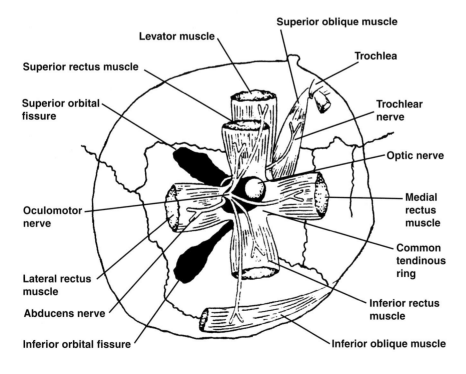

FIGURE 10-8. Annulus of Zinn. Orbital apex with the globe removed. The relationship between the superior orbital fissure and the common tendinous ring is shown.

Labels in figure:
Levator muscle
Superior oblique muscle
Superior rectus muscle
Trochlea
Superior orbital fissure
Trochlear nerve
Optic nerve
Oculomotor nerve
Medial rectus muscle
Common tendinous ring
Lateral rectus muscle
Abducens nerve
Inferior rectus muscle
Inferior orbital fissure
Inferior oblique muscle

FIGURE 10-9. Insertions of the rectus muscles forming the spiral of Tillaux.

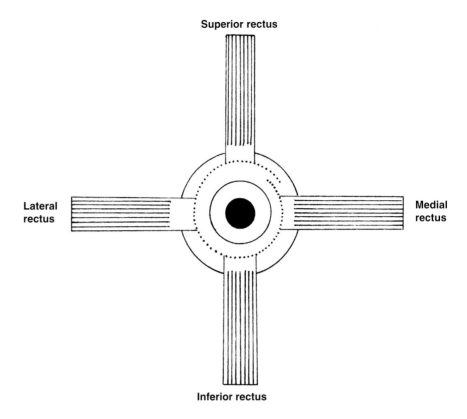

Superior rectus

Lateral rectus

Medial rectus

Inferior rectus

no signs of this condition are visible in the fundus, but pain with extreme eye movement can be one of the early presenting signs.[2, 17] The optic nerve sheath is supplied with a dense sensory nerve network and, because of the close association of muscle and optic nerve sheaths, eye movement can cause stretching of the optic nerve sheath, resulting in the sensation of pain.[26]

The area enclosed by the tendinous ring is called the **oculomotor foramen**, and several blood vessels and nerves pass through the foramen, having entered the orbit either through the optic canal or the superior orbital fissure (see Figure 10-8). The optic nerve and ophthalmic artery enter the oculomotor foramen from the optic canal; the superior and inferior divisions of the oculomotor nerve, the abducens nerve, and the nasociliary nerve enter the oculomotor foramen from the superior orbital fissure (see Figure 10-8). These structures lie within the muscle cone, the area enclosed by the four rectus muscles and the connective tissue joining them. Thus, the motor nerve to each rectus muscle can enter the surface of the muscle that lies within the muscle cone.

In 1887, Motais described a common muscle sheath between the rectus muscles enclosing the space within the muscle cone, as cited by Eggers.[6] More recently, dissections by Koorneef[27] revealed no definitive, continuous muscle sheath between the rectus muscles in the retrobulbar region.

The lacrimal and frontal nerves and the superior ophthalmic vein lie above the ring tendon, and the inferior ophthalmic vein lies below. They are outside the muscle cone.

Insertions of the Rectus Muscles: The Spiral of Tillaux

The four rectus muscles insert into the globe anterior to the equator. A line connecting the rectus muscle insertions forms a spiral as described by Tillaux and cited by Eggers.[6] This spiral starts at the medial rectus, the insertion that is closest to the limbus, and proceeds to the inferior rectus, lateral rectus and, finally, the superior rectus, the insertion farthest from the limbus (Figure 10-9). In a recent study, variations were found from person to person in specific measurements, but the **spiral of Tillaux** always was respected.[28] The tendons of insertion pierce Tenon's capsule and merge with scleral fibers. A sleeve of the capsule covers the tendon for a short distance, and the muscle can slide freely within this sleeve.[6, 12]

Medial Rectus Muscle

The **medial rectus muscle** is the largest of the extraocular muscles, its size probably is due to the frequency of its use in convergence.[17] Its origin is from both the upper and lower parts of the common tendon *and* from the sheath of the optic nerve. The insertion of the medial rectus is some 5.5 mm from the limbus, and the tendon is approximately 3.7 mm long (Table 10-2).[6] The insertion

TABLE 10-2. Rectus Muscle Tendon Measurements

Muscle	Tendon length (mm)	Distance from limbus (mm)	Tendon width (mm)
Medial rectus	3.7	5.5	10.3
Lateral rectus	8.8	6.9	9.2
Superior rectus	5.8	7.7	10.8
Inferior rectus	5.5	6.5	9.8

Source: Adapted from HM Eggers. Functional Anatomy of the Extraocular Muscles. In W Tasman, EA Jaeger (eds), Duane's Foundations of Clinical Ophthalmology. Philadelphia: Lippincott, 1994;1.

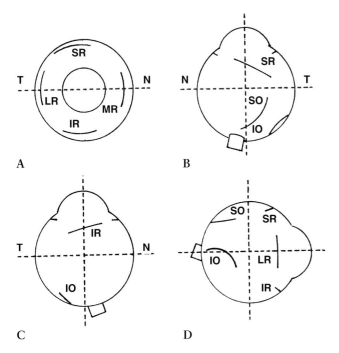

FIGURE 10-10. Insertions of the extraocular muscles. The globe viewed from (A) in front, (B) above, (C) below, and (D) the lateral side. (LR = lateral rectus; MR = medial rectus; SR = superior rectus; IR = inferior rectus; SO = superior oblique; IO = inferior oblique; N = nasal; T = temporal.)

line lies vertically such that the horizontal plane of the eye approximately bisects it (Figure 10-10). The superior oblique muscle, ophthalmic artery, and nasociliary nerve lie above the medial rectus. Fascial expansions from the sheath of the muscle run to the medial wall of the orbit and form the well-developed medial check ligament (see Figure 8-11). The medial rectus is innervated by the inferior division of cranial nerve III, the oculomotor nerve, which enters the muscle on its lateral surface.

Lateral Rectus Muscle

The **lateral rectus muscle** has its origin on both limbs of the common tendinous ring *and* the spina recti lateralis, a prominence on the greater wing of the sphenoid bone. The insertion parallels that of the medial rectus and is

approximately 6.9 mm from the limbus, the length of the tendon being approximately 8.8 mm.[6]

The lacrimal artery and nerve run along the superior border of the muscle. The ciliary ganglion, the abducens nerve, and the ophthalmic artery lie medial to the lateral rectus between it and the optic nerve. Fascial expansions from the muscle sheath attach to the lateral wall of the orbit and form the lateral check ligament (see Figure 8-11). The lateral rectus is innervated by cranial nerve VI, the abducens nerve, which enters on the medial side of the muscle.

Superior Rectus Muscle

The **superior rectus muscle** has its origin on the superior part of the common tendinous ring *and* the sheath of the optic nerve.[17] The muscle passes forward beneath the levator muscle; the sheaths enclosing these two muscles are connected to each other, allowing coordination of eye movement with eyelid position and resulting in elevation of the eyelid with upward gaze. An additional band of this tissue connects to the superior conjunctival fornix.

The insertion of the superior rectus is some 7.7 mm from the limbus[6] and is curved slightly, with the convex side forward. The line of the insertion is oblique, with the nasal side closer to the limbus than the temporal side (see Figure 10-10). The tendon length is approximately 5.8 mm.[6] A line drawn from the origin to the insertion along the muscle will form an angle of approximately 23 degrees with the sagittal axis.

The frontal nerve runs above the superior rectus and levator muscles, and the nasociliary nerve and the ophthalmic artery lie below. The tendon of insertion for the superior oblique muscle runs below the anterior part of the superior rectus muscle (see Figure 10-7).

The superior rectus is innervated by the superior division of the oculomotor nerve, which enters the muscle on its inferior face. Branches pass either through the muscle or around it to innervate the levator.

Inferior Rectus Muscle

The **inferior rectus muscle** has its origin on the lower limb of the tendinous ring; its insertion is some 6.5 mm from the limbus in an arc, convex side forward, with the nasal side nearer the limbus; the tendon length is approximately 5.5 mm.[6] The inferior rectus approximately parallels the superior rectus, making an angle of 23 degrees with the sagittal axis.

Below the inferior rectus lies the floor of the orbit, and above it is the inferior division of the oculomotor nerve. Anteriorly, the inferior oblique muscle comes between the inferior rectus and the orbital floor (see Figure 10-7). Fascial attachments from the sheath to the inferior eyelid tissue allow coordination of eye movements with eyelid position, assuring lowering of the lid on downgaze. The sheaths of these two inferior muscles unite to contribute to the suspensory ligament of Lockwood (see Figure 8-10). The inferior rectus is innervated by the inferior division of cranial nerve III—the oculomotor—which enters the muscle on its superior surface.

Superior Oblique Muscle

The **superior oblique muscle** has its origin on the lesser wing of the sphenoid bone, medial to the optic canal near the frontoethmoid suture.[15] The muscle courses forward and passes through the trochlea, a U-shaped piece of cartilage attached to the orbital plate of the frontal bone (see Figure 10-7). The tendon of insertion actually begins approximately 1 cm behind the trochlea. Normally, no connective adhesions exist between these two structures, allowing the tendon to slide easily through the trochlea.[2]

The superior oblique muscle is the longest and thinnest of the extraocular muscles, owing to its long tendon of insertion (2.5 cm long).[17] The tendon of insertion changes direction as it passes through the trochlea to run in a posterior direction. It lies inferior to the superior rectus muscle and attaches in the superior, posterior, lateral quadrant of the globe (see Figure 10-10).[29] The insertion of the superior oblique muscle is fan-shaped, concave forward, and oblique.

The trochlea is considered the physiologic or effective origin of the superior oblique muscle in determining muscle action, as it acts as a pulley and changes the direction of muscle pull. In considering the action of the superior oblique, a line is drawn from the trochlea to the insertion rather than from the anatomic origin to the insertion. A line drawn from the physiologic origin to the insertion makes an angle of approximately 55 degrees with the visual axis.[29] The superior oblique muscle lies above the medial rectus, with the nasociliary nerve and the ophthalmic artery lying between them. Innervation is by the trochlear nerve—cranial nerve IV—which enters the posterior area of the muscle.

Inferior Oblique Muscle

The **inferior oblique muscle** has its origin on the maxillary bone just posterior to the inferior medial orbital rim and

TABLE 10-3. Extraocular Muscle Innervation

Muscle	Nerve
Medial rectus	Inferior division of oculomotor (CN III)
Lateral rectus	Abducens (CN VI)
Superior rectus	Superior division of oculomotor (CN III)
Inferior rectus	Inferior division of oculomotor (CN III)
Superior oblique	Trochlear (CN IV)
Inferior oblique	Inferior division of oculomotor (CN III)

CN = cranial nerve.

lateral to the nasolacrimal canal.[30] The inferior oblique is the only extraocular muscle to have its anatomic origin in the anterior orbit. The muscle runs from the medial corner of the orbit to the lateral aspect of the globe, its length approximately paralleling the tendon of insertion of the superior oblique muscle.

The insertion is on the posterior portion of the globe on the lateral side, mostly inferior, lying just outer to the macular area.[2, 17] The insertion is curved concave downward. The muscle makes an angle of approximately 51 degrees with the visual axis.[29] Above the inferior oblique are the inferior rectus and globe, and below it lies the floor of the orbit.

The inferior oblique is innervated by the inferior division of the oculomotor nerve, which enters the muscle on its upper surface. Table 10-3 lists the motor innervation of the extraocular muscles.

Check Ligaments

Dense connective-tissue septa between the extraocular muscle sheaths and between the sheaths and the orbital bones form a rather complex, highly organized network that contributes to the framework supporting the globe within the orbit. The horizontal rectus muscles are anchored to the periorbita at the anterior of the orbital walls via the medial and lateral check ligaments. The medial check ligament is attached to the bones of the medial orbital wall, and the lateral check ligament is attached to the lateral tubercle on the zygomatic bone of the lateral wall, both ligaments being posterior to the orbital septum. The medial check ligament is better developed than is the lateral.[27] Traditionally, these ligaments were described as "brakes" that limit the extent of movement of the globe—that is, in abduction the medial check ligament stops lateral movement of the globe when extension of the medial rectus muscle starts to exert pull on the relatively inelastic ligament.

Current evidence suggests that the extraocular muscles are constrained by connective-tissue septa that connect muscle to muscle and periodically connect individual muscles to the orbital walls along a significant portion of

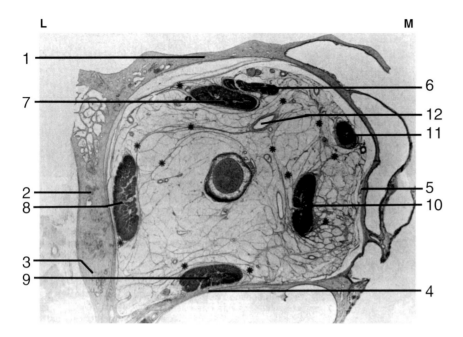

FIGURE 10-11. Frontal section (60 µm) of a right orbit in the retrobulbar area, 2.1 mm from the back of the eyeball. (1) frontal bone; (2) greater wing of sphenoid bone; (3) zygomatic bone; (4) maxilla; (5) ethmoid bone; (6) superior levator palpebrae muscle; (7) superior rectus muscle; (8) lateral rectus muscle; (9) inferior rectus muscle; (10) medial rectus muscle; (11) superior oblique muscle; (12) superior ophthalmic vein; (*) connective-tissue septa. (M = medial; L = lateral.) (H&E/Mayer, ×3.) (Reprinted with permission from L Koornneef. Human orbital connective tissue. Arch Ophthalmol 1977;95:1272.)

the muscle length.[31, 32] According to dissection studies by Koornneef, intermuscular septa include those joining lateral rectus, inferior rectus, and medial rectus; medial rectus and superior rectus; lateral rectus and superior rectus; medial rectus to the superior oblique and the orbital roof and floor; medial rectus to the periorbita of the ethmoid; superior oblique to the frontoethmoid angle; inferior rectus to the orbital floor; lateral rectus to the lateral wall; and levator to adjacent periorbita.[27] The presence and orientation of these septa vary from front to back. Figure 10-11 shows a representation of the septa within the orbit. The considerable amount of attachment between muscle and bone can cause limitations in eye movement.[27]

ISOLATED AGONIST MODEL

One of the earliest models developed to explain eye movement is the isolated agonist model described by Duane.[33] This straightforward model has been used widely in the clinical evaluation of extraocular muscles and can be used to describe the movement around the axes that occurs with contraction of each muscle. However, it is important to remember that during eye movements, all six extraocular muscles are in some state of contraction or relaxation, and it is strictly hypothetical to discuss the movement of the eye as if only one muscle contracts. In each of these descriptions the eye begins in primary position.

Movements from Primary Position

Horizontal Rectus Muscles

The medial rectus lies parallel to the sagittal axis and perpendicular to the vertical axis; therefore, it has only one action, which is rotation around the vertical axis in a nasal direction—adduction. The lateral rectus also lies parallel to the sagittal axis and perpendicular to the vertical axis; contraction causes rotation in a temporal direction—abduction (Figure 10-12).

Vertical Rectus Muscles

The action of the superior rectus is more complex, as it lies at an angle to each of the axes; with the insertion above the origin and on the anterior of the eye, movement around the horizontal axis causes elevation. The muscle insertion is lateral to the origin, so movement around the vertical axis causes adduction; the oblique insertion on the superior surface of the globe causes intorsion on contraction (Figure 10-13A). The primary action is said to be elevation; adduction and intorsion are secondary.

The primary action of the inferior rectus is depression, because the insertion is below the origin and on the anterior of the globe. Secondary actions are adduction, as the insertion is lateral to the origin and extorsion is due to the oblique insertion on the inferior surface of the globe (see Figure 10-13B).

Oblique Muscles

The primary action of the superior oblique muscle is intorsion.[6, 15, 34–36] This action results from the oblique insertion on the lateral, posterior, superior quadrant (Table 10-4); contraction rotates the eye around the sagittal axis, causing intorsion. The secondary actions are depression and abduction.[6, 15, 34–36] Depression occurs because the insertion is posterior to the physiologic origin; contraction of the muscle pulls the back of the eye up, and the anterior pole moves down. Because the insertion is lateral to the trochlea, contraction of the superior

FIGURE 10-12. (A) Adduction on contraction of medial rectus muscle with eye in primary position. (B) Abduction on contraction of lateral rectus muscle with eye in primary position. (L = lateral; M = medial.)

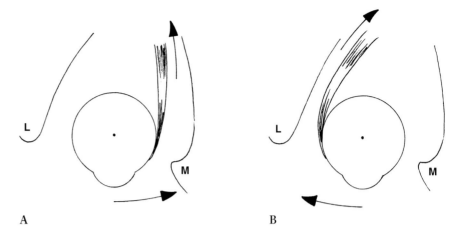

FIGURE 10-13. (A) Globe movement around each of Fick's axes on contraction of superior rectus muscle, with the eye in primary position: (*1*) elevation, movement around the *X*-axis; (*2*) adduction, movement around the *Z*-axis; (*3*) intorsion, movement around the *Y*-axis. (B) Globe movement around each of Fick's axes on contraction of inferior rectus muscle, with the eye in primary position: (*1*) depression, movement around the *X*-axis; (*2*) adduction, movement around the *Z*-axis; (*3*) extorsion, movement around the *Y*-axis. (L = lateral; M = medial.)

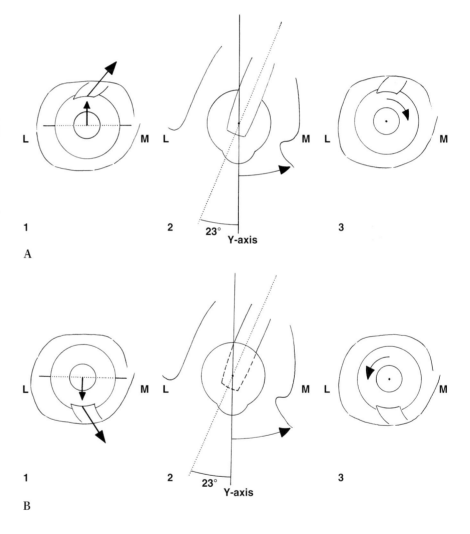

oblique pulls the back of the globe medially, thus moving the anterior pole laterally (see Figure 10-14A).

The primary action of the inferior oblique—extorsion—occurs because the muscle wraps around the lower portion of the globe and the insertion is lateral to the origin. Secondary actions are elevation and abduction.[6, 15,] [34-36] As the insertion is on the posterior of the eye and above the origin, contraction pulls the back of the eye down, elevating the front. Abduction occurs because the insertion on the back of the eye is pulled toward the medial side; thus, the anterior pole is moved laterally in abduction (see Figure 10-14B). (Warwick,[17] in *Eugene*

TABLE 10-4. Origin, Insertion, and Action of the Extraocular Muscles

Muscle	Origin	Insertion	Primary action	Secondary action
Medial rectus	Common ring tendon and optic nerve sheath	Anterior globe	Adduction	None
Lateral rectus	Common ring tendon and greater wing of sphenoid	Anterior globe	Abduction	None
Superior rectus	Common ring tendon and optic nerve sheath	Superior, anterior globe	Elevation	Adduction, intorsion
Inferior rectus	Common ring tendon	Inferior, anterior globe	Depression	Adduction, extorsion
Superior oblique	Anatomic: lesser wing of sphenoid Physiologic: trochlea	Superior, posterior, lateral globe	Intorsion	Depression, abduction
Inferior oblique	Medial maxillary bone	Posterior, lateral globe	Extorsion	Elevation, abduction

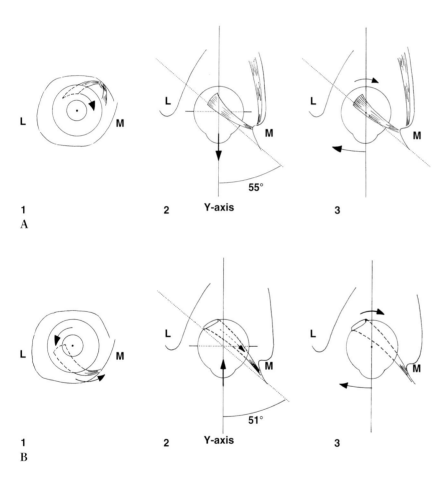

FIGURE 10-14. (A) Globe movement around each of Fick's axes on contraction of superior oblique muscle, with the eye in primary position: (*1*) intorsion, movement around the Y-axis; (*2*) depression, movement around the X-axis; (*3*) abduction, movement around the Z-axis. (B) Globe movement around each of Fick's axes on contraction of inferior oblique muscle, with the eye in primary position: (*1*) extorsion, movement around the Y-axis; (*2*) elevation, movement around the X-axis; (*3*) abduction, movement around the Z-axis. (L = lateral; M = medial.)

Wolff's Anatomy of the Eye and Orbit offers the contrasting view that the primary action of the superior oblique is depression, that of the inferior oblique is elevation, and the torsional actions are secondary.)

Movements from Secondary Positions

As the position of the globe changes, the relationship between the muscle origin and insertion changes relative to the axes, and contraction of a muscle will have a different effect than that which occurs when the eye is in primary position. If the eye is elevated, contraction of the horizontal rectus muscles no longer causes strictly adduction or abduction but also will cause a slight elevation; if the eye is depressed, contraction will cause further depression.[37]

In a vector analysis, when a force acts along an axis, movement occurs only in the direction of that axis. If a force acts at a right angle to an axis, no movement

FIGURE 10-15. The relationship between the line of muscle movement and Fick's axes when the eye is in a secondary position. (A) When the eye is adducted 67 degrees (putting the plane of the muscle at almost right angles to the Y-axis), contraction of the superior rectus muscle cannot cause elevation. (B) When the eye is abducted 23 degrees (putting the plane of the muscle parallel to the Y-axis), contraction of the superior rectus muscle causes only elevation. (L = lateral; M = medial.)

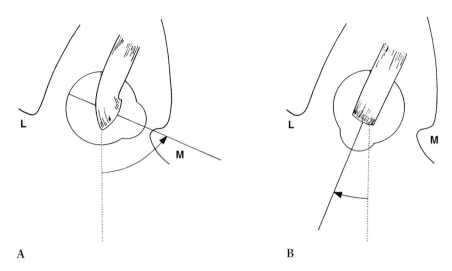

FIGURE 10-16. The relationship between the line of muscle movement and Fick's axes when the eye is in a secondary position. (A) When the eye is abducted 35 degrees (putting the plane of the muscle at an almost right angle to the Y-axis), contraction of the superior oblique muscle cannot cause depression. (B) When the eye is adducted 55 degrees (putting the plane of the muscle parallel to the Y-axis), contraction of the superior oblique muscle almost exclusively causes depression. (L = lateral; M = medial.)

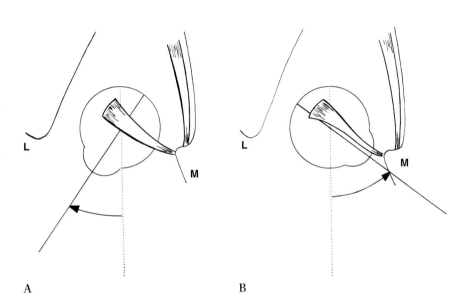

is possible in the direction of that axis. These principles are applied to muscle contraction of the vertical rectus and oblique muscles in the following discussion.

Vertical Rectus Muscles

With the eye abducted approximately 23 degrees from primary position, the vertical rectus muscles parallel the sagittal axis, and only vertical movement will occur. In this position, contraction of the superior rectus will cause only elevation, and contraction of the inferior rectus will cause only depression (Figure 10-15).[33]

As the eye adducts, it approaches a position wherein the plane of the vertical rectus muscles will be at a right angle to the sagittal axis; this occurs at approximately 67 degrees adduction (which may be physically impossible because of the connective-tissue constraints of the orbit).

If the muscle plane of the vertical rectus muscles is at a right angle to the sagittal axis, contraction of the superior or inferior rectus muscle will not cause vertical movement (see Figure 10-15).[33]

Oblique Muscles

As the eye adducts 51–55 degrees, the plane of the oblique muscles becomes parallel to the sagittal axis. In this position, the superior oblique will cause depression, and the inferior oblique will cause elevation. When the eye is abducted 35–39 degrees, the plane of the oblique muscles makes a right angle with the sagittal axis, and the obliques cannot cause vertical movement (Figure 10-16).[33]

This analysis is used in the clinical assessment of extraocular muscle function. As the eye increases in abduction, the elevating and depressing abilities of the vertical rectus muscles increase. As the eye increasingly moves into adduction, the elevating and depressing abilities of the oblique muscles increase.

Agonist and Antagonist Muscles

In any position of gaze, the innervation of all extraocular muscles is controlled carefully, and each muscle is in some stage of contraction or relaxation. No single muscle acts alone; they work together as agonists, antagonists, or synergists. In all these movements, fine motor control should provide for smooth, continuous movements. According to Sherrington's law of reciprocal innervation, contraction of a muscle is accompanied by a simultaneous and proportional relaxation of the antagonist.[38] In adduction, the increased contraction of the medial rectus is accompanied by the increased relaxation of the antagonist lateral rectus.

When the superior rectus muscle and the inferior oblique muscle contract at the same time, the adduction action of the superior rectus and the abduction action of the inferior oblique, and the intorsion of the superior rectus and the extorsion of the inferior oblique, will counteract each other. The resultant eye movement is elevation; they are synergists in elevation. Jampel[39] demonstrated this in a study in which the superior rectus and the inferior oblique muscles were stimulated simultaneously, and the eye moved directly up.

When the superior oblique and the inferior rectus muscles were stimulated simultaneously, the eye moved directly downward.[39] The superior oblique and the inferior rectus are synergists in depression. The superior oblique is the antagonist for the inferior oblique in vertical movements and torsional movements but is synergistic for abduction.

In primary position, the muscles are in a balanced state, each exerting contraction sufficient to keep the eye centered in the palpebral fissure. If one muscle is inactive, the eye will be deviated from primary position in the direction of the pull of the affected muscle's antagonist. If the medial rectus muscle is paralyzed, the eye, in primary position, will be positioned temporally due to the *apparent* overaction of the lateral rectus.

✍ CLINICAL COMMENT: EXTRAOCULAR
        MUSCLE ASSESSMENT
    Assessment of eye position and movements can be an important tool in determining the integrity of the extraocular muscles and their associated nerves. The practitioner first notes the position of each eye while directing the patient to fixate on a target straight ahead. An eye that is deviated toward the nose would be indicative of an underactive lateral rectus; the medial rectus is unopposed by the lateral rectus. Figure 10-17A is a useful diagram that

shows the direction of pull of each muscle when the eye is in primary position.

Ocular motility testing will give further information on the contractile abilities of the muscles. Evaluation of horizontal eye movement is straightforward. If the eye cannot adduct, the problem lies with the medial rectus; if the eye cannot move into the abducted position, the problem lies with the lateral rectus.

With the more complex movements of the other muscles, the most reliable way to determine a dysfunctional muscle is to put the eye into a position in which one muscle is the primary actor. In the adducted position, the oblique muscles are the primary elevator and depressor; in the abducted position, the vertical rectus muscles are the primary elevator and depressor. This arrangement can be represented by the H-diagram shown in Figure 10-17B. Thus, when doing ocular motility testing, it is important to move the eyes to such a position as to isolate the vertical abilities of these muscles.

The usual manner of performing ocular motility testing follows. Using a small target, usually a bead, the patient is instructed to follow the target. The horizontal ability is determined first by moving the bead to the far left and to the far right, noting any inability of either eye to follow.

Then, in left gaze, the bead is elevated to determine the ability of the left superior rectus (the left eye is abducted) and the right inferior oblique (the right eye is adducted). The bead is depressed to determine the ability of the left inferior rectus and the right superior oblique.

In right gaze, the bead is elevated to determine the ability of the right superior rectus (the right eye is abducted) and the left inferior oblique (the left eye is adducted). The bead is depressed to determine the ability of the right inferior rectus and the left superior oblique.

✍ CLINICAL COMMENT: BROWN'S SUPERIOR
        OBLIQUE SHEATH SYNDROME
    Inability to elevate the eye in the adducted position usually is caused by a dysfunctional inferior oblique muscle; however, such a limitation could be caused also by an immobile superior oblique muscle (Figure 10-18). This situation was described by Brown.[40] Using electromyography, he determined that a patient with inability to elevate the eye in adduction had a functional inferior oblique muscle but that the movement of the superior oblique through the trochlea was restricted. The superior oblique could not lengthen when the inferior oblique contracted.[40] In congenital Brown's syndrome, the cause could be a short or anchored tendon; in acquired Brown's syndrome, the cause could be an

FIGURE 10-17. (A) The direction of movement of the eye on contraction of each muscle, with the eye in primary position. (Curved arrows represent torsional movements.) For example, with the eye in primary position, if the superior rectus muscle contracts, the eye will move up and in and intort. (SR = superior rectus; MR = medial rectus; IR = inferior rectus; SO = superior oblique; LR = lateral rectus; IO = inferior oblique.) (B) The muscles that cause vertical movement when the eye is either adducted or abducted. For example, in adduction, the muscle that causes elevation is the inferior oblique (IO). (SR = superior rectus; IR = inferior rectus; SO = superior oblique.)

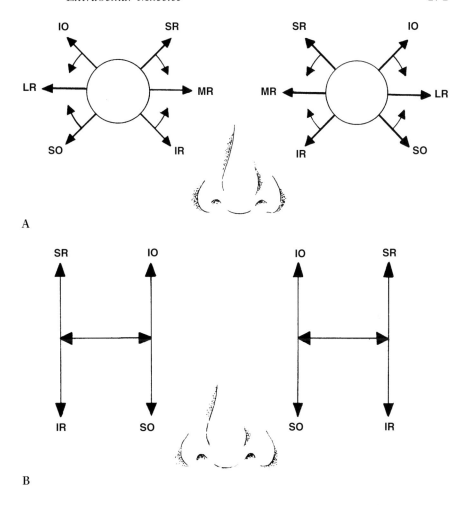

A

B

accumulation of fluid or tissue between the trochlea and the tendon.[34, 41]

CLINICAL COMMENT: LONG-STANDING IMMOBILITY

In assessing ocular motility and determining the damaged muscle, it may be difficult to determine the dysfunctional muscle, especially if the injury is long-standing. As a muscle becomes inactive, it can become immobile and can neither contract nor stretch, in effect influencing the abilities of the other extraocular muscles to move the eye.

Hyperthyroidism (Grave's Disease)
Enlargement of the extraocular muscles produced by Grave's disease is caused by chronic inflammatory infiltration of the muscles with glycoprotein and mucopolysaccharide deposition, resulting in proptosis.[2] In addition, restricted ocular motility is evident; however, as fibrosis of the muscles can occur, limiting muscle activity, evaluation of the restricted movement may not depict the correct dysfunctional muscle. For example, if the medial rectus is fibrotic, eye movement may be restricted in the lateral direction because the medial rectus is

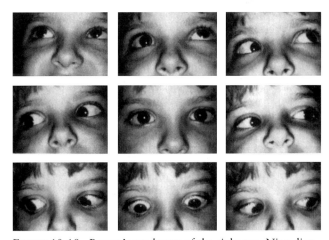

FIGURE 10-18. Brown's syndrome of the right eye. Nine diagnostic action gaze positions. Note the marked limitation of elevation in the fully adducted position. (Reprinted with permission from KK Saldana, MW Rouse. Differential diagnosis of an isolated inferior oblique paresis vs. Brown's syndrome: a case report. J Am Optom Assoc 1993;64[5]:354.)

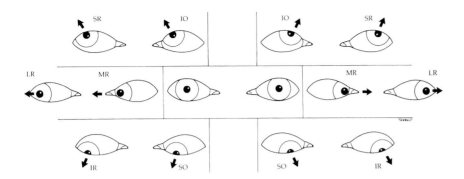

FIGURE 10-19. Six cardinal positions of gaze and yoke muscles. (SR = superior rectus; IO = inferior oblique; LR = lateral rectus; MR = medial rectus; IR = inferior rectus; SO = superior oblique.) (Reprinted with permission from JJ Kanski. Clinical Ophthalmology [3rd ed]. Oxford: Butterworth–Heinemann, 1995;429.)

unable to elongate and acts as a check on lateral movement. Restriction may appear to be impairment of the lateral rectus but actually may be due to the fibrotic medial rectus.

Forced Duction Test

If a fibrotic muscle is suspected, a forced duction test can be performed. Under topical anesthesia, the practitioner grasps the conjunctiva near the limbus and attempts to move the eye in a direction opposite from the suspected restriction. Resistance will be met if the cause is fibrosis; however, if the muscle is paralyzed, the eye can be moved. For instance, if the lateral rectus is suspect, the practitioner would attempt to move the eye medially. If the lateral rectus is fibrotic, resistance to movement occurs; if it is paralyzed, the eye can be moved with the forceps.[35]

Yoke Muscles

Yoke muscles are those muscles of the two eyes acting together to cause binocular movements (Figure 10-19). Hering's law of equal innervation states that the innervation to the muscles of the two eyes is equal and simultaneous. Thus, the movements of the two eyes normally are symmetric.[42] In dextroversion, equal and simultaneous innervation is supplied to the yoke muscles—the right lateral rectus and left medial rectus; in convergence, equal and simultaneous innervation is supplied to the yoke muscles—the right medial rectus and left medial rectus.

PAIRED ANTAGONIST MODEL

A later model by Boeder[37] analyzes the actions of the extraocular muscles as antagonist pairs. Figure 10-20 shows the path that the anterior pole of the eye traces with contraction of these pairs. The vertical pair of muscles have as primary actions elevation and depression and secondary actions of adduction and torsion. Adduction increases with medial movement, as do the torsional effects. In abduction, both muscles must relax.[37]

The primary actions of the paired obliques are intorsion and extorsion. The oblique muscle tendons insert obliquely into the globe, and the torsional effects do not diminish with horizontal movement because the insertion does not act as a unit. In adduction, the medial fibers of the superior oblique tendon exert greater contractile force and, in abduction, the lateral fibers are shortened.[42] In adduction, the lateral fibers of the inferior oblique tendon are shortened and, in abduction, the medial fibers contract.[39]

The contraction of one muscle is associated with lengthening of its antagonist. This state of relaxation or extension is considered an activity equivalent to contraction. In all positions of gaze, all muscles are in some state of activity. An analysis of the change of length of each muscle during a simple horizontal excursion shows that as the medial rectus contracts, the lateral rectus lengthens, and vice versa. The vertical rectus muscles behave as one, both contracting in adduction and lengthening in abduction. The obliques co-contract in abduction but, in adduction, the superior oblique lengthens, and the inferior oblique shortens (Figure 10-21).[37]

COMPLEXITY OF THE OBLIQUE MUSCLES

Some controversy exists over the horizontal abilities of the inferior oblique muscle. The relationship of the muscle plane of the inferior oblique with the vertical axis determines whether the inferior oblique is an adductor or an abductor. If the muscle plane lies in front of the vertical axis, the inferior oblique will aid in adduction; with increasing lateral movement of the eye, a point will be reached at which the inferior oblique plane is put behind the vertical axis, causing it then to aid in abduction.[29] Animal studies in which the muscles are stimulated directly either singularly or collectively seem to support this view.[39, 43] When the superior oblique and inferior oblique were stimulated simultaneously, no ocular movement occurred; in some positions, these two muscles appeared to be complete antagonists, and abduction did not occur. These observations do not change the model used clinically: In adduction, the obliques are responsible for elevation and depression and, in abduction, the vertical recti are responsible for elevation and depression.

FIGURE 10-20. Traces of the line of fixation with activity of each of the three muscle pairs in various positions of gaze. (Reprinted with permission from P Boeder. The co-operation of extraocular muscles. Am J Ophthalmol 1961;51:469.)

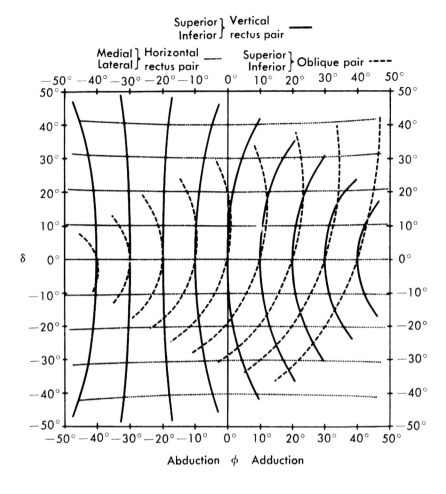

FIGURE 10-21. Changes in muscle length of all extraocular muscles occurring in a horizontal rotation. (LR = lateral rectus; SO = superior oblique; IO = inferior oblique; IR = inferior rectus; SR = superior rectus; MR = medial rectus.) (Reprinted with permission from P Boeder. The co-operation of extraocular muscles. Am J Ophthalmol 1961;51:469.)

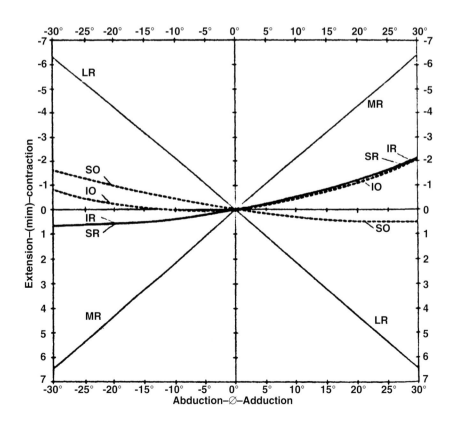

INNERVATION AND BLOOD SUPPLY

Innervation

The medial rectus, inferior rectus, and inferior oblique muscles are innervated by the inferior division of the oculomotor nerve; the superior rectus is innervated by the superior division of the oculomotor nerve; the lateral rectus is supplied by the abducens nerve; and the superior oblique is innervated by the trochlear nerve (see Table 10-3 and Figure 10-8).

Blood Supply

The extraocular muscles are supplied by two muscular branches from the ophthalmic artery: The superior (lateral) branch supplies the superior and lateral rectus and the superior oblique muscles, and the inferior (medial) branch supplies the inferior and medial rectus and the inferior oblique muscles.[2, 44] Other arteries make various contributions to the extraocular muscle blood supply, namely the lacrimal, supraorbital, and infraorbital arteries. These vessels and the muscles they supply are described in Chapter 11.

REFERENCES

1. Guyton AC. Textbook of Medical Physiology (8th ed). Philadelphia: Saunders, 1991;76.

2. Doxanas MT, Anderson RL. Clinical Orbital Anatomy. Baltimore: Williams & Wilkins, 1984;116.

3. Honda H, Asakura S. Calcium-triggered movement of regulated actin in vitro. A fluorescence microscopy study. J Mol Biol 1989;205(4):677.

4. Bagni MA, Cecchi G, Colomo F, et al. Tension and stiffness of frog muscle fibres at full filament overlap. J Muscle Res Cell Motil 1990;11:371.

5. Smith DA. The theory for sliding filament models for muscle contraction. J Theor Biol 1990;146(4):433.

6. Eggers HM. Functional Anatomy of the Extraocular Muscles. In W Tasman, EA Jaeger (eds), Duane's Foundations of Clinical Ophthalmology (Vol 1). Philadelphia: Lippincott, 1994;1.

7. Wirtschafter JD. Neuroanatomy of the Ocular Muscles. In MJ Reeh, JL Wobig, JD Wirtschafter (eds), Ophthalmic Anatomy. San Francisco: American Academy of Ophthalmology, 1981;267.

8. Namba T, Nakamura T, Grob D. Motor nerve endings in human extraocular muscle. Neurology 1968;18:403.

9. Hess A. Further morphological observations of "en plaque" and "en grappe" nerve endings on mammalian extrafusal muscle fibers with the cholinesterase technique. Rev Can Biol 1962;21:241.

10. Brandt DE, Leeson CR. Structural differences of fast and slow fibers in human extraocular muscle. Am J Ophthalmol 1966;62:478.

11. Brenin GM. The structure and function of extraocular muscle—an appraisal of the duality concept. Am J Ophthalmol 1971;71(1):1.

12. Peachy L. The Structure of the Extraocular Muscle Fibers of Mammals. In P Bach-y-Rita, CC Collins, JE Hyde (eds), The Control of Eye Movements. New York: Academic, 1971;47.

13. Scott AB, Collins CC. Division of labor in human extraocular muscle. Arch Ophthalmol 1973; 90:319.

14. Montagnani S, De Rosa P. Morphofunctional features of human extrinsic ocular muscles. Doc Ophthalmol 1989;72(2):119.

15. Burde RM, Feldon SE. The Extraocular Muscles. In WM Hart Jr (ed), Adler's Physiology of the Eye (9th ed). St. Louis: Mosby, 1992;101.

16. Cooper S, Daniel PM. Muscle spindles in human extrinsic eye muscles. Brain 1949;72:1.

17. Warwick R. Eugene Wolff's Anatomy of the Eye and Orbit (7th ed). Philadelphia: Saunders, 1976;248.

18. Alpern M. Movements of the Eyes (Part 1). In H Dawson (ed), The Eye (Vol 3). New York: Academic, 1962;36.

19. Walls GL. The evolutionary history of eye movements. Vision Res 1962;2:69.

20. Linwong M, Herman SJ. Cycloduction of the eyes with head tilt. Arch Ophthalmol 1971;85:570.

21. Jampel RS. Ocular torsion and the function of the vertical extraocular muscles. Am J Ophthalmol 1975;77:292.

22 Duke-Elder S. Textbook of Ophthalmology (Vol 4). St. Louis: Mosby, 1949;3945.

23. Diamond SG, Markham CH. Ocular counterrolling as an indicator of vestibular otolith function. Neurology 1983;33:1460.

24. Collewijin H, Van der Steer J, Ferman L, et al. Human ocular counterroll: assessment of static and dynamic properties from electromagnetic scleral coil recordings. Exp Brain Res 1985;59:185.

25. Ott D, Eckmiller R. Ocular torsion measured by TV—and scanning laser ophthalmoscopy during horizontal pursuit in humans and monkeys. Invest Ophthalmol Vis Sci 1989;30(12):2512.

26. Burton H. Somatic Sensations from the Eye. In WM Hart Jr (ed), Adler's Physiology of the Eye (9th ed). St. Louis: Mosby, 1992;185.

27. Koorneef L. Orbital Connective Tissue. In: Jakobiec FA (ed), Ocular Anatomy, Embryology, and Teratology. Philadelphia: Harper & Row, 1982;27:835.

28. de-Gottrau P, Gajisin S. Anatomic, histologic, and morphometric studies of the ocular rectus muscles and their relation to the eye globe and Tenon's capsule [abstract]. Klin Monatsbl Augenheilkd 1992;200(5):515.

29. Krewson WE. Comparison of the oblique extraocular muscles. Arch Ophthalmol 1944;32:204.

30. Wobig JL. The Extrinsic Ocular Muscles. In MJ Reeh, JL Wobig, JD Wirtschafter (eds), Ophthalmic

Anatomy. San Francisco: American Academy of Ophthalmology, 1981;33.

31. Miller JM. Functional anatomy of normal human rectus muscles. Vision Res 1989;29(2):223.

32. Miller JM, Demer JL, Rosenbaum AL. Effects of transposition surgery on rectus muscle paths by magnetic resonance imaging. Ophthalmology 1993;100(4):475.

33. Duane A. The monocular movements. Arch Ophthalmol 1936;8:531.

34. Leigh RJ, Zee DS. The Neurology of Eye Movements. Philadelphia: Davis, 1983;145, 170.

35. von Noorden GK, Maumenee AE. Atlas of Strabismus (2nd ed). St. Louis: Mosby, 1973;6, 112

36. Kanski JJ. Clinical Ophthalmology (3rd ed). Oxford: Butterworth–Heinemann, 1994;428.

37. Boeder P. The co-operation of extraocular muscles. Am J Ophthalmol 1969;51:469.

38. Sherrington CS. Experimental note on two movements of the eyes. J Physiol (Lond) 1984;17:27.

39. Jampel RS. The fundamental principle of the action on the oblique ocular muscles. Am J Ophthalmol 1970;69:623.

40. Brown HW. Congenital Structural Muscle Anomalies. In ED Allen (ed), Strabismus Ophthalmic Symposium. St. Louis: Mosby, 1950;250.

41. Helveston EM, Merriam WW, Ellis FD, et al. The trochlea, a study of the anatomy and physiology. Ophthalmology 1982;89:124.

42. Hering E. Theory of Binocular Vision. New York: Plenum, 1977.

43. Jampel RS. The action of the superior oblique muscle. Arch Ophthalmol 1966;75:535.

44. Hayreh SS. The ophthalmic artery: III. Branches. Br J Ophthalmol 1962;46:212.

Orbital Blood Supply

Circulation to the head and neck is supplied by the common carotid artery that divides into two vessels, the internal carotid and the external carotid. The internal carotid artery supplies the structures within the cranium, including the eye and related structures. The external carotid artery supplies the superficial areas of the head and neck and provides a small portion of the circulation to the ocular adnexa.

INTERNAL CAROTID ARTERY

The **internal carotid artery** runs upward through the neck and enters the skull through the carotid canal located in the petrous portion of the temporal bone. The artery leaves the canal and enters the cavernous sinus, where it runs forward along the medial wall beside the sphenoid bone; then it exits through the roof of the sinus. Within the sinus, the abducens nerve is closely adherent to the border of the internal carotid.[1] Throughout its pathway—up the neck, into the skull, and through the cavernous sinus—the internal carotid is surrounded by a plexus of sympathetic nerves from the superior cervical ganglion (Plate 11-1). The second and third cranial nerves accompany the vessel as it leaves the sinus; the optic nerve lies medial and the oculomotor nerve lies lateral to the internal carotid. The ophthalmic artery branches from the internal carotid artery just as it passes medial to the anterior clinoid process of the sphenoid bone.

✍ CLINICAL COMMENT: SCLEROSIS OF THE INTERNAL CAROTID ARTERY

In some postmortem studies, compression of the optic nerve caused by sclerosis of the internal carotid artery was found, with pathologic changes, such as atrophy, evident in the optic nerve. Visual field defects may be caused by this compression and should be one of the differential diagnoses when optic nerve head atrophy accompanies a field defect.[2]

OPHTHALMIC ARTERY

The **ophthalmic artery** enters the orbit within the dural sheath of the optic nerve and passes through the optic canal, below and lateral to the nerve (Figure 11-1). Once in the orbit, it emerges from the meningeal sheath, runs inferolateral to the optic nerve for a short distance, and then crosses either above or below it; the ophthalmic artery, together with the nasociliary nerve, runs toward the medial wall of the orbit.[3] The artery continues forward between the medial rectus and superior oblique muscles, giving off branches to various areas. Just posterior to the superior medial orbital margin, it divides into its terminal branches, the supratrochlear and dorsonasal arteries. In general, the intraorbital arteries are located in the adipose compartments and perforate the connective-tissue septa as they pass between sections.[4] The ophthalmic artery is the main blood supply to the globe and adnexa but is supplemented by a few branches from the external carotid supply.

Throughout its rather tortuous course, many branches emerge: (1) central retinal artery, (2) lacrimal artery, (3) ciliary arteries (usually two), (4) ethmoid arteries (usually two), (5) supraorbital artery, (6) muscular arteries (usually two), (7) medial palpebral arteries (superior and inferior), (8) supratrochlear artery, and (9) dorsonasal artery.

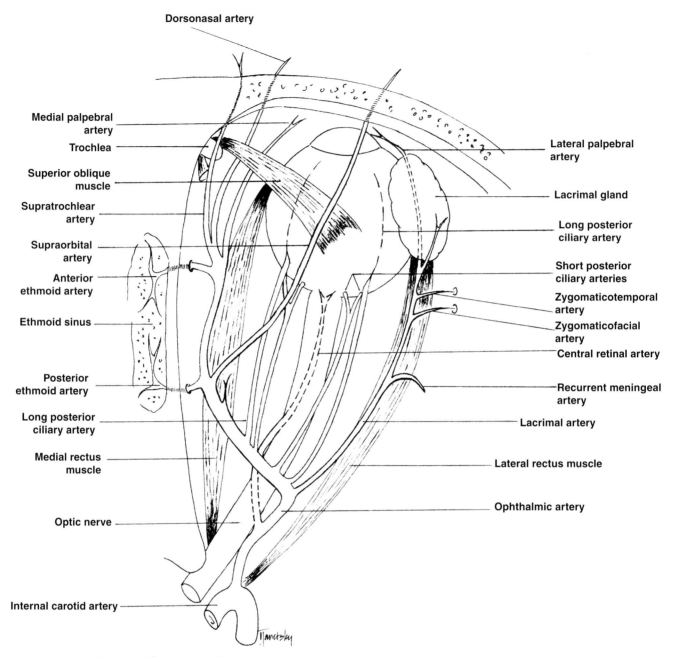

FIGURE 11-1. Orbit viewed from above, illustrating the branches of the ophthalmic artery.

Marked variability is evident in the order of the origin of the branches of the ophthalmic artery, and the sequence appears to correlate with whether the artery crosses above or below the optic nerve. The most common patterns of distribution are shown in Table 11-1.[5] A great many anatomic variations can occur in the branches and their courses; the most commonly reported are included here.

Central Retinal Artery

One of the first branches of the ophthalmic artery, the **central retinal artery** (Figure 11-2), is among the small-est branches. It leaves the ophthalmic artery as it lies below the optic nerve. The central retinal artery runs forward for a short distance before entering the meningeal sheath of the nerve some 10–12 mm behind the globe. While within the optic nerve, it provides branches to the nerve and pia mater.[5] (Often, these branches are called **collateral branches**.) As the central retinal artery runs forward within the optic nerve, a sympathetic nerve plexus (the nerve of Tiedemann) surrounds the artery.[6] The central retinal artery passes through the lamina cribrosa and enters the optic disc just nasal to center, branching superiorly and inferiorly. These branches divide into nasal and temporal branches,

TABLE 11-1. Order of Origin of Branches of Ophthalmic Artery

Order of origin	Sequence of branches when ophthalmic artery crosses above optic nerve	Sequence of branches when ophthalmic artery crosses below optic nerve
1	Central retinal and medial posterior	Lateral posterior ciliary
2	Lateral posterior ciliary	Central retinal
3	Lacrimal	Medial muscular
4	Muscular to superior rectus and levator	Medial posterior ciliary
5	Posterior ethmoid and supraorbital, jointly or separately	Lacrimal
6	Medial posterior ciliary	Muscular to superior rectus and levator
7	Medial muscular	Posterior ethmoid and supraorbital, jointly or separately
8	Muscular to superior oblique and medial rectus, jointly or separately	Muscular to superior oblique and medial rectus, jointly or separately
9	To areolar tissue	Anterior ethmoid
10	Anterior ethmoid	To areolar tissue
11	Medial palpebral or inferior medial palpebral	Medial palpebral or inferior medial palpebral
12	Superior medial palpebral	Superior medial palpebral
Terminal	Dorsonasal and supratrochlear	Dorsonasal and supratrochlear

Source: Adapted from SS Hayreh. The ophthalmic artery: III. Branches. Br J Ophthalmol 1962;46:212.

then continue to branch dichotomously within the retinal nerve fiber layer. The retinal blood vessels are discussed in Chapter 4.

✍ CLINICAL COMMENT: RETINAL VENOUS
       BRANCH OCCLUSION
The branches of the central retinal artery and vein are joined in a common connective-tissue sheath at the point where the vessels cross each other. Generally, the artery crosses over the vein and, in such disease processes as arterial sclerosis, may compress the vein at the crossing, causing at first a deflection of the vessel, which in time may progress to a venous occlusion. Restriction of flow in the vein results in retinal edema and hemorrhage in the area surrounding the occlusion.

Lacrimal Artery

One of the largest branches, the **lacrimal artery**, leaves the ophthalmic artery just after it enters the orbit (see Figure 11-1); sometimes, though rarely, it branches before the ophthalmic artery enters the optic canal.[7] The lacrimal artery and the lacrimal nerve run forward along the upper border of the lateral rectus muscle. Within the orbit, the lacrimal artery may supply branches to the lateral rectus muscle.

A **recurrent meningeal artery** (see Figure 11-1) might branch from the lacrimal artery and course back, leaving the orbit through the lateral aspect of the superior orbital fissure and forming an anastomosis with the middle meningeal artery, a branch from the external carotid artery circulation.[8] Other branches, the **zygomaticotemporal artery** and the **zygomaticofacial artery**, exit the orbit through foramina of the same name within the zygomatic bone (see Figure 11-1) and anastomose with branches from the external carotid in the temporal fossa and on the face.

The lacrimal artery continues forward to supply the lacrimal gland. Terminal branches pass through the gland, pierce the orbital septum, and enter the lateral side of the upper and lower eyelids to form the **lateral palpebral arteries** (Figure 11-3). These anastomose with branches from the medial palpebral arteries and form vessel arches called the **palpebral arcades**. Other terminal branches enter the conjunctiva and form a capillary network.

Posterior Ciliary Arteries

The **posterior ciliary arteries** are branches of the ophthalmic artery, and much variation can occur in their distribution.[9] The **short posterior ciliary arteries** arise as 1 or 2 branches that then form 10–20 branches. They enter the sclera in a ring around the optic nerve and form the arterial network within the choroidal stroma (Figure 11-4). Other branches from the short posterior ciliary arteries anastomose to form the **circle of Zinn** (see Figure 11-2), which encircles the optic nerve at the level of the choroid. A capillary bed, the peripapillary choroidal network, supplies the superficial optic disc and is formed by branches from the short posterior ciliary arteries, with

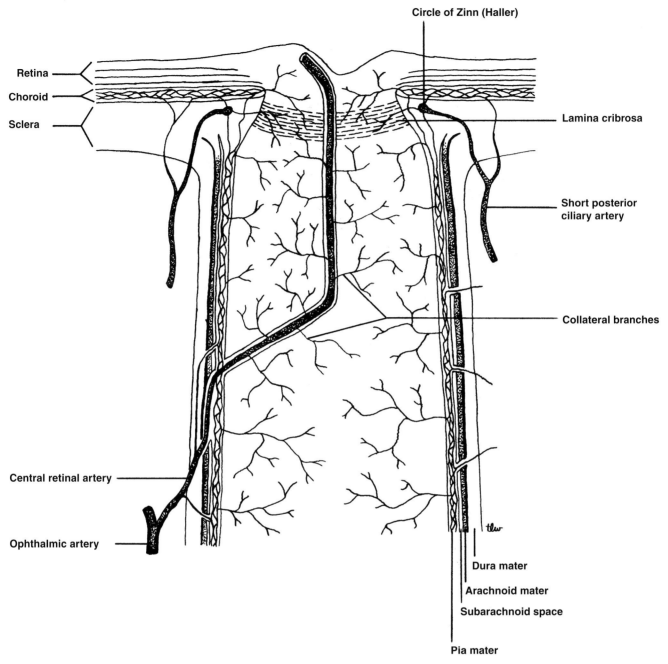

FIGURE 11-2. Longitudinal section of the optic nerve.

variable contributions from the central retinal artery and the pial vessels.[10, 11]

🖎 CLINICAL COMMENT: CILIORETINAL ARTERY

A cilioretinal artery may arise either from the vessels entering the choroid or from the circle of Zinn; thus, this vessel, located within the retina, arises from the ciliary circulation and not from the retinal supply. A cilioretinal artery is found in perhaps 15% of the population and usually enters the retina from the temporal side of the optic disc to supply the macular area (Figure 11-5).[12] If occlusion of the

central retinal artery occurs, the direct blood supply to the macular area will be maintained in those persons with such a cilioretinal artery.

Two long branches of the posterior ciliary arteries enter the sclera, one lateral and one medial to the ring of short ciliary arteries. These are the **long posterior ciliary arteries**, which run between the sclera and the choroid to the anterior globe (see Figure 11-4). Here they enter the ciliary body and branch superiorly and inferiorly. These branches anastomose with each other and with the anterior ciliary arteries to form a circular blood vessel, the

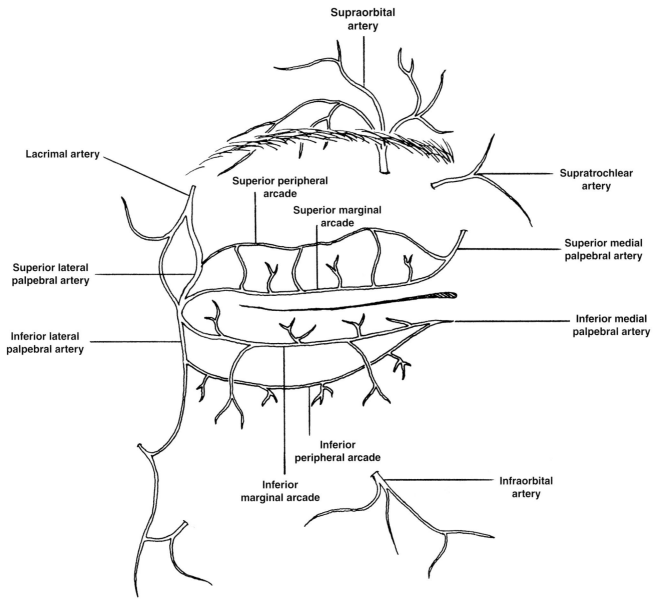

Figure 11-3. Palpebral arteries.

major arterial circle of the iris (Plate 11-2). This circular artery is located in the ciliary stroma near the iris root and is the source of the radial vessels found in the iris. Before forming the major circle, branches from the long posterior ciliary arteries supply the ciliary body and the anterior choroid, where they form a network that anastomoses with the choroidal vessels from the short posterior ciliary arteries (see Figure 11-4).

Ethmoid Arteries

As the ophthalmic artery courses near the medial wall, two branches arise and enter the ethmoid bone (see Figure 11-1). The **posterior ethmoid artery** passes through the posterior ethmoid canal to supply the posterior eth-

moid sinus and the sphenoid sinus; it sends branches into the nasal cavity to supply the upper part of the nasal mucosa. The **anterior ethmoid artery** generally is larger and passes through the anterior ethmoid canal and supplies the anterior and middle ethmoid sinuses, the sphenoid sinus, the frontal sinus, the nasal cavity, and the skin of the nose.

Supraorbital Artery

The **supraorbital artery** arises from the ophthalmic artery as it lies medial to the optic nerve (see Figure 11-1). This vessel runs upward to a position above the superior extraocular muscles, turns anteriorly, and runs with the supraorbital nerve between the periorbita of the orbital

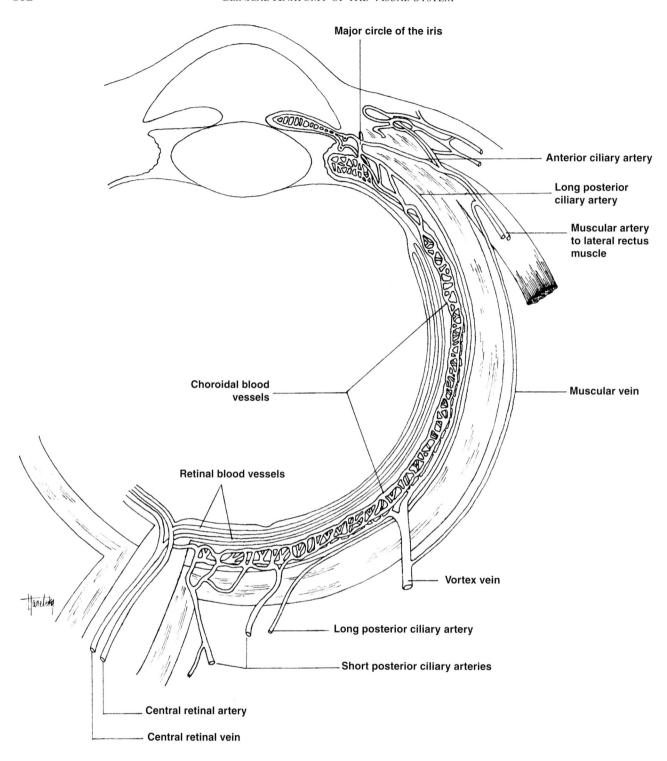

FIGURE 11-4. Horizontal section of the eye showing ciliary circulation. (Redrawn with permission from D Vaughan, T Asbury. General Ophthalmology. Norwalk, CT: Appleton & Lange, 1980.)

roof and the levator muscle. It passes through the supraorbital notch or foramen, often dividing into two branches to supply the skin and the muscles of the forehead and scalp (see Figure 11-3). Terminal branches anastomose with the artery from the opposite side, with the supratrochlear artery, and with the anterior temporal artery from the external carotid. While the supraorbital artery is in the orbit, it sends branches to the superior rectus, superior oblique, and levator muscles, and to the periorbita.

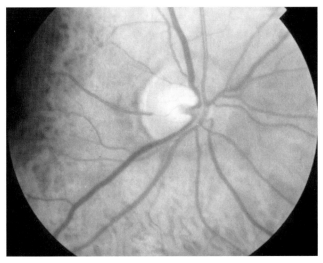

FIGURE 11-5. Fundus photograph of the right eye, showing a temporal cilioretinal artery. (Courtesy of Family Vision Center, Pacific University, Forest Grove, OR.)

TABLE 11-2. Extraocular Muscle Blood Supply

Muscle	Arterial supply
Medial rectus	Medial (inferior) muscular
Lateral rectus	Lateral (superior) muscular
	Lacrimal
Superior rectus	Lateral (superior) muscular
	Lacrimal
	Supraorbital
Inferior rectus	Medial (inferior) muscular
	Infraorbital
Superior oblique	Lateral (superior) muscular
	Supraorbital
Inferior oblique	Medial (inferior) muscular
	Infraorbital

Muscular Arteries

Much variation occurs in the vessels supplying the muscles and, in any individual, any combination of the vessels named here might be present. In one common presentation, the muscular arteries come off the ophthalmic artery as two branches, the **lateral** (or **superior**) and the **medial** (or **inferior**). The lateral (superior) branch supplies the lateral rectus, the superior rectus, the superior oblique, and the levator muscles.[6, 7] The medial (inferior) branch supplies the medial rectus, the inferior rectus, and the inferior oblique muscles. Additional branches supplying the muscles may come from other sources. The lacrimal artery supplies the lateral and superior rectus muscles. The supraorbital artery supplies the superior rectus, superior oblique, and levator muscles. The infraorbital artery supplies the inferior rectus and inferior oblique muscles (Table 11-2).

Anterior Ciliary Arteries

The **anterior ciliary arteries** branch from the vessels supplying the rectus muscles. These arteries exit the muscles near the muscle insertions, run forward along the tendons a short distance, then loop inward to pierce the sclera just outer to the limbus (see Figure 11-4). An accumulation of pigment may be evident at the point at which the artery enters the sclera. Branches enter the episclera to form a network of vessels before entering the uvea. The anterior ciliary arteries then enter the ciliary body and anastomose with the branches of the long posterior ciliary arteries, forming the major circle of the iris (Figure 11-6). Generally, two anterior ciliary arteries emanate from each of the rectus muscles, with the exception of the lateral rectus, which provides only one such artery. Before entering the eyeball, the anterior ciliary arteries

send branches into the conjunctiva, forming a network of vessels in the limbal conjunctiva (see Figure 11-6).

CLINICAL COMMENT: RED EYE

Inflammations generate an increase of the blood supply to the affected area, causing hyperemia. In cases of a red eye, an understanding of the organization of the blood supply in the limbal area can help in differentiating a less serious process, such as conjunctivitis, from a more serious situation, such as uveitis. In conjunctivitis and mild corneal involvement, the superficial blood vessels are injected, giving the conjunctiva a bright red color that often increases toward the fornix. The vessels move with conjunctival movement and can be blanched with a topical vasoconstrictor. In uveitis, the deeper scleral and episcleral vessels are injected, giving the circumlimbal area a purplish or rose-pink color.[13] These vessels do not move with the conjunctiva and are not blanched with a topical vasoconstrictor.

Medial Palpebral Arteries

Two **medial palpebral arteries** branch either directly from the ophthalmic or from the dorsonasal artery near the trochlea of the superior oblique muscle. They pierce the orbital septum on either side of the medial palpebral ligament and enter the superior and inferior eyelids (see Figure 11-3). These branches run through the eyelid and form arches between the orbicularis muscle and the tarsal plate. They anastomose with branches from the lacrimal artery and form the vessels known as the **palpebral arcades.** Usually, two arcades occur in each lid: the marginal arcade, which runs near the marginal edge of the tarsal plate, and the peripheral arcade, which runs

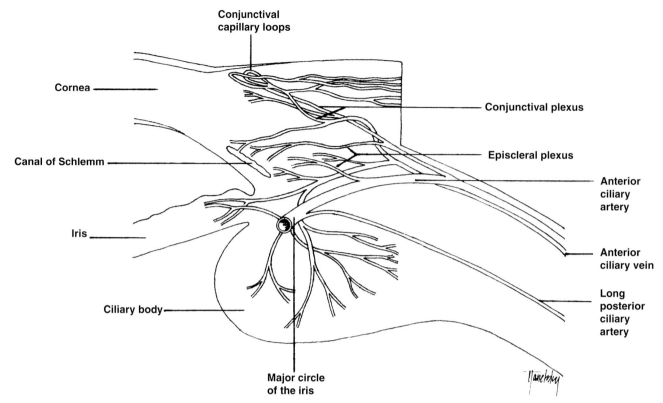

FIGURE 11-6. Section through ciliary body and limbal area, showing the blood supply.

near the peripheral edge of the tarsal plate. These provide the blood supply for the eyelid structures. Additional branches from the medial palpebral arteries supply the structures in the medial canthus.

Supratrochlear Artery

One of the terminal branches of the ophthalmic artery—the **supratrochlear artery**—pierces the orbital septum at the superior, medial corner of the orbit (see Figure 11-3). It passes with the supratrochlear nerve upward to supply the skin of the forehead and scalp and the muscles of the forehead. It forms anastomoses with the supraorbital artery, the opposite supratrochlear, and the anterior temporal artery of the external carotid supply.

Dorsonasal Artery

The other terminal branch of the ophthalmic artery, the **dorsonasal artery (dorsal nasal artery)**, also leaves the orbit by piercing the orbital septum below the trochlea above the medial palpebral ligament. It sends vessels to supply the lacrimal sac, then runs alongside the nose to anastomose with the angular artery from the external carotid supply.

EXTERNAL CAROTID ARTERY

The other branch of the common carotid—the **external carotid artery**—passes upward through the tissue of the neck. Only those few branches of this artery that supply the globe and orbit are discussed. The branches from the internal and external carotid arteries that supply the ocular structures, and their most common anastomoses, are shown in the flowchart in Figure 11-7.

Facial Artery

The **facial artery** arises from the external carotid near the angle of the mandible, runs along the posterior edge of the lower jaw, and curves upward over the outside of the jaw and across the cheek to the angle of the mouth. It ascends along the side of the nose and sends a terminal branch, the **angular artery**, to the medial canthus (Figure 11-8). The angular artery supplies the lacrimal sac, the medial part of the lower lid, and the skin of the cheek. Some branches anastomose with the infraorbital artery and some with the dorsonasal artery.

Superficial Temporal Artery

The **superficial temporal artery** is a terminal branch of the external carotid artery (see Figure 11-8). Branches of the superficial temporal artery that supply areas near the orbit are the anterior temporal, the zygomatic, and the transverse facial arteries.[14] The **anterior temporal artery** supplies the skin and muscles of the forehead and anastomoses with the supraorbital

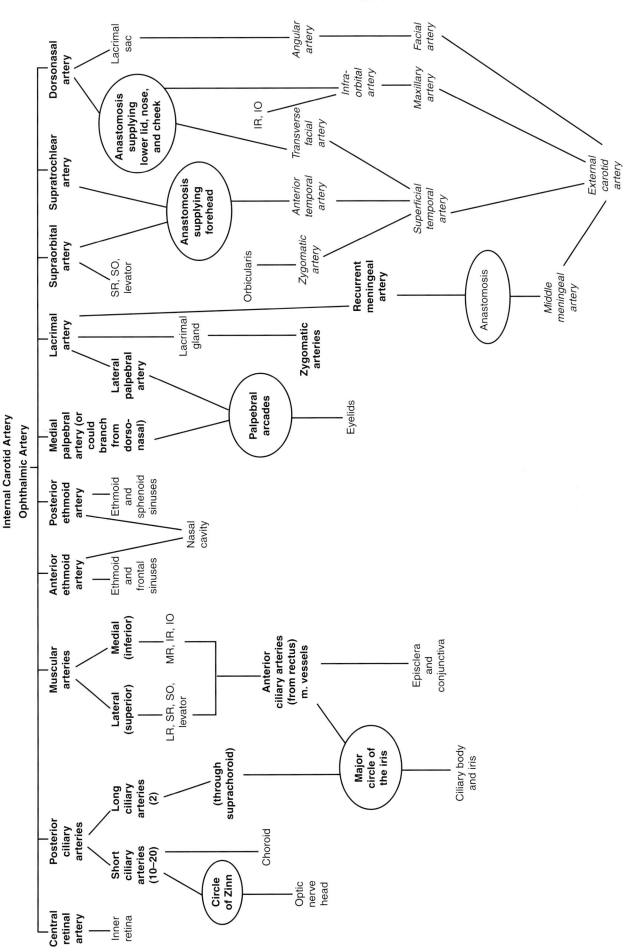

FIGURE 11-7. Flowchart of the internal carotid artery. (LR = lateral rectus; MR = medial rectus; SR = superior rectus; SO = superior oblique; IR = inferior rectus; IO = inferior oblique.)

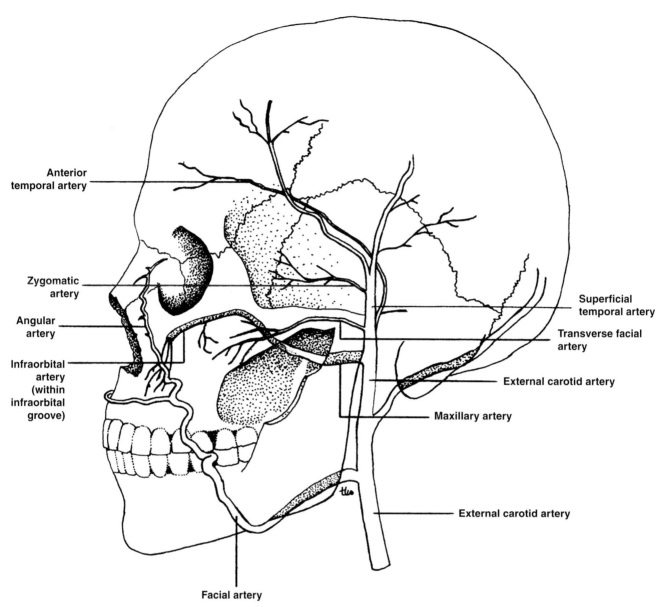

FIGURE 11-8. The branches of the external carotid artery that supply the ocular adnexa. (Redrawn with permission from CD Clemente. Anatomy: A Regional Atlas of the Human Body. Munich: Urban and Schwarzenberg, 1987. Copyright 1987, Lea & Febiger.)

and supratrochlear arteries. The **zygomatic artery** extends above the zygomatic arch and supplies the orbicularis muscle. The **transverse facial artery** supplies the skin of the cheek and anastomoses with the infraorbital artery.

✍ CLINICAL COMMENT: TEMPORAL ARTERITIS

Temporal arteritis (or giant cell arteritis) is an inflammatory condition that can affect large arteries but is found primarily in the arteries in the temporal or occipital region. The disease often is accompanied by swelling, redness, and tenderness in the temporal area. Ocular symptoms, such as vision loss, may occur. Biopsy of the superficial temporal artery often

is necessary to confirm the diagnosis before treatment is begun.[15]

Maxillary Artery

The other branch of the external carotid that supplies areas in proximity to the orbit is the **maxillary artery**. It passes through the infratemporal fossa and then upward, medial to the mandibular joint toward the maxillary bone (see Figure 11-8). Within the infratemporal fossa, the maxillary artery shows some variability in both its branching pattern and in its topographic relations with other structures.[16–18] It runs along the pterygopalatine fossa and enters the orbit through the inferior orbital fissure as the **infraorbital artery**.

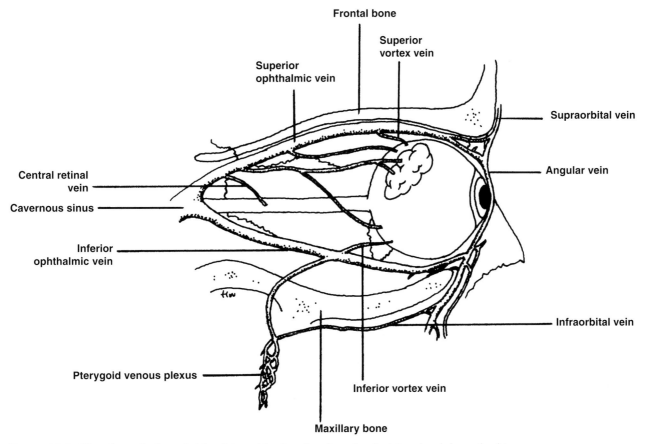

FIGURE 11-9. View from the lateral side of the orbit, showing the veins draining the globe and orbit.

The artery then runs forward through the maxillary bone within the infraorbital canal and exits via the infraorbital foramen (see Figure 11-3). It supplies the lower eyelid and lacrimal sac, and it anastomoses with the angular artery and the dorsonasal artery.[14] While in the infraorbital canal, the infraorbital artery supplies the inferior rectus and inferior oblique muscles and sends some branches to the maxillary sinus and to the teeth of the upper jaw.

VEINS OF THE ORBIT

The veins of the orbit have no valves; thus, the direction of blood flow may change and is determined by pressure gradients.[3] Over a large part of their path, the veins are embedded within the connective-tissue septa that compartmentalize the orbit.[4] Unlike the parallel routes of veins and arteries in most of the body, many orbital veins follow a course that differs from the corresponding arteries.[7,19] The orbit has a single ophthalmic artery but two ophthalmic veins. The superior and inferior ophthalmic veins primarily drain into the cavernous sinus.

Superior Ophthalmic Vein

The **superior ophthalmic vein** is formed by the joining of the angular and supraorbital veins within the orbit (Figure 11-9). The **supraorbital vein** enters the orbit through the supraorbital notch, and the **angular vein** passes through the orbital septum above the medial palpebral ligament.

The superior ophthalmic vein, the larger of the two ophthalmic veins, runs with the ophthalmic artery and, as it passes posteriorly, receives blood from veins that drain the superior orbital structures. It passes below the superior rectus muscle and crosses the optic nerve to the upper part of the superior orbital fissure, where it leaves the orbit to empty into the cavernous sinus.

The veins that drain into the superior ophthalmic vein are the anterior and posterior ethmoid veins, the muscular veins draining the superior and medial muscles, the lacrimal vein, the central retinal vein, and the upper vortex veins.

Central Retinal Vein

The venous branches located in the retinal tissue come together and exit the eyeball as a single **central retinal vein**. This vessel leaves the optic nerve approximately 10–12 mm behind the lamina cribrosa alongside the central retinal artery. It emerges from the meningeal sheath of the optic nerve and either joins the superior ophthalmic vein or exits the orbit and drains directly into the cavernous sinus.

✍ CLINICAL COMMENT: PAPILLEDEMA

The sheaths that surround the optic nerve are continuous with the meningeal sheaths of the brain. The subarachnoid space, located within these layers, contains cerebrospinal fluid. Thus, the fluid that surrounds the optic nerve is continuous with the fluid found throughout the cranial cavity. With increased intracranial pressure, the central retinal vein might be compressed as it crosses the subarachnoid space on its exit from the optic nerve. The central retinal artery is not affected, because it has a thicker sheath and is not compressed as easily as is the vein.[20] The resultant blockage causes congestion of the retinal veins and edema of the retina. Edema of the optic nerve head (papilledema) will be evident as blurred disc margins, with hemorrhages sometimes evident as well.

Vortex Veins

The **vortex veins**, of which there are four or five, drain the choroid; usually, one is located in each quadrant (see Plate 11-2). They exit the globe 6 mm posterior to the equator.[6] The vortex veins can be seen with an indirect ophthalmoscope and a dilated pupil.

Inferior Ophthalmic Vein

The **inferior ophthalmic vein** begins as a plexus near the anterior floor of the orbit. It drains blood from the lower and lateral muscles, the inferior conjunctiva, the lacrimal sac, and the lower vortex veins. It may form two branches, one that empties into either the superior ophthalmic vein[19, 21] or the cavernous sinus and one that empties into the **pterygoid venous plexus** (see Figure 11-9). The branch that empties into the pterygoid plexus exits the orbit through the inferior orbital fissure, and the other branch passes through the superior orbital fissure either to join the superior ophthalmic vein or to empty directly into the cavernous sinus.

Anterior Ciliary Veins

The **anterior ciliary veins** receive branches from the conjunctival capillary network and then accompany the anterior ciliary arteries, pierce the sclera, and join with the muscular veins.

Infraorbital Vein

The **infraorbital vein** is formed by several veins that drain the face. It enters the infraorbital foramen and, along with the infraorbital artery and nerve, passes posteriorly through the infraorbital canal and groove. It receives branches from some structures in the inferior part of the orbit and may communicate with the inferior ophthalmic vein. The infraorbital vein drains into the pterygoid venous plexus (see Figure 11-9).

Cavernous Sinus

The **cavernous sinus** is a relatively large venous channel formed by a splitting of the dura mater on each side of the body of the sphenoid bone. The cavernous sinus extends from the medial end of the superior orbital fissure to the petrous portion of the temporal bone. The internal carotid artery and the abducens nerve are located medially within the sinus covered by the endothelial lining of the sinus. The oculomotor, ophthalmic, and maxillary nerves are found within the lateral wall of the cavernous sinus (Figure 11-10). The cavernous sinus drains into the superior petrosal sinus located along the upper crest of the petrous portion of the temporal bone and into the inferior petrosal sinus located in the groove between the petrous portion and the occipital bone. Both drain either directly or indirectly into the internal jugular vein.

LYMPHATIC DRAINAGE

No lymphatic vessels occur in the globe proper; lymphatics are found in the conjunctiva and the eyelids. The lymphatics that drain the medial aspects of the lids and the medial canthal structures (including the lacrimal sac) empty into the submandibular lymph nodes; those that drain the lateral eyelids and the lacrimal gland empty into the parotid lymph nodes in the preauricular area (Figure 11-11).[7, 21]

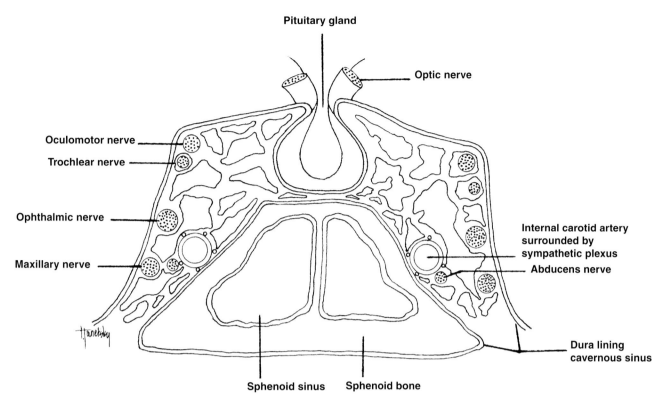

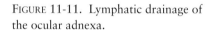

FIGURE 11-10. Coronal section through the sphenoid bone and cavernous sinus, showing the nerves that pass through the sinus en route to and from the orbit.

FIGURE 11-11. Lymphatic drainage of the ocular adnexa.

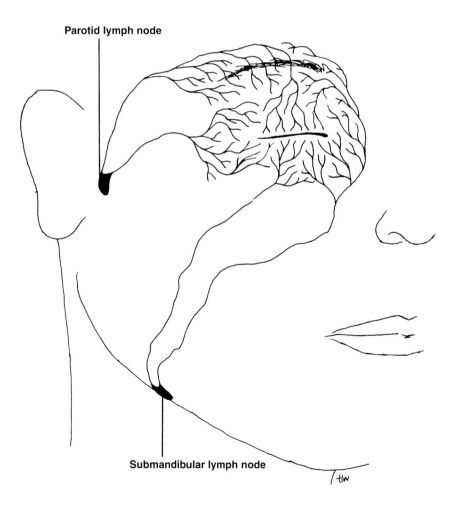

REFERENCES

1. Nuza AB, Taner D. Anatomical variations of the intracavernous branches of the internal carotid artery with reference to the relationship of the internal carotid artery and sixth cranial nerve. Acta Anat (Basel) 1990;138(3):238.

2. Liu XJ. Pathological changes of the optic nerve from compression by the internal carotid artery [abstract]. Chung Hua Yen Ko Tsa Chih 1990;26(6):364.

3. Hayreh SS. The ophthalmic artery: II. Intraorbital course. Br J Ophthalmol 1962;46:165.

4. Koorneef L. Orbital Connective Tissue. In FA Jakobiec (ed), Ocular Anatomy, Embryology, and Teratology. Philadelphia: Harper & Row, 1982;835.

5. Hayreh SS. The ophthalmic artery: III. Branches. Br J Ophthalmol 1962;46:212.

6. Warwick R. Eugene Wolff's Anatomy of the Eye and Orbit (7th ed). Philadelphia: Saunders, 1976; 92,146,406.

7. Doxanas MT, Anderson RL. Clinical Orbital Anatomy. Baltimore: Williams & Wilkins, 1984;153.

8. Diamond MK. Homologies of the meningeal-orbital arteries of humans: a reappraisal. J Anat 1991; 178:223.

9. Yoshii I, Ikeda A. A new look at the blood supply of the retro-ocular space. Anat Rec 1992;233:321.

10. Hayreh SS. Blood supply of the optic nerve head and its role in optic atrophy, glaucoma, and oedema of the optic disc. Br J Ophthalmol 1969;53:721.

11. Hayreh SS. Pathogenesis of cupping of the optic disc. Br J Ophthalmol 1974;58:863.

12. Hayreh SS. The central artery of the retina: its role in the blood supply of the optic nerve. Br J Ophthalmol 1963;47:651.

13. Catania LJ. Primary Care of the Anterior Segment. East Norwalk, CT: Appleton & Lange, 1988;194.

14. Tucker SM, Lindberg JV. Vascular anatomy of the eyelids. Ophthalmology 1994;101:1118.

15. Berkow R (ed). The Merck Manual (14th ed). Rahway, NJ: Merck, 1982;557.

16. Morton AL, Khan A. Internal maxillary artery variability in the pterygopalatine fossa. Otolaryngol Head Neck Surg 1991;104(2):204.

17. Ortug G, Moriggl B. The topography of the maxillary artery within the infratemporal fossa [abstract]. Anat Anz 1991;172(3):197.

18. Pretterklieber ML, Skopakoff C, Mayr R. The human maxillary artery reinvestigated: topographical relations in the infratemporal fossa. Acta Anat (Basel) 1991;142(4):281.

19. Murakami K, Murakami G, Komatsu A, et al. Gross anatomical study of veins in the orbit [abstract]. Nippon Ganka Gakkai Zasshi 1991;95(1):31.

20. Whiting AS, Johnson LN. Papilledema: clinical clues and differential diagnosis. Am Fam Phys 1992; 45(3):125.

21. Wobig JL. The Blood Vessels and Lymphatics of the Orbit and Lid. In JL Wobig, MJ Reeh, JD Wirtschafter (eds), Ophthalmic Anatomy. San Francisco: American Academy of Ophthalmology, 1981;77.

Cranial Nerve Innervation of Ocular Structures

The orbital structures are innervated by cranial nerves (CN) II, III, IV, V, VI, and VII (Table 12-1). Motor functions of the striated muscles are controlled by CN III, the oculomotor nerve; CN IV, the trochlear nerve; CN VI, the abducens nerve; and CN VII, the facial nerve. CN V, the trigeminal nerve, carries the sensory supply of the orbital structures. CN II, the optic nerve, carries visual information and is discussed in Chapter 14. Sensory and motor innervation of the orbit, including pathways, functions, and presenting signs of dysfunction, are discussed here.

THE NERVOUS SYSTEM

Information comes into the central nervous system (CNS) via afferent fibers. Afferent sensory fibers usually have specialized nerve endings that respond to such sensations as touch, pressure, temperature, or pain.

Information processing occurs within the brain or spinal cord and involves communication between different areas of the CNS via fiber tracts. A fiber tract also may be called a **fasciculus**, a **peduncle**, or a **brachium**. The portion of the cranial nerve from the cell body in the nucleus to the exit from the brainstem is the fascicular part of the nerve.

Efferent fibers, either somatic or autonomic, carry information from the CNS to the target structures: muscles, organs, or glands. The efferent pathway in the somatic system generally consists of a fiber that runs the distance from the CNS to the target muscle. The autonomic pathway, which is discussed in Chapter 13, generally has a synapse within its pathway.

AFFERENT PATHWAY: ORBITAL SENSORY INNERVATION

The eye is richly supplied with sensory nerves that carry sensations of touch, pressure, warmth, cold, and pain. Sensations from the cornea, iris, conjunctiva, and sclera consist primarily of pain; even very light touch of the cornea is registered as irritation or pain.[1]

Trigeminal Nerve

The fibers of the trigeminal nerve (CN V) serving ocular structures are sensory and originate in the innervated structures. The description of the pathways of these nerves begins at the involved structures and follows the nerves as they join to become larger nerves, come together in the ganglion of the fifth cranial nerve, and then exit the ganglion and enter the pons. It is hoped that this presentation, though unconventional, will enable the reader to keep in mind the actual direction of the action potential and, thus, the information flow in these fibers. Plate 12-1 shows the branches and paths of the trigeminal nerve within the orbit.

Ophthalmic Division of the Trigeminal Nerve

Nasociliary Nerve. Sensory fibers from the structures of the medial canthal area—the caruncle, the canaliculi, the lacrimal sac, the medial aspect of the eyelids, and the skin at the side of the nose—join to form the **infratrochlear**

TABLE 12-1. Orbital Cranial Nerves

Cranial nerve	Origin	Destination	Function
II, Optic	Retinal ganglion cells	Lateral geniculate body	Sensory: sight

III, Oculomotor: inferior division	Midbrain	Medial rectus muscle
		Inferior rectus muscle
		Inferior oblique muscle
		Ciliary ganglion
			Motor: adduction
			  depression, adduction, extorsion
			  elevation, abduction, extorsion
			Parasympathetic: motor to iris
			  sphincter and ciliary muscle for
			  miosis and accommodation

III, Oculomotor: superior division	Midbrain	Superior rectus muscle
		
		Superior palpebral levator
		  muscle
			Motor: elevation, adduction,
			  intorsion
			Motor: elevation of eyelid

IV, Trochlear	Midbrain	Superior oblique muscle	Motor: depression, abduction, intorsion
VI, Abducens	Pons	Lateral rectus muscle	Motor: abduction

VII, Facial	Pons	Frontalis, procerus, corrugator,
		  orbicularis muscles
		Sphenopalatine ganglion
			Motor: facial expressions,
			  closure of eyelids
			Parasympathetic: secretomotor to
			  lacrimal gland for lacrimation

nerve. This nerve penetrates the orbital septum, enters the orbit below the trochlea, and runs along the upper border of the medial rectus muscle, becoming the nasociliary nerve as other branches join it (Figure 12-1).

Sensory fibers from the skin along the center of the nose, the nasal mucosa, and the ethmoid sinuses form the **anterior ethmoid nerve**; fibers from the ethmoid sinuses and the sphenoid sinus form the **posterior ethmoid nerve**. The ethmoid nerves enter the orbit with their companion arteries through foramina within the frontoethmoid suture.[2] Both nerves join the nasociliary nerve as it runs along the medial aspect of the orbit (see Figure 12-1).

Corneal sensory innervation is dense, estimated to be three to four times as dense as other epithelial tissue innervation.[1] Three networks of nerves are formed: One is located in the corneal epithelium, another (the subepithelial plexus) is in the anterior stroma, and the third is in the middle of the stroma (Figure 12-2). No nerves are found in posterior stroma, Descemet's membrane, or endothelium. The fibers from these plexus come together in peripheral stroma and radiate out into the limbus as 70–80 branches; they become myelinated in the last 2 mm of the cornea.[3]

Some of these branches join with nerves from other anterior segment structures to form two **long ciliary nerves**. These long ciliary nerves, one on the lateral side and one on the medial side of the globe, course between the choroid and sclera to the back of the eye, where they leave the globe at points approximately 3 mm on each side of the optic nerve (Figure 12-3). (In addition to afferent fibers, the long ciliary nerves transmit sympathetic

fibers to the dilator muscle of the iris.) The two long ciliary nerves then join the nasociliary nerve.

✍ CLINICAL COMMENT: (SCLERAL) NERVE LOOPS
(OF AXENFELD)
A slight variation can occur in the pathway of the long ciliary nerve, in which the fibers loop into the sclera from the suprachoroidal space, forming a dome-shaped elevation some 2 mm from the limbus, on either the nasal or the temporal side. Often, this raised area is pigmented—usually blue or black—and it should be differentiated from a melanoma.[4] Sometimes, the nerve loop is painful when touched, a characteristic that should aid in its diagnosis.[3]

The other branches radiating from the cornea into the limbus join other sensory nerves from the anterior segment; they enter the choroid, join with the choroidal nerves, then course to the back of the eye, where they leave as 6–10 **short ciliary nerves** (see Figure 12-3). The short ciliary nerves exit the sclera in a ring around the optic nerve in company with the short posterior ciliary arteries and enter the ciliary ganglion (see Figure 12-1). The sensory fibers do not synapse but pass through the ganglion, leaving as the **sensory root of the ciliary ganglion**, which then joins the nasociliary nerve. (The short ciliary nerves carry sympathetic and parasympathetic fibers in addition to sensory fibers.)

Thus, the nasociliary nerve is formed by the joining of the infratrochlear nerve, the anterior and posterior ethmoid nerves, the long ciliary nerves, and the sensory root of the ciliary ganglion (see Figure 12-1). The nasociliary

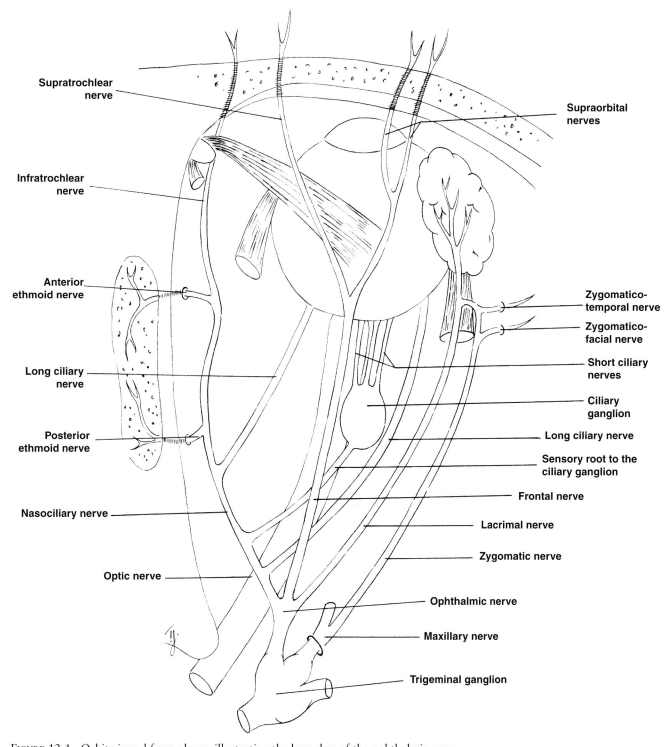

FIGURE 12-1. Orbit viewed from above, illustrating the branches of the ophthalmic nerve.

nerve exits the orbit by passing through the common tendinous ring and the superior orbital fissure into the cranial cavity.

✍ CLINICAL COMMENT: HERPES ZOSTER

Herpes zoster is an acute CNS infection caused by the varicella zoster virus. Signs and symptoms include pain and rash in the distribution area supplied by sensory nerves.[5] It is believed that the virus lies dormant in a sensory ganglion and, on becoming activated, migrates down the sensory pathway to the skin.[6] An eruption of herpes zoster is more common in the elderly but may occur at any age and may be related to a delayed hypersensitivity reaction.[7] Approxi-

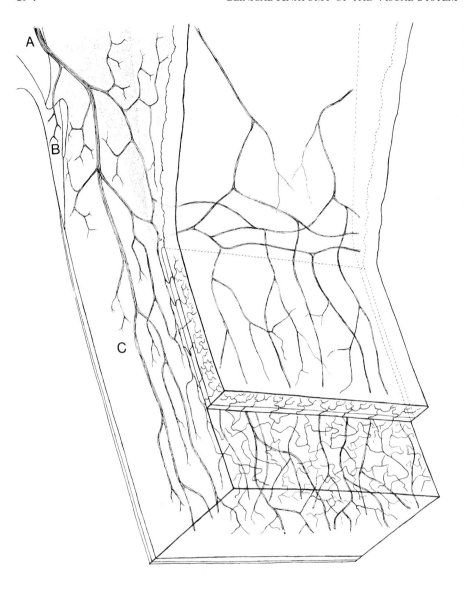

FIGURE 12-2. Innervation of the limbus and cornea. The long ciliary nerve (*A*) supplies the limbal region, then sends branches into the cornea. Nerves also supply the trabecular meshwork (*B*) and the region of the canal of Schlemm. Note the paucity of nerves in the deep cornea (*C*) and their absence in the region of Descemet's membrane. (Reprinted with permission from MJ Hogan, JA Alvarado, JE Weddell. Histology of the Human Eye. Philadelphia: Saunders, 1971;63.)

mately 10% of all cases affect the ophthalmic division of the trigeminal nerve.[8] Involvement of the tip of the nose often indicates that the eye also will be involved, reflecting the distribution of the nasociliary branches. This association of ocular involvement with zoster affecting the tip of the nose is Hutchinson's sign.[9]

Frontal Nerve.   Sensory fibers from the skin and muscles of the forehead and upper eyelid come together and form the **supratrochlear nerve**. This nerve enters the orbit by piercing the superior medial corner of the orbital septum (Figure 12-4).

Sensory fibers from the skin and muscles of the forehead and upper eyelid form a second nerve—the **supraorbital nerve**—lateral to the supratrochlear nerve (see Figure 12-4). The supraorbital nerve enters the orbit as one or two branches; one branch enters through the supraorbital notch, accompanying the supraorbital artery. The supraorbital nerve joins the supratrochlear nerve midway in the

orbit and forms the frontal nerve (see Figure 12-1). The frontal nerve courses back through the orbit between the levator muscle and the periorbita, exiting the orbit through the superior orbital fissure above the common tendinous ring.

Lacrimal Nerve.   Sensory fibers from the lateral aspect of the upper eyelid and temple area come together and enter the lacrimal gland; they join the sensory fibers that serve the gland itself to form the **lacrimal nerve**. The lacrimal nerve leaves the gland and runs posteriorly along the upper border of the lateral rectus muscle (see Plate 12-1). It receives a branch from the zygomatic nerve containing the autonomic innervation of the lacrimal gland. The lacrimal nerve exits the orbit through the superior orbital fissure above the muscle cone.

Ophthalmic Nerve Formation

After exiting the orbit, the nasociliary nerve, the lacrimal nerve, and the frontal nerve join and form the ophthalmic

FIGURE 12-3. Posterior sclera. Posterior portion of globe, showing the optic nerve passing through the posterior scleral foramen, the long and short ciliary arteries and nerves passing through the posterior apertures, and the vortex veins passing through the middle apertures.

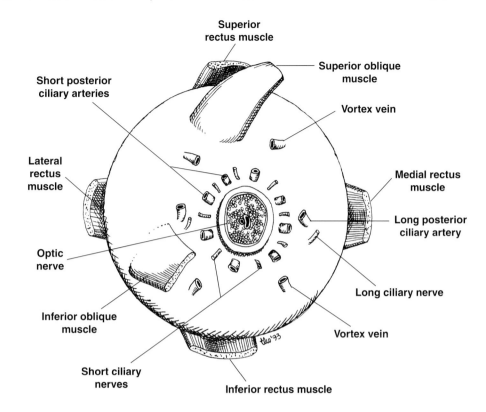

FIGURE 12-4. Palpebral nerves.

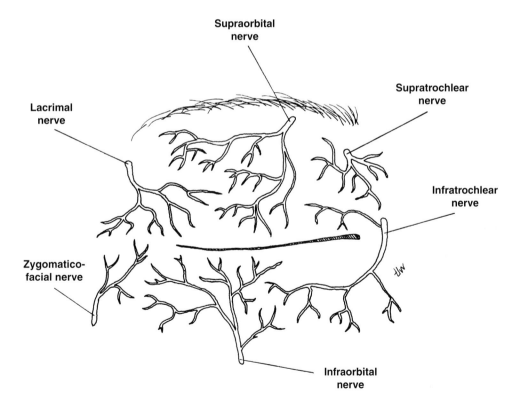

division of the trigeminal nerve (see Figure 12-1). The **ophthalmic nerve** then enters the lateral wall of the cavernous sinus. While within the wall of the sinus, the nerve receives sensory fibers from the oculomotor, trochlear, and abducens nerves. Some of these fibers probably carry proprioceptive information from the extraocular muscles.[10]

Maxillary Division of the Trigeminal Nerve

Branches of the maxillary division of the trigeminal nerve are shown in Plate 12-2.

Infraorbital Nerve. The **infraorbital nerve**, formed by sensory fibers from the cheek, upper lip, and lower eyelid, enters the maxillary bone through the infraorbital foramen. It runs posteriorly through the infraorbital canal and groove; while in the maxillary bone, branches join from the upper teeth and maxillary sinus. As the nerve leaves the infraorbital groove, it exits the orbit via the inferior orbital fissure and joins other fibers in forming the maxillary nerve.

✍ CLINICAL COMMENT: REFERRED PAIN
Referred pain is pain felt in an area remote from the actual site of involvement; however, the two areas usually are connected by a sensory nerve network. Frequently, the pathways of the trigeminal nerve are involved in referred pain. A common example is a momentary severe bilateral frontal headache sometimes experienced when an individual eats ice cream.[3] An abscessed tooth can cause pain described by a patient as ocular pain and should be suspected when no orbital cause for the pain can be found.

Zygomatic Nerve. Sensory fibers from the lateral aspect of the forehead enter the orbit through a foramen in the zygomatic bone as the zygomaticotemporal nerve. Fibers from the lateral aspect of the cheek and lower eyelid enter the orbit through a foramen in the zygomatic bone as the zygomaticofacial nerve.[9] These two nerves join to become the **zygomatic nerve** and course along the lateral orbital wall, exiting the orbit through the inferior orbital fissure and joining with the maxillary nerve (see Plate 12-2).

Maxillary Nerve Formation

Having been formed by the joining of the infraorbital nerve, the zygomatic nerve, and nerves from the roof of the mouth, the upper teeth and gums, and the mucous membranes of the cheek, the **maxillary nerve** traverses the area between the maxilla and the sphenoid bone. As it passes near the pterygopalatine fossa, it receives some autonomic fibers from the sphenopalatine ganglion (see Plate 12-2). (These autonomic fibers are destined for the lacrimal gland; they are discussed in Chapter 13.) The maxillary nerve enters the skull through the foramen rotundum.

Mandibular Division of the Trigeminal Nerve

The mandibular nerve innervates the lower face and contains both sensory and motor fibers. It enters the skull via the foramen ovale.

Trigeminal Nerve Formation

As these three divisions—the ophthalmic, maxillary, and mandibular—enter the skull, they run posteriorly within the lateral wall of the cavernous sinus[11, 12] (see Plate 12-1) and enter the **trigeminal ganglion (Gasserian ganglion, semilunar ganglion)**, where they synapse (Figure 12-5). The ganglion, flattened and semilunar in shape, is located lateral to the internal carotid artery and the posterior portion of the cavernous sinus. The motor fibers of the mandibular division, which innervate the muscles of mastication, pass along the lower edge of the ganglion.[13] Only the sensory fibers synapse within the ganglion.

The fibers leave the trigeminal ganglion and enter the lateral aspect of the pons as either the sensory root or the motor root of the trigeminal nerve. The sensory root carries information from the structures of the face and head, including all orbital structures. After entering the brain stem, these fibers form an ascending and a descending tract, both terminating in the sensory nuclei of the trigeminal nerve (see Figure 12-5). The ascending tract terminates in the principal sensory nucleus in the pons; it registers the sensations of touch and pressure.[1] The descending tract, which carries pain and temperature sensations, courses through the pons and medulla to the elongated nucleus of the spinal tract.[1] The tract extends into the second cervical segment of the spinal cord.[14] Information from the trigeminal nuclei is relayed to the thalamus.

✍ CLINICAL COMMENT: OCULOCARDIAC REFLEX
The oculocardiac reflex consists of bradycardia (slowed heart beat), nausea, and faintness and can be elicited by pressure on the globe or stretch on the extraocular muscles (e.g., during ocular surgery).[15–17] Fibers from the trigeminal spinal nucleus project into the reticular formation near the vagus nerve nuclei and can activate vagus synapses precipitating this reflex. The motor aspect of the reflex can be blocked by retrobulbar anesthesia or intravenous or intramuscular atropine.[1, 9, 18]

EFFERENT PATHWAY: MOTOR NERVES

The cranial nerves that supply striated muscles of the orbit and adnexa are the oculomotor nerve, the trochlear nerve,

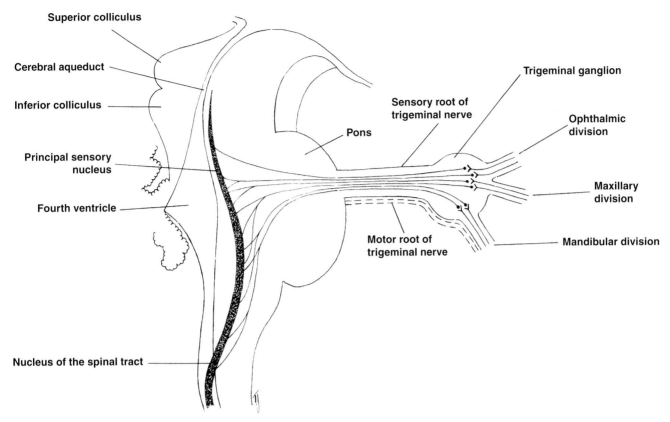

FIGURE 12-5. Sagittal section through brain stem, showing divisions, ganglion, motor and sensory roots, and nuclei of cranial nerve V.

the abducens nerve, and the facial nerve. The motor innervation within the orbit is shown in Plate 12-3.

Oculomotor Nerve: Cranial Nerve III

The **oculomotor nerve** innervates the superior rectus, the medial rectus, the inferior rectus, the inferior oblique, and the superior palpebral levator muscles. It also provides a route along which the autonomic fibers travel to innervate the iris sphincter muscle, the ciliary muscle, and the smooth muscles of the eyelid.

Oculomotor Nucleus

The **oculomotor nucleus** is located in the midbrain, ventral to the cerebral aqueduct, at the level of the superior colliculus (Figure 12-6). It extends in a column from the posterior edge of the floor of the third ventricle to the trochlear nucleus.[2, 9]

A definitive area or subnucleus within the oculomotor nucleus controls each muscle. The proposed arrangement of the subnuclei are postulated primarily on the basis of animal models.[18–21] The nucleus for the medial rectus is located toward the lower border of the oculomotor nucleus; the inferior rectus nucleus lies toward the upper border, with the nucleus for the inferior oblique between. The nucleus of the superior rectus lies in the medial and

caudal two-thirds of the oculomotor nucleus. Each of these subnuclei are found in the right and left oculomotor nucleus. The nucleus for the levator is single and is located centrally in the caudal area (Figure 12-7).

Fibers to the inferior rectus, the inferior oblique, and the medial rectus muscles supply the ipsilateral eye; fibers innervating the superior rectus muscle decussate and supply the contralateral eye. The decussating fibers pass through the opposite superior rectus nucleus; thus, damage to the right oculomotor nucleus might have bilateral superior rectus muscle involvement.[21–24] The centrally placed caudal nucleus provides innervation for both levator muscles.

An autonomic nucleus (the Edinger-Westphal nucleus) supplies parasympathetic innervation to the ciliary and iris sphincter muscles. It is located in the rostral, ventral portion of the oculomotor nucleus (see Figure 12-7).[24, 25]

Oculomotor Nerve Pathway

Fibers from each of the individual nuclei join, forming the fascicular part of the nerve that passes through the red nucleus and the cerebral peduncle. These fibers emerge from the interpeduncular fossa on the anterior aspect of the midbrain as the oculomotor nerve. The nerve passes between the superior cerebellar and poste-

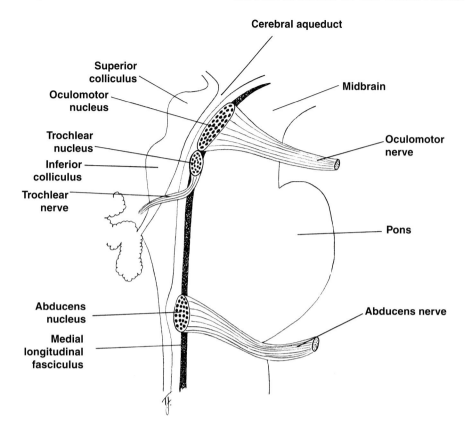

FIGURE 12-6. Sagittal section through brain stem, showing oculomotor, trochlear, and abducens nuclei.

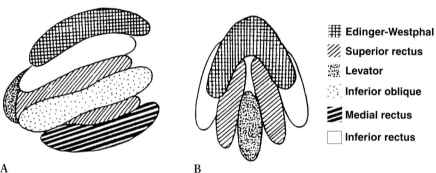

A   B

FIGURE 12-7. Oculomotor nerve nuclei. (A) Lateral view. (B) Dorsal view.

⊞ Edinger-Westphal
▨ Superior rectus
▥ Levator
⋰ Inferior oblique
◤ Medial rectus
☐ Inferior rectus

rior cerebral arteries as it runs forward, lateral to, and slightly inferior to the posterior communicating artery of the circle of Willis (Figure 12-8). The nerve pierces the roof of the cavernous sinus and runs within its lateral wall above the trochlear nerve (Figure 12-9).[2, 11] While in the cavernous sinus, the oculomotor nerve sends small sensory branches to the ophthalmic nerve and receives sympathetic fibers from the plexus around the internal carotid artery.[2, 14]

The oculomotor nerve exits the sinus and enters the orbit through the superior orbital fissure, having divided into a superior and inferior division; both are located within the oculomotor foramen. The superior branch runs medially above the optic nerve and enters the superior rectus on its inferior surface; additional fibers either pierce the muscle or pass around its border to innervate the levator (Figure 12-10).[26]

The inferior branch runs below the optic nerve and divides into three branches. One branch enters the medial rectus on its lateral surface, and one enters the inferior rectus on its upper surface. The third branch gives off parasympathetic fibers that form the parasympathetic root to the ciliary ganglion; then it runs along the lateral border of the inferior rectus, crossing it to enter the inferior oblique muscle near its midpoint (see Figure 12-10).[3, 27, 28]

Trochlear Nerve: Cranial Nerve IV

The **trochlear nerve** innervates the superior oblique muscle.

Trochlear Nucleus

The **trochlear nucleus** is located in the midbrain, anterior to the cerebral aqueduct and below the oculomo-

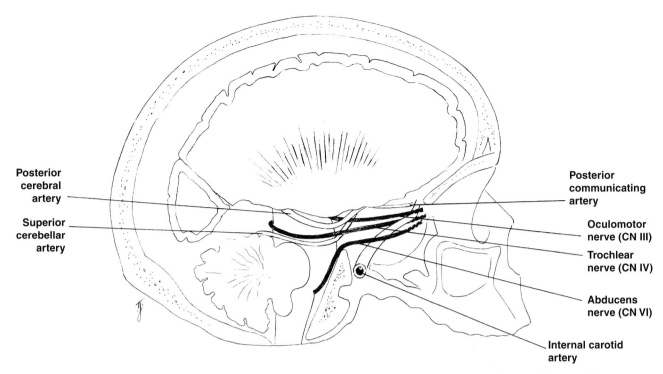

FIGURE 12-8. Sagittal section through brain, showing relationship between cranial nerves III, IV, and VI and the neighboring blood vessels.

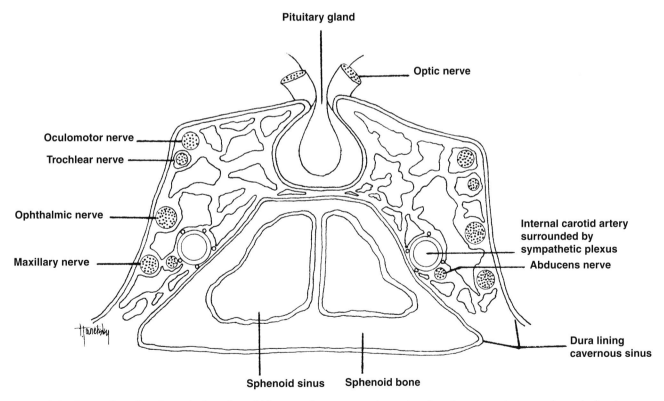

FIGURE 12-9. Coronal section through the sphenoid bone and cavernous sinus, showing the nerves that pass through the sinus en route to and from the orbit.

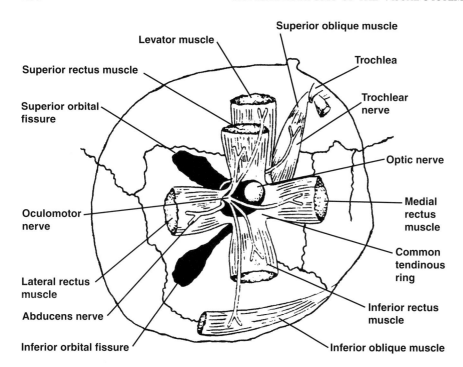

FIGURE 12-10. Orbital apex with the globe removed. The relationship between the superior orbital fissure and the common tendinous ring is shown.

tor nucleus, at the level of the inferior colliculus (see Figure 12-6). The fibers travel dorsally and decussate. CN IV is the only cranial nerve to cross; thus, the trochlear nucleus innervates the contralateral superior oblique muscle.

Trochlear Nerve Pathway

Of the cranial nerves, the trochlear nerve is the only one that leaves the dorsal aspect of the CNS. It is the most slender of the cranial nerves, and its attachment is very delicate. (The small diameter of the nerve probably reflects the fact that it supplies only one muscle, that muscle being the most slender of the extraocular muscles.) As the trochlear nerve emerges from the dorsal midbrain below the inferior colliculus, it decussates and curves around the cerebral peduncle at the upper border of the pons, approximately paralleling the superior cerebellar and posterior cerebral arteries. It passes between these two vessels and runs forward lateral to the oculomotor nerve (see Figure 12-8).

The trochlear nerve enters the wall of the cavernous sinus and lies between the oculomotor nerve and the ophthalmic division of the trigeminal (see Figure 12-9).[3, 11] While in the sinus, it sends sensory fibers to the ophthalmic nerve. It enters the orbit through the superior orbital fissure above the common tendinous ring, outside the muscle cone (see Figure 12-10). The trochlear nerve runs with the frontal nerve to the medial side of the orbit above the levator and superior

rectus muscles and enters the upper surface of the superior oblique muscle.[9]

Abducens Nerve: Cranial Nerve VI

The **abducens nerve** innervates the lateral rectus muscle.

Abducens Nucleus

The **abducens nucleus** is located near the midline of the pons beside the floor of the fourth ventricle (see Figure 12-6). The fibers from the nucleus pass through the pons and exit in the groove between the pons and the medulla oblongata.

Abducens Nerve Pathway

In its long, tortuous, intracranial course, the abducens nerve runs along the occipital bone at the base of the skull and up along the posterior slope of the petrous portion of the temporal bone, makes a sharp bend over the petrous ridge (see Figure 12-8), and enters the cavernous sinus.[3, 9, 29] Within the sinus, it lies near the lateral wall of the internal carotid artery[12] (see Figure 12-9); it gives off small branches, possibly proprioceptive fibers, to the ophthalmic nerve. The abducens nerve enters the orbit through the superior orbital fissure within the common tendinous ring and innervates the lateral rectus muscle on the medial surface (see Figure 12-10).

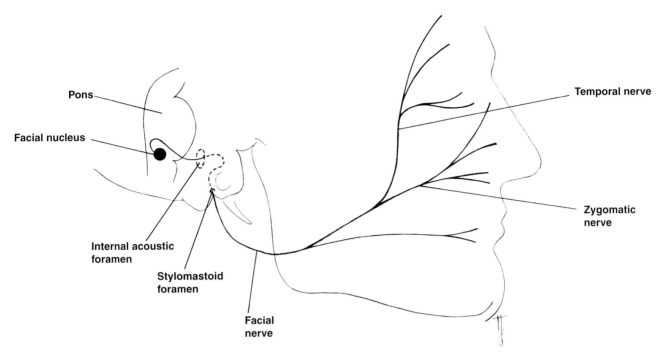

FIGURE 12-11. Facial nerve pathway. Motor pathway of facial nerve to orbital structures.

Superior Orbital Fissure

The trochlear, frontal, and lacrimal nerves and the superior ophthalmic vein are located in the superior orbital fissure *above* the muscle cone. The superior and inferior divisions of the oculomotor nerve, the abducens nerve, and the nasociliary nerve are located within the superior orbital fissure *and* the common tendinous ring. The inferior ophthalmic vein lies below the fissure and the tendinous ring (see Figure 8-8).

Control of Eye Movements

Communication among areas of the CNS is necessary to produce controlled and coordinated eye movements. The **corticonuclear tract** contains fibers that run from the cerebral hemispheres to the nuclei of CNs III, IV, and VI; the **tectobulbar tract** connects the superior colliculus to the CNs III, IV, and VI nuclei. The **medial longitudinal fasciculus** extends from the midbrain into the spinal cord and connects the vestibular nucleus, the oculomotor nucleus, the abducens nucleus, and the trochlear nucleus, providing a connection between eye movement control and the vestibular apparatus (see Figure 12-6).

Facial Nerve: Cranial Nerve VII

The **facial nerve** has two roots; the large motor root innervates the facial muscles, and the smaller root contains sensory and parasympathetic fibers. The sensory fibers carry taste sensations from the tongue. The parasympathetic nerves supply secretomotor fibers to various glands of the face; those supplying the lacrimal gland are discussed in Chapter 13.

Facial Nucleus

The motor nucleus of the facial nerve is located in the reticular formation of the pons. The upper segment of the nucleus supplies the frontalis, procerus, corrugator superciliaris, and orbicularis muscles, and the lower segment supplies the remaining facial muscles.[30, 31]

Facial Nerve Pathway

The fibers leave the facial nucleus, arch around the abducens nucleus, and emerge as the facial nerve from the brainstem at the lower border of the pons. The facial nerve enters the internal acoustic foramen in the petrous portion of the temporal bone and runs through a canal within the bone. While in the temporal bone, parasympathetic fibers en route to the lacrimal gland are given off as the greater petrosal nerve.[30, 31] The motor fibers of the facial nerve emerge through the stylomastoid foramen, pass below the external auditory canal, travel over the mandibular ramus, and divide into several branches (Figure 12-11). The upper two—the temporal and zygomatic branches—supply the frontalis, procerus, corrugator, and orbicularis muscles.

✍ CLINICAL COMMENT: CRANIAL NERVE DAMAGE
Injury to sensory cranial nerve fibers results in anesthesia, a loss of sensation in the innervated area.

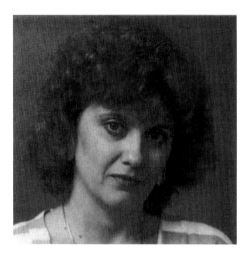

FIGURE 12-12. Patient tilts head toward the left shoulder and turns head to the left and down, owing to right superior oblique dysfunction. (Reprinted with permission from JB Eskridge. Evaluation and diagnosis of incomitant ocular deviations. J Am Optom Assoc 1989;60[5]:378.)

Injury to a cranial motor nerve causes either a partial loss (paresis) or a total loss (paralysis) of muscle function. Paresis or paralysis of an extraocular muscle can result in diplopia if the involvement is acquired; in congenital involvement, diplopia usually is not a complaint, because the brain has learned to disregard the double image, resulting in suppression.

Nerve fibers can be damaged by a compromise of the blood supply caused by vascular diseases, such as hypertension, atherosclerosis, or diabetes mellitus, or by space-occupying lesions, such as aneurysms, hemorrhages, or tumors, that exert pressure on the nerve fibers. The location of the involvement will influence the presenting signs and symptoms.

In various studies of isolated extraocular nerve paralysis, the sixth cranial nerve was reported to be affected most often, and the fourth cranial nerve was affected least often.[32, 33] The tortuosity and length of the abducens nerve make it susceptible to compression and stretching injuries and may explain why it is damaged so frequently.[11]

A number of clinical signs and symptoms accompany damage to the motor nerves that innervate the extraocular muscles. Muscle paresis or paralysis will be evident in testing ocular motility (as described in Chapter 10). In acquired extraocular muscle impairment, a patient often attempts to minimize diplopia by carrying the head in a compensatory position. If a horizontal deviation is present, the head will be turned to the right or left. With a vertical deviation, the head is raised or lowered and, if a torsional deviation occurs, the head is tilted toward the shoulder. With right superior

oblique involvement, the head will be turned to the left, positioned down, and tilted toward the left shoulder (Figure 12-12).[34, 35]

✍ CLINICAL COMMENT: OCULOMOTOR DAMAGE

Midbrain Involvement

A lesion in the midbrain can affect the entire oculomotor nucleus or selectively affect only some subnuclei; however, such definitive damage is unusual.[22] If the lesion affects the entire oculomotor nucleus, the muscles involved are the ipsilateral medial rectus, inferior rectus, and inferior oblique, the contralateral superior rectus, and both levator muscles. The ipsilateral superior rectus might be involved also, as the decussating fibers pass through the contralateral superior rectus nucleus.[22] The trochlear nucleus is near the oculomotor nucleus, and if it too is involved, the contralateral superior oblique muscle will be involved.

Intracranial Involvement

The oculomotor nerve lies near several blood vessels in its intracranial path and frequently is involved in an aneurysm of the posterior communicating artery.[36] An aneurysm of the superior cerebellar artery or the posterior cerebral artery could impinge also on the nerve, damaging fibers.

Once the oculomotor nerve exits the midbrain, all its fibers supply the ipsilateral eye, and the dysfunction is unilateral. Damage to the nerve results in ptosis because of paralysis of the levator; in primary position, the eye is positioned out, owing to the unopposed action of the superior oblique and lateral rectus muscles (Figure 12-13). (As the superior oblique muscle is unaffected, the eye also should be positioned down, but clinically this is not always evident.[37]) The eye cannot adduct and, in the abducted position, cannot move up or down (Figure 12-14).[2] In paralysis of the iris sphincter and ciliary muscle, the pupil will be dilated, and accommodation will not occur.

Incomplete lesions of the oculomotor nerve are possible. In external ophthalmoplegia, the extraocular muscles are paralyzed, and the intrinsic muscles are spared; internal ophthalmoplegia occurs when the internal muscles are paralyzed and the extraocular muscles are spared. Sparing of the circumferential portion of the nerve may account for normal pupillary responses usually seen with diabetic ophthalmoplegia.[22, 38, 39]

Cavernous Sinus Involvement

The lateral wall of the cavernous sinus contains the oculomotor nerve as well as the trochlear, ophthalmic, and maxillary nerves. A lesion that affects all these nerves would leave only the lateral rectus

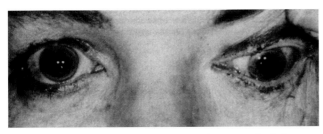

FIGURE 12-13. Complete third-nerve palsy. Note the left ptosis, exotropia, hypotropia, and dilated pupil. (Reprinted with permission from JD Bartlett, SD Jaanus. Clinical Ocular Pharmacology [2nd ed]. Boston: Butterworth–Heinemann, 1989;449.)

muscle still functioning. The eye would be positioned out in primary gaze and could move only from the lateral position to the midline. Anesthesia of the areas of the face served by the ophthalmic and maxillary nerves would be present in addition to the impaired ocular motility.

Orbital Involvement

Both divisions of the oculomotor nerve are located within the muscle cone, together with the abducens and nasociliary nerves. A retrobulbar tumor or inflammation involving these nerves would leave only the superior oblique muscle functional. In primary position, the eye would be positioned downward and outward slightly and would be fairly immobile. Decreased corneal sensitivity could be present, owing to nasociliary nerve involvement.

FIGURE 12-14. Third-nerve paralysis. Right-sided paralysis of (A) levator palpebrae (ptosis), (B) medial rectus, (C) inferior rectus, and (D) superior rectus muscles. (Reprinted with permission from DG Cogan. Neurology of the Ocular Muscles [2nd ed]. Springfield, IL: Thomas, 1972;59.)

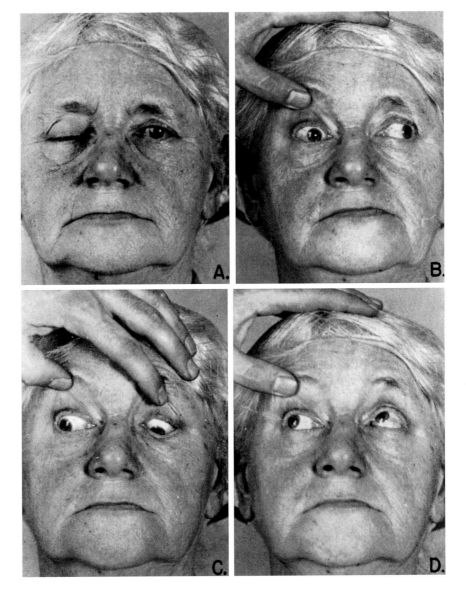

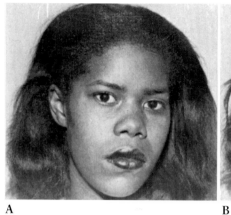
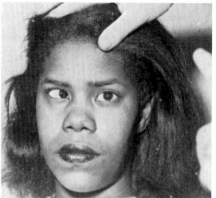

A   B

FIGURE 12-15. Paralysis of the left lateral rectus muscle showing (A) compensatory turning to the left and (B) inability to turn the left eye to the left. (Reprinted with permission from DG Cogan. Neurology of the Ocular Muscles [2nd ed]. Springfield, IL: Thomas, 1972;79.)

✍ CLINICAL COMMENT: TROCHLEAR DAMAGE

When the superior oblique muscle is affected by trochlear nerve damage, the eye is elevated in primary gaze and is unable to move down in the adducted position. The head may be tilted toward the opposite shoulder to compensate for the unopposed extortion of the inferior oblique muscle (see Figure 12-12).[3] The condition that most often affects CN IV is trauma.[40, 41]

Midbrain Involvement

Damage to the trochlear nucleus will affect the contralateral superior oblique muscle. Due to the proximity of the oculomotor nucleus, a lesion could affect both cranial nerve nuclei.

Intracranial Involvement

For the most part, the trochlear nerve follows the same path as that followed by the oculomotor nerve and is susceptible to the same injuries. Damage to the trochlear nerve affects the ipsilateral superior oblique muscle.

Cavernous Sinus Involvement

A lesion in the lateral wall of the cavernous sinus could affect the trochlear nerve. It could affect also the oculomotor, ophthalmic, and maxillary nerves.

Orbital Involvement

The trochlear nerve lies above the muscle cone near the frontal nerve, and injury affecting both could impair the superior oblique muscle and cause decreased sensitivity of the areas of the skin and scalp innervated by the branches of the frontal nerve.

✍ CLINICAL COMMENT: ABDUCENS DAMAGE

Damage to the abducens nerve results in paralysis of the lateral rectus muscle; because of the unopposed action of the medial rectus muscle, a convergent strabismus is evident.[42] The eye will be unable to abduct (Figure 12-15). The patient might try to compensate for the diplopia by turning the face toward the paralyzed side.[3]

Pons Involvement

Both the abducens and facial nuclei are located in the pons, and the fasciculus of the facial nucleus arches around the abducens nucleus. Damage here could affect the lateral rectus and the muscles of the forehead and the orbicularis. Symptoms might include inability to abduct the eye and an incomplete closure of the eyelid.

Intracranial Involvement

The tortuous course of the abducens nerve renders it particularly susceptible to increased intracranial pressure that causes the brainstem to be displaced posteriorly, stretching the nerve over the bony prominence of the temporal bone.[9, 29, 32] Fractures of the base of the skull and aneurysms of the basilar and carotid arteries can involve the abducens nerve.

Cavernous Sinus Involvement

The abducens nerve is located near the internal carotid artery within the cavernous sinus. Often, it is the first nerve affected with an aneurysm of that vessel.

Orbital Involvement

The abducens nerve is located within the muscle cone. It accompanies the two divisions of the oculomotor and the nasociliary nerve (as discussed previously).

REFERENCES

1. Burton H. Somatic Sensations from the Eye. In WM Hart Jr (ed), Adler's Physiology of the Eye (9th ed). St. Louis: Mosby, 1992;71.

2. Warwick R. Eugene Wolff's Anatomy of the Eye and Orbit (7th ed). Philadelphia: Saunders, 1976;275.

3. Wirtschafter JD. The Peripheral Courses of the Third, Fourth, Fifth, Sixth, and Seventh Cranial Nerves. In MJ Reeh, JL Wobig, JD Wirtschafter (eds), Ophthalmic Anatomy. San Francisco: American Academy of Ophthalmology, 1981;234.

4. Catania LJ. Primary Care of the Anterior Segment. East Norwalk, CT: Appleton & Lange, 1988;74.

5. Berkow R (ed). The Merck Manual (14th ed). Rahway, NJ: Merck, 1982;187.

6. Bartlett JD, Jaanus SD. Clinical Ocular Pharmacology (2nd ed). Boston: Butterworth–Heinemann, 1989;544.

7. Schlaegel TF. Uveitis Associated with Viral Infections. In TD Duane, EA Jaeger (eds), Clinical Ophthalmology. Philadelphia: Harper & Row, 1982;10.

8. Kanski JJ. Clinical Ophthalmology (3rd ed). London: Butterworth–Heinemann, 1994;111.

9. Doxanas MT, Anderson RL. Clinical Orbital Anatomy. Baltimore: Williams & Wilkins, 1984;131.

10. Feldon SE, Burde RM. The Oculomotor System. In WM Hart Jr (ed), Adler's Physiology of the Eye (9th ed). St. Louis: Mosby, 1992;134.

11. Umansky J, Nathan H. The lateral wall of the cavernous sinus: with special reference to the nerves related to it. J Neurosurg 1982;56:228.

12. Nuza AB, Taner D. Anatomical variations of the intracavernous branches of the internal carotid artery with reference to the relationship of the internal carotid artery and sixth cranial nerve. Acta Anat 1990;138:238.

13. Beck RW, Smith CH. Trigeminal Nerve. In W Tasman, EA Jaeger (eds), Duane's Foundations of Clinical Ophthalmology (Vol 1). Philadelphia: Lippincott, 1994;1.

14. Warwick R, Williams PL (eds). Gray's Anatomy (35th ed). Philadelphia: Saunders, 1973;1001, 1006.

15. Stott DG. Reflex bradycardia in facial surgery. Br J Plast Surg 1989;42(5):595.

16. Eustis HS, Eiswirth CC, Smith DR. Vagal responses to adjustable sutures in strabismus correction. Am J Ophthalmol 1992;114(3):307.

17. Hampl KF, Marsch SC, Schneider M, et al. Vasovagal heart block following cataract surgery under local anesthesia. Ophthalmic Surg 1993;24(6):422.

18. Chong JL, Tan SH. Oculocardiac reflex in strabismus surgery under general anesthesia. Singapore Med J 1990;31(1):38.

19. Warwick R. Representation of the extraocular muscles in the oculomotor nucleus of the monkey. J Comp Neurol 1953;98:449.

20. Warwick R. Oculomotor Organization. In MB Bender, The Oculomotor System. New York: Harper & Row, 1964;173.

21. Castro O, Johnson LN, Mamourian AC. Isolated inferior oblique paresis from brain stem infarction.

22. Brazis PW. Localization of lesions of the oculomotor nerve: recent concepts. Mayo Clin Proc 1991;66(10):1029.

23. Bienfans DC. Crossing axons in the third nerve nucleus. Invest Ophthalmol 1975;12:927.

24. Marinkovic S, Marinkovic Z, Filipovic B. The oculomotor nuclear complex in humans. Microanatomy and clinical significance. Neurology 1989;38(2):135.

25. Jampel RS, Mindel J. The nucleus for accommodation in the midbrain of the macaque. Invest Ophthalmol 1967;6:40.

26. Sacks JG. Peripheral innervation of the extraocular muscles. Am J Ophthalmol 1983;95:520.

27. Krewson W. Comparison of the oblique extraocular muscles. Arch Ophthalmol 1944;32:204.

28. Reeh MJ, Wobig JL, Wirtschafter JD. Ophthalmic Anatomy. San Francisco: American Academy of Ophthalmology, 1981;75.

29. Umansky F, Valarezo A, Elidan J. The microsurgical anatomy of the abducens nerve in its intracranial course. J Neurosurg 1991;75(2):294.

30. Monkhouse WS. The anatomy of the facial nerve. Ear Nose Throat J 1990;69:677.

31. Proctor B. The anatomy of the facial nerve. Otolaryngol Clin North Am 1991;24:479.

32. Rucker CW. The causes of paralysis of the third, fourth, and sixth cranial nerves. Am J Ophthalmol 1966;63:1293.

33. Rush JA, Younge BR. Paralysis of cranial nerves III, IV, and VI. Arch Ophthalmol 1981;99:76.

34. Eskridge JB. Evaluation and diagnosis of incomitant ocular deviations. J Am Optom Assoc 1989;60(5):375.

35. Rubin MM. Trochlear nerve palsy simulating an orbital blowout fracture. J Oral Maxillofac Surg 1992;50:1238.

36. Troost BT, Glaser JS. Aneurysms, Arteriovenous Communications and Related Vascular Malformations. In JS Glaser (ed), Neuro-Ophthalmology. Hagerstown, MD: Harper & Row, 1978;319.

37. Jampel RS. Ocular torsion and the function of the vertical extraocular muscles. Am J Ophthalmol 1975;79:292.

38. Goldstein JE, Cogan DG. Diabetic ophthalmoplegia with special reference to the pupil. Arch Ophthalmol 1960;64:592.

39. Gray LG. A clinical guide to third nerve palsy. Rev Optom 1994;1:86.

40. Burger LJ. Kalvin NH, Smith JL. Acquired lesions of the fourth cranial nerve. Brain 1970;93:567.

41. Young BR, Sutla F. Analysis of trochlear nerve palsies. Diagnosis, etiology, and treatment. Mayo Clin Proc 1977;52:11.

42. Galetta SL, Smith JL. Chronic isolated sixth nerve palsies. Arch Neurol 1989;46:79.

Arch Neurol 1990;47:235.

SUGGESTED READING

Warwick R, Williams PL (eds). Gray's Anatomy (35th ed). Philadelphia: Saunders, 1973;998.

Wobig JL. The Orbital Nerves. In MJ Reeh, JL Wobig, JD Wirtschafter (eds), Ophthalmic Anatomy. San Francisco: American Academy of Ophthalmology, 1981;73.

Tiffin P, MacEwen C, Craig E, et al. Acquired palsy of the oculomotor, trochlear, and abducens nerves. Eye 1996;10:377.

Autonomic Innervation of Ocular Structures

The autonomic nervous system innervates smooth muscles, glands, and heart, and consists of two parts: the sympathetic system, which, when stimulated, prepares the body to face an emergency, and the parasympathetic system, which maintains and restores the resting state. Balance is maintained between these two systems and is particularly evident in those structures innervated by both. The ocular structures innervated by the autonomic nervous system are the iris muscles, the ciliary muscle, the smooth muscles of the eyelids, the choroidal and conjunctival blood vessels, and the lacrimal gland.

AUTONOMIC PATHWAY

The sympathetic pathway originates in the lateral gray column of the thoracic and upper lumbar segments (T-1 through L-2) of the spinal cord; sympathetic innervation for ocular structures originates in segments T-1 through T-3. The parasympathetic pathway originates in the midbrain, pons, medulla, and sacral spinal cord; parasympathetic innervation of ocular structures originates in the midbrain and pons.

The autonomic efferent pathway consists of two neurons. The cell body of the first, the preganglionic neuron, is located in the brain or spinal cord, whereas the cell body of the second, the postganglionic neuron, is in a ganglion outside the central nervous system. The preganglionic fiber, which generally is myelinated, terminates in an autonomic ganglion, where a synapse occurs. The postganglionic fiber, which usually is nonmyelinated, exits the ganglion and innervates the target structure. Sympathetic ganglia usually are located near the spinal column, whereas parasympathetic ganglia are located near the target structure.

Ocular structures supplied by the sympathetic system are the iris dilator, the smooth muscle of the lids, the lacrimal gland, and the choroidal and conjunctival blood vessels. Many investigators have documented sympathetic innervation to the ciliary muscle as well.[1-5] Ocular structures supplied by the parasympathetic system are the iris sphincter, the ciliary muscle, the lacrimal gland, and the choroidal blood vessels. Plates 11-1, 12-2, and 12-3 show the sympathetic and parasympathetic pathways to the orbital structures.

Sympathetic Pathway to Ocular Structures

Sympathetic fibers are controlled by the hypothalamus via a pathway that terminates in the lateral column of the cervical spinal cord. The fiber from the preganglionic neuron leaves the spinal cord in the vicinity of T-1 to T-3 through the ventral root and enters the sympathetic ganglion chain located adjacent to the vertebrae (Figure 13-1). These **preganglionic fibers** then ascend in the sympathetic chain to a synapse in the **superior cervical ganglion**, located near the second and third vertebrae.[6, 7]

The **postganglionic fibers** leave the ganglion, form the carotid plexus around the internal carotid artery, and enter the skull through the carotid canal. The network of fine sympathetic fibers destined for orbital structures leaves the plexus in the cavernous sinus and takes multiple pathways to the target structures. Those most commonly described in the literature will be presented here.

Some of these sympathetic fibers travel with the ophthalmic division of the trigeminal nerve from the cavernous sinus into the orbit.[8] Once in the orbit, the sympathetic fibers follow the nasociliary nerve and then

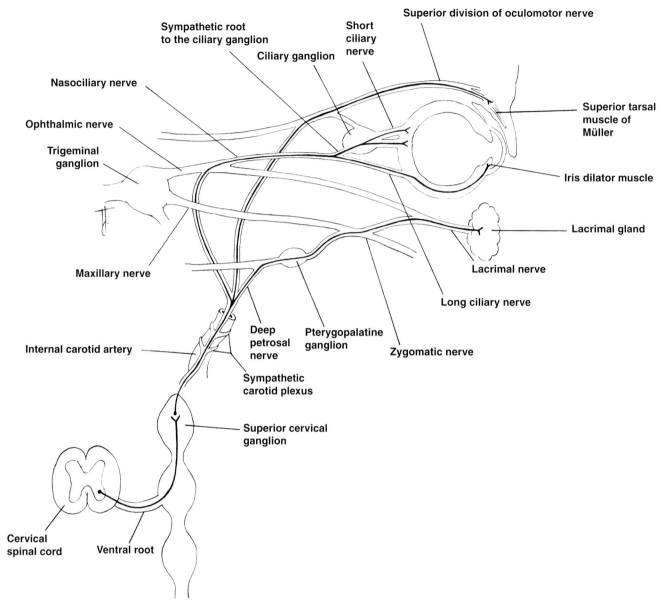

FIGURE 13-1. Sympathetic innervation to ocular structures.

travel with the long ciliary nerves to innervate the iris dilator and the ciliary muscle (see Figure 13-1).[8–11]

Other fibers from the carotid plexus follow this same route to the nasociliary nerve and then branch to the ciliary ganglion as the sympathetic root; these fibers pass through the ganglion without synapsing. They enter the globe as the short ciliary nerves to innervate the choroidal blood vessels. Alternately, the sympathetic root to the ciliary ganglion may emanate directly from the internal carotid plexus. The pathway to the conjunctival vasculature may be via either the long or short ciliary nerves.

Still other fibers from the carotid plexus join the oculomotor nerve and travel with it into the orbit to innervate the smooth muscle of the upper eyelid. These fibers follow the same path as the superior division of the oculomotor nerve (see Figure 13-1).[8]

Sympathetic stimulation activates the iris dilator, causing pupillary dilation and thereby increasing retinal illumination, and exhibits a small inhibitory effect on the ciliary muscle in some people.[1–3, 5, 12, 13] It also causes vasoconstriction of the choroidal and conjunctival vessels and widening of the palpebral fissure by stimulating the smooth muscle of the eyelids.

Parasympathetic Pathway to Ocular Structures

The preganglionic neuron in the parasympathetic pathway to the intrinsic ocular muscles is located in the midbrain in the **parasympathetic accessory third-nerve nucleus**, also called the **Edinger-Westphal nucleus**. The **preganglionic fibers** leave the nucleus with the motor

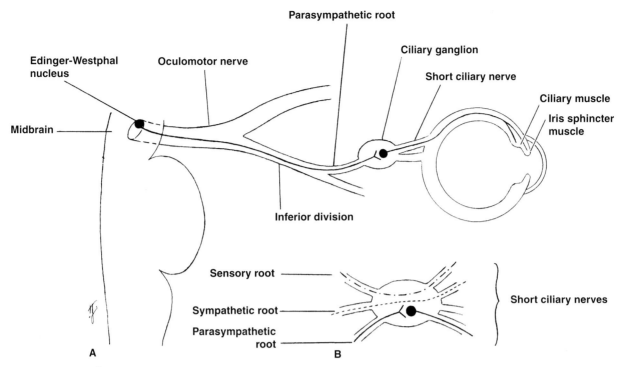

FIGURE 13-2. (A) Parasympathetic innervation to the ciliary muscle and iris sphincter muscle. (B) Sensory, sympathetic, and parasympathetic fibers are found in the ciliary ganglion, though only the parasympathetic fibers synapse. Each short ciliary nerve carries the three types of fibers.

fibers of the oculomotor nerve and follow the inferior division of that nerve into the orbit.[14] The parasympathetic fibers leave the inferior division and enter the ciliary ganglion as the parasympathetic root (Figure 13-2).[15-17]

The **ciliary ganglion** is a small, somewhat flat structure, 2 mm long and 1 mm high, located within the muscle cone between the lateral rectus muscle and the optic nerve, approximately 1 cm anterior to the optic canal.[9, 18] Three roots are located at the ganglion's posterior edge: the parasympathetic root, described earlier; the sensory root, which carries sensory fibers from the globe and joins with the nasociliary nerve; and the sympathetic root, which supplies the choroidal blood vessels. Only the parasympathetic fibers synapse in the ciliary ganglion; the sensory and sympathetic fibers pass through without synapsing (see Figure 13-2).

The short ciliary nerves, located at the anterior edge of the ciliary ganglion, carry sensory, sympathetic, and parasympathetic fibers. The **postganglionic parasympathetic fibers**, which are myelinated,[15] exit the ganglion in the short ciliary nerves, enter the globe, and travel to the anterior segment of the eye to innervate the sphincter and ciliary muscles. Most of the fibers innervate the ciliary body; only approximately 3% supply the iris sphincter.[15, 16]

Parasympathetic stimulation causes pupillary constriction, thus decreasing retinal illumination and reducing chromatic and spherical aberrations. It also causes contraction of the ciliary muscle, enabling the eye to focus on near objects in accommodation.

✐ CLINICAL COMMENT: IRIS EQUILIBRIUM
The iris contains muscles innervated by both autonomic systems. The parasympathetic system innervates the sphincter, and the sympathetic system innervates the dilator. The size of the pupil changes constantly, reflecting this balance. For instance, during sleep, the pupils are small because the sympathetic system shuts down and the parasympathetic system predominates.

✐ CLINICAL COMMENT: INHIBITION
OF CILIARY MUSCLE
The parasympathetic innervation of the ciliary body and parasympathetic control of accommodation is widely accepted. However, the concept of dual innervation, though still somewhat controversial, has been documented,[19, 20] and many investigators, using pharmacologic,[21, 22] electrophysiologic,[23] and anatomic[15, 24, 25] evidence, have demonstrated the presence of both sympathetic receptors and fibers in animals and humans. The sympathetic effect appears

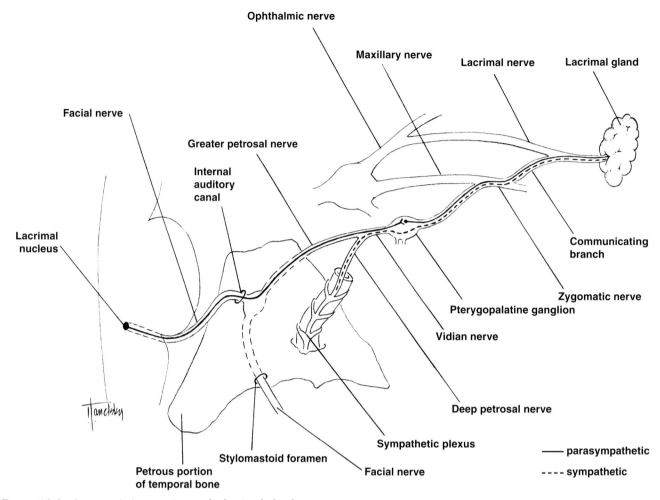

FIGURE 13-3. Autonomic innervation to the lacrimal gland.

to be a small, slow inhibition that is a function of the level of parasympathetic activity.[1–5, 13]

Autonomic Innervation to the Lacrimal Gland

The efferent autonomic pathway to the lacrimal gland follows a complex route. Fibers controlling the parasympathetic innervation originate in the lacrimal nucleus of the pons. These preganglionic fibers exit the pons with the motor fibers of the facial nerve, enter the internal auditory canal, and pass through the geniculate ganglion of the facial nerve without synapsing. They leave the ganglion as the **greater petrosal nerve**, which exits the petrous portion of the temporal bone.[26] The greater petrosal nerve is joined by the **deep petrosal nerve**, composed of sympathetic postganglionic fibers from the carotid plexus. The greater petrosal and the deep petrosal nerves together form the **vidian nerve (nerve of the pterygoid canal)** (Figure 13-3).

The vidian nerve enters the pterygopalatine ganglion, where the parasympathetic fibers synapse. The **ptery-** gopalatine ganglion (also called the **sphenopalatine ganglion**) lies in the upper portion of the pterygopalatine fossa (see Plate 11-1). It is a parasympathetic ganglion because it contains parasympathetic cell bodies and synapses; sympathetic fibers pass through without synapsing.

The autonomic fibers (all of which are now postganglionic) leave the ganglion, join with the maxillary branch of the trigeminal nerve, pass into the zygomatic nerve, and then form a communicating branch to the lacrimal nerve (see Figure 13-3). An alternate pathway bypasses the zygomatic nerve and travels from the ganglion directly to the gland.[27] The parasympathetic fibers that innervate the lacrimal gland are of the secretomotor type and so cause increased secretion. The sympathetic fibers innervate the blood vessels of the gland and cause vasoconstriction. Sympathetic stimulation might indirectly cause decreased production of lacrimal gland secretion owing to the restricted blood flow. Parasympathetic stimulation causes increased lacrimation. (A flowchart of the common autonomic nervous pathways to orbital structures is shown in Figure 13-4.)

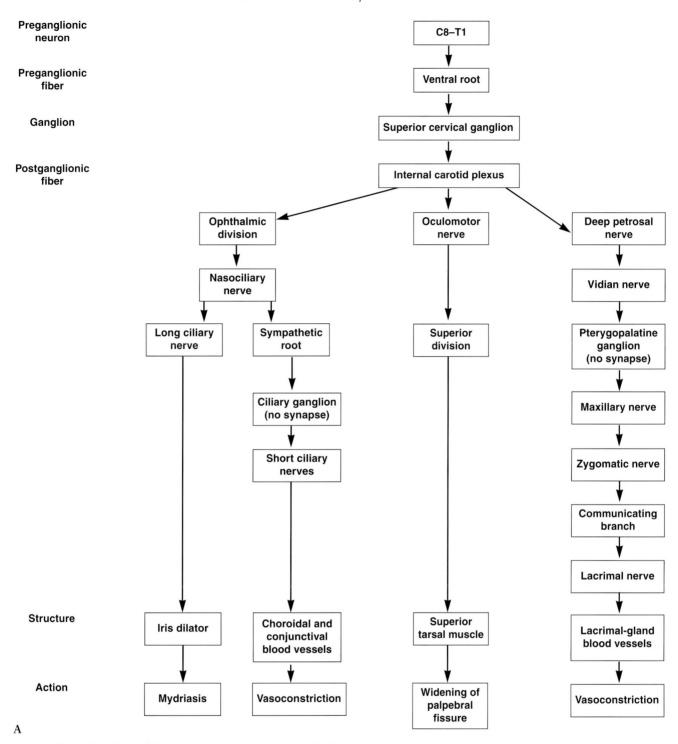

FIGURE 13-4. Flowchart of the autonomic nervous system. (A) Sympathetic innervation.

Sympathetic fibers from the zygomatic nerve also branch into the lower eyelid to innervate Müller's muscle of the lower lid.[28]

Parasympathetic innervation to the choroidal blood vessels is believed to emanate directly from the sphenopalatine ganglion via a network of fine nerves, the rami oculares.[29] Parasympathetic activation presumably causes vasodilation, which might raise intraocular pressure.[27, 30]

Irritation of any branch of the trigeminal nerve activates a reflex afferent pathway, precipitating increased lacrimation.[7, 31]

✍ CLINICAL COMMENT: CORNEAL REFLEX
Corneal touch will initiate the three-part corneal reflex: lacrimation, miosis, and a protective blink (Figure 13-5). The pain sensation elicited by the

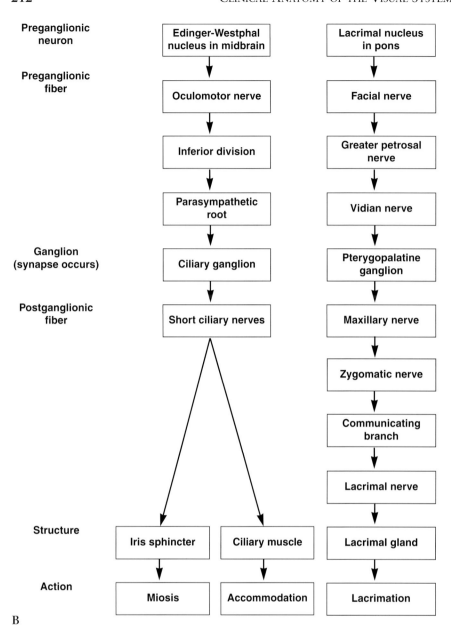

FIGURE 13-4. *(continued)* (B) Parasympathetic innervation.

touch travels to the trigeminal ganglion. Communication from the trigeminal ganglion to the Edinger-Westphal nucleus causes activation of the sphincter muscle. Communication to the facial nerve nucleus activates the motor pathway to the orbicularis muscle, causing the blink, and communication to the lacrimal nucleus and the parasympathetic pathway to the lacrimal gland stimulates increased lacrimation (see Figure 13-5).

PHARMACOLOGIC RESPONSES OF THE INTRINSIC MUSCLES

Pharmacologic agents can alter autonomic responses. Topical ophthalmic drugs, which readily pass through the cornea, can be used to activate the intrinsic ocular muscles. A brief, basic discussion of neurotransmitters and drug types, relative to iris musculature, will be presented. Specific drugs that induce mydriasis or miosis, and those used in the differential diagnosis of certain pupillary abnormalities will be discussed. Nonetheless, the reader is encouraged to review a text on pharmacology for complete, detailed information.

Neurotransmitters

When an action potential reaches the terminal end of an axon, a neurotransmitter is released that activates either the next fiber in the pathway or the target structure, the effector. In the sympathetic pathway, the neurotransmitter released by the preganglionic fiber is **acetylcholine** and the neurotransmitter released by the postganglionic

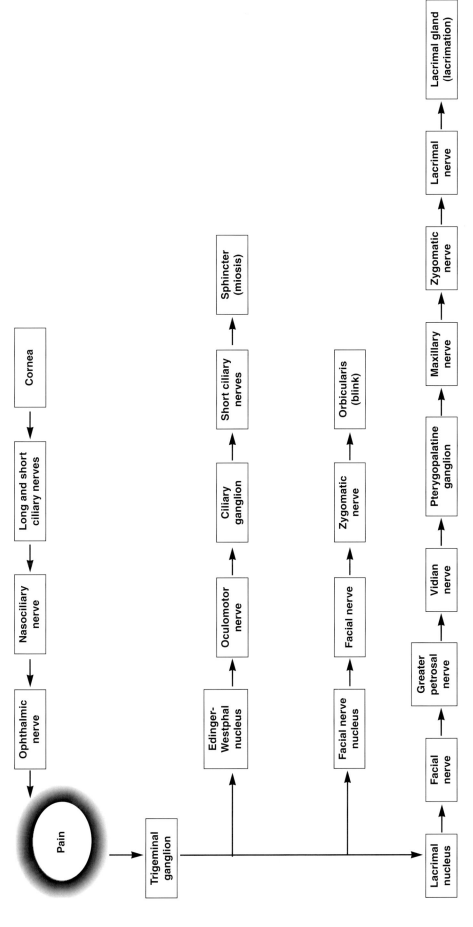

FIGURE 13-5. Pathways involved when pain from the cornea results in the reflex actions of miosis, blink, and lacrimation.

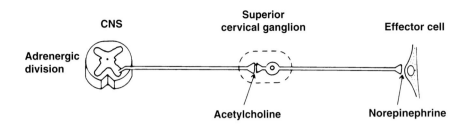

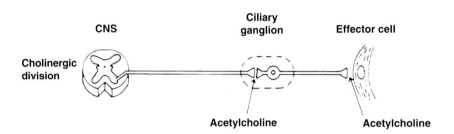

FIGURE 13-6. Autonomic neurotransmitters at their sites of action. (CNS = central nervous system.) (Reprinted with permission from JD Bartlett, SD Jaanus. Clinical Ocular Pharmacology [2nd ed]. Boston: Butterworth–Heinemann, 1989;71.)

fiber is **norepinephrine**. In the parasympathetic system, both the preganglionic and postganglionic fibers secrete acetylcholine (Figure 13-6). Fibers that release acetylcholine are called **cholinergic** and fibers that release norepinephrine are called **adrenergic**.

The neurotransmitter binds to effector sites on the muscle and initiates a contraction. The neurotransmitter then is released from the muscle and either is inactivated or is taken back up by the nerve ending, thus preventing continual muscle spasm; further muscle contraction should occur only with another action potential and release of additional transmitter. At the cholinergic neuromuscular junction, cholinesterase hydrolyzes and inactivates acetylcholine; at the adrenergic neuromuscular junction, norepinephrine is recycled by being taken back up into the nerve ending.

Drugs: Agonists and Antagonists

A drug that replicates the action of a neurotransmitter is called an **agonist**. A **direct-acting agonist** usually is similar structurally to the transmitter and duplicates the action of the neurotransmitter by acting on the receptor sites of the effector. An **indirect-acting agonist** causes the action to occur either by exciting the nerve fiber, thereby causing release of the transmitter, or by preventing the recycling or re-uptake of the transmitter, thus allowing it to continue its activity. **Antagonists** either block the receptor sites or block the release of the neurotransmitter, thus preventing action of the effector.

Ophthalmic Agonist Agents

Epinephrine and phenylephrine are direct-acting adrenergic agonists that bind to sites on the dilator muscle,

causing contraction (Figure 13-7).[32] Hydroxyamphetamine and cocaine are indirect-acting adrenergic agonists. Hydroxyamphetamine causes the release of norepinephrine from the nerve ending, thus indirectly initiating muscle contraction. Cocaine prevents the re-uptake of norepinephrine by the nerve ending; thus, norepinephrine remains at the neuromuscular junction and can continue to activate the dilator (see Figure 13-7).[32]

Pilocarpine is a direct-acting cholinergic agonist that directly stimulates the sites on the iris sphincter and ciliary muscle, causing contraction (Figure 13-8).[32] Physostigmine is an indirect-acting cholinergic agonist that inhibits cholinesterase.[32] Therefore, acetylcholine is not broken down but remains in the junction, and the sphincter and ciliary muscle contraction continue in a spasm (see Figure 13-8).

Ophthalmic Antagonist Agents

Dapiprazole is an adrenergic antagonist that blocks receptor sites, thereby preventing norepinephrine from activating the dilator muscle. Atropine, cyclopentolate, and tropicamide are cholinergic antagonists that compete with acetylcholine by blocking sphincter and ciliary muscle sites, thereby inhibiting miosis and accommodation (Figure 13-9).[32]

✍ CLINICAL COMMENT: DRUG-INDUCED MYDRIASIS
  For maximum dilation to occur, the dilator muscle should be activated and the sphincter muscle should be inhibited. This end is achieved by the combination of a direct-acting adrenergic agonist with a cholinergic antagonist. A common procedure for a dilated fundus examination involves the use of 2.5% phenylephrine and 1% tropicamide. Phenylephrine-induced mydriasis

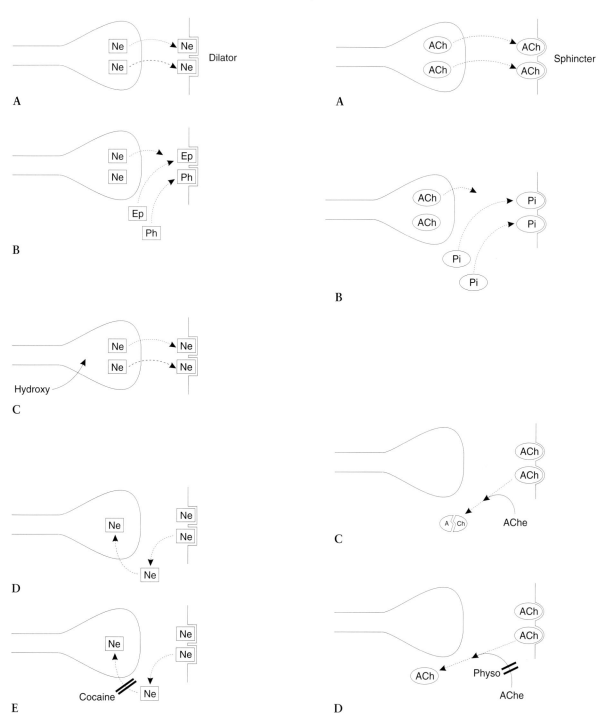

FIGURE 13-7. Adrenergic neuromuscular junction and actions of adrenergic agonists. (A) Norepinephrine (Ne) is released by the axon terminal and binds to sites on the iris dilator muscle, causing contraction. (B) Epinephrine (Ep) and phenylephrine (Ph) are direct-acting adrenergic agonists that bind to those same sites on the iris dilator muscle, causing contraction. (C) Hydroxyamphetamine (Hydroxy) is an indirect-acting adrenergic agonist that acts on the nerve fiber, causing the release of Ne. (D) Once it is released from the effector site, Ne is taken back up by the nerve ending. (E) Cocaine is an indirect-acting adrenergic agonist. It prevents the re-uptake of Ne, allowing it to remain in the neuromuscular junction and rebind to the effector site.

FIGURE 13-8. Cholinergic neuromuscular junction and actions of cholinergic agonists. (A) Acetylcholine (ACh) is released by the axon terminal and binds to the sites on the iris sphincter muscle, causing contraction. (B) Pilocarpine (Pi) is a direct-acting cholinergic agonist that binds to those sites on the iris sphincter muscle, causing contraction. (C) Once it is released from the effector site, ACh is broken down by acetylcholinesterase (AChe), which prevents it from rebinding to the site. (D) Physostigmine (Physo) is an indirect-acting cholinergic agonist. It inhibits AChe, allowing ACh to remain active in the neuromuscular junction.

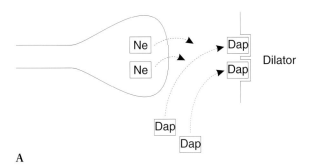

A

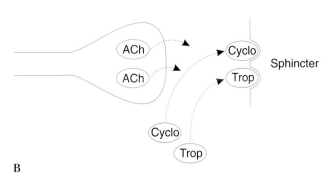

B

FIGURE 13-9. Actions of adrenergic and cholinergic antagonists at the neuromuscular junction. (A) Dapiprazole (Dap) is an adrenergic antagonist that blocks the receptor sites of the iris dilator muscle, preventing norepinephrine (Ne) from binding and causing muscle contraction. (B) Cyclopentolate (Cyclo) and tropicamide (Trop) are cholinergic antagonists that block the receptor sites of the iris sphincter muscle, preventing acetylcholine (ACh) from binding and causing muscle contraction.

can be reversed with dapiprazole, which blocks the dilator receptor sites and prevents phenylephrine activity.

ACCOMMODATION-CONVERGENCE REACTION (NEAR-POINT REACTION)

The **accommodation-convergence reaction** is not a true reflex but rather a synkinesis or an association of three occurrences: convergence, accommodation, and miosis. As an object is brought near along the midline, the medial rectus muscles contract to move the image onto the fovea; the ciliary muscle contracts to keep the near object in focus; and the sphincter muscle constricts to decrease the size of the pupil, thereby improving depth of field.

Each of these actions can occur without the others. If plus lenses are placed in front of each eye, pupillary constriction and convergence occur without accommodation. If a base-in prism is placed in front of each eye, pupillary constriction and accommodation occur without convergence.[33]

The afferent pathway for this reaction follows the visual pathway to the striate cortex. From the striate cortex, information is sent to the frontal eye fields, which communicate with the oculomotor nucleus and the Edinger-Westphal nucleus through the internal capsule (Figure 13-10). The efferent pathway, via the oculomotor nerve, innervates the medial rectus muscles, and the parasympathetic pathway innervates the ciliary muscle and iris sphincter.

PUPILLARY LIGHT PATHWAY

An understanding of the pupillary light pathway can be an important tool in diagnosing clinical problems with pupillary manifestations. Shining a bright light into an eye normally will initiate pupillary constriction. The afferent fibers that carry this information are called **pupillary fibers,** to distinguish them from visual fibers, which carry visual information. It remains uncertain whether there are two separate sets of fibers or whether the pupillary fibers are branches of the visual fibers.[33]

In either case, the afferent pupillary light pathway parallels the visual pathway as far as the posterior optic tract, with the nasal fibers crossing in the chiasm. The pupillary fibers exit in the posterior third of the optic tract and travel in the superior brachium to the **pretectal nucleus,** located in the midbrain near the superior colliculus. The fibers synapse, leave the pretectal nucleus, and travel to both Edinger-Westphal nuclei, being distributed approximately equally to both.[33] The tract carrying the fibers from the pretectal area to the oculomotor parasympathetic nucleus is the **tectotegmental tract.** The fibers that travel to the opposite Edinger-Westphal nucleus cross in the **posterior commissure** (Figure 13-11). Thus, the optic tract carries fibers from both eyes, and the tectotegmental tract carries fibers from both pretectal nuclei.

The efferent parasympathetic pathway from the Edinger-Westphal nucleus to the sphincter and ciliary muscles was described previously under *Parasympathetic Pathway to Ocular Structures.* As the third nerve leaves the midbrain, the pupillomotor fibers generally lie in a superior position, but as the nerve leaves the cavernous sinus and enters the orbit, the pupillomotor fibers move into an inferior position and travel in the inferior division of the oculomotor nerve.[33]

✍ CLINICAL COMMENT: THE PUPILLARY LIGHT RESPONSE

In assessment of the pupillary light pathway, both the direct response and the consensual response are tested. When a bright light is directed into the eye, both a direct response—constriction of the ipsilateral iris—and a consensual response—constriction of the contralateral iris—occur. The consensual

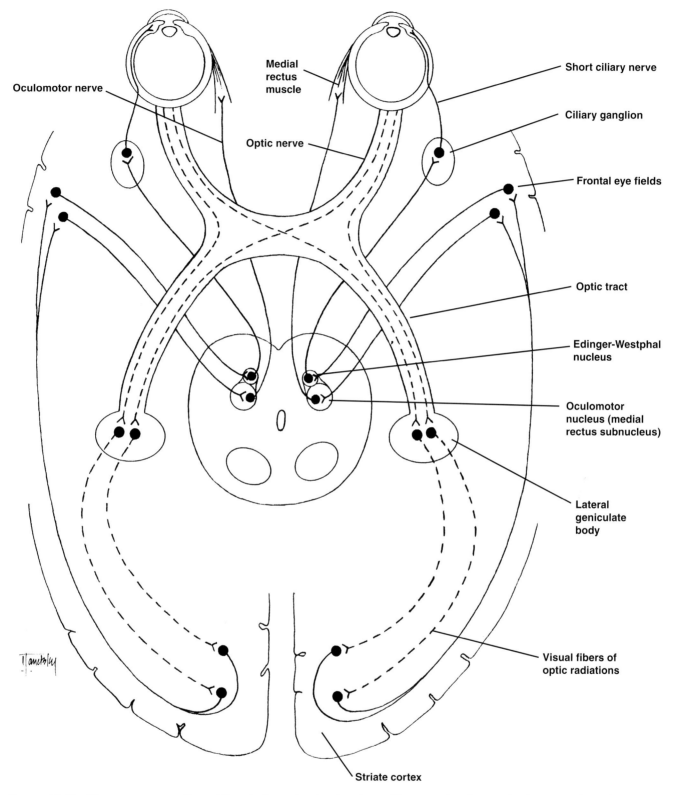

FIGURE 13-10. The near response. Dotted lines indicate the visual pathway fibers carrying the visual information from the eye to the visual cortex. Solid lines indicate the pathway from the striate cortex to the frontal eye fields, then to the oculomotor nucleus, and from there to the medial rectus, ciliary, and sphincter muscles. (See text for further details.)

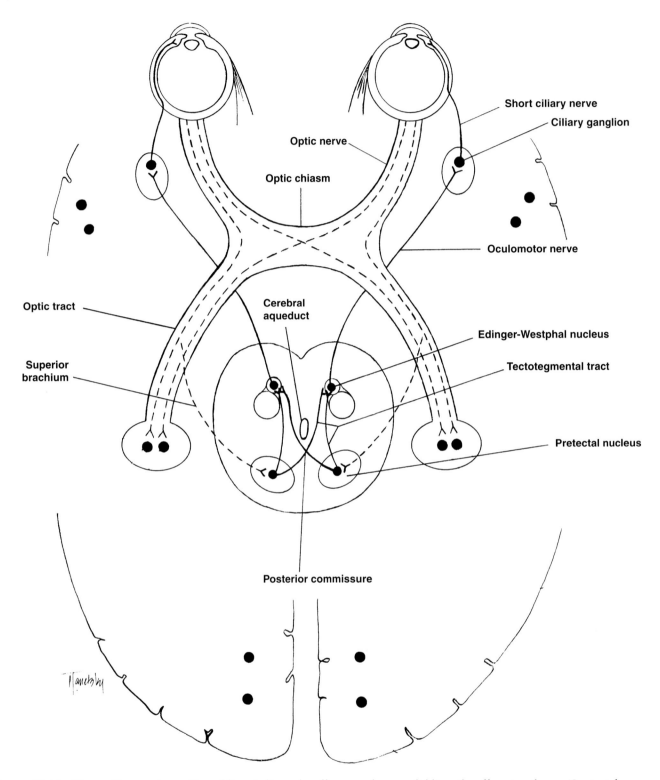

FIGURE 13-11. The pupillary pathway. Dotted lines indicate the afferent pathway, solid lines the efferent pathway. (See text for further details.)

response occurs because of the two crossings of the fibers in the pathway: The nasal retinal fibers cross in the chiasm, and some fibers from the pretectal nucleus cross in the posterior commissure.

Disruption in the Afferent Pathway

A disruption in the afferent pathway will result in poor direct and consensual responses. For example, in the presence of a disruption in the right afferent pathway, a light directed into the right eye will cause little or no response in both the right and left eyes, although both responses would be normal if the light were directed into the left eye. If the damage to the afferent pathway is complete (i.e., all the fibers from one eye are affected), there would be no direct and no consensual response when light is directed into the affected eye. More commonly, only some fibers are damaged such that the abnormal pupillary responses might be recognized only when compared to the normal pupillary responses; hence, the term **relative afferent pupillary defect** (RAPD) is applied.

Disruption can occur anywhere in the afferent pathway—retina, optic nerve, chiasm, optic tract, or superior brachium. The swinging-flashlight test can be used to determine the presence of an RAPD. Damage posterior to the crossing in the chiasm might not be evident with the swinging-flashlight test unless the damage affects a great number of fibers from one eye and significantly fewer fibers from the other eye.[34]

✍ CLINICAL COMMENT:
SWINGING-FLASHLIGHT TEST
The patient is asked to fixate on a distant object, and then the practitioner swings a light from eye to eye, several times rhythmically, taking care to illuminate each pupil for an equal length of time (approximately 1–2 seconds). If both pathways are normal, little or no change in pupil size will be noted; the eye will not recover from the consensual response before it is subjected to the direct light beam. The normal, symmetric response is characterized by equal pupillary constriction in both eyes when the light is presented to either eye. An abnormal response is characterized by larger pupils when the light is directed into the affected eye than when the light is directed into the normal eye (Figure 13-12).

As the intensity of the light increases, stronger constrictions occur with light presented to a normal eye. There is, however, a threshold beyond which no increase occurs. A very bright light can be used for detecting subtle defects; however, the luminance level should be recorded because a future change in the measured RAPD might reflect only a different light condition.[35, 36]

✍ CLINICAL COMMENT: AFFERENT PUPILLARY DEFECT IN CATARACT
It would appear likely that a dense cataract would cause an RAPD because less light penetrates a cataract to stimulate the retina. However, in a clinical situation, a dense cataract has been found to cause an RAPD in the contralateral eye.[37, 38] Light scattered back to the retina from the lens opacity probably produces an enhanced pupillary response, which is manifested as an RAPD of the contralateral eye.

✍ CLINICAL COMMENT: OPTIC NEURITIS
The most common site of damage in an RAPD is the optic nerve. Ninety percent of patients with optic neuritis exhibit an RAPD during some stage of the disease.[33]

Disruption Within the Central Nervous System

A lesion in the midbrain can involve the pretectal nucleus or the tectotegmental tract. Damage to the pretectal nucleus might not cause a pupillary defect as fibers from the other pretectal nucleus still supply both of the parasympathetic nuclei.

Damage to the tectotegmental tract, if limited to one side, results in a pupil that does not react either directly or consensually but that does constrict in the near response because the pathway for the near reaction does not include the tectotegmental tract. This pupillary response commonly is called the **Argyll-Robertson pupil** and is said to show a light-near dissociation.[39] Because the pathway from the frontal eye fields is intact and the efferent path is viable, the sphincter and ciliary muscle still will constrict to a near object.[40] In the Argyll-Robertson pupil, the affected side shows no direct or consensual response, and the retained near response exceeds the best direct-light response (Figure 13-13). Diabetic neuropathy, alcoholic neuropathy, or neurosyphilis is suspected in a complete Argyll-Robertson pupil that involves both sides.

Disruption in the Efferent Pathway

A lesion in the efferent pathway will cause the eye to show poor direct and consensual pupillary responses and can involve other ocular structures. Damage in the oculomotor nucleus or nerve could involve the superior rectus, medial rectus, inferior rectus, inferior oblique, or levator muscles, and so the patient should be examined for related ocular motility impairment.

Damage to the ciliary ganglion or the short ciliary nerves could be caused by local injury or disease and results in a **tonic pupil**, which is characterized by poor pupillary light response and loss of accommoda-

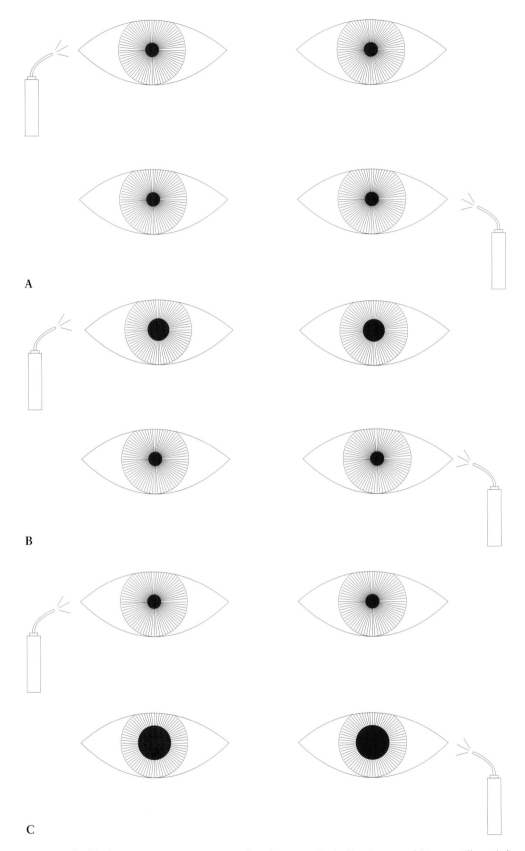

FIGURE 13-12. Swinging-flashlight test. (A) Response is equal and symmetric, indicating no relative pupillary defect. (B) Response is unequal, both pupils growing larger as light is directed into the right eye, indicating a grade 1+ relative afferent pupillary defect right eye. (C) Unequal pupillary response in which both pupils enlarge as light is directed into the left eye, indicating a grade 3+ relative afferent pupillary defect left eye.

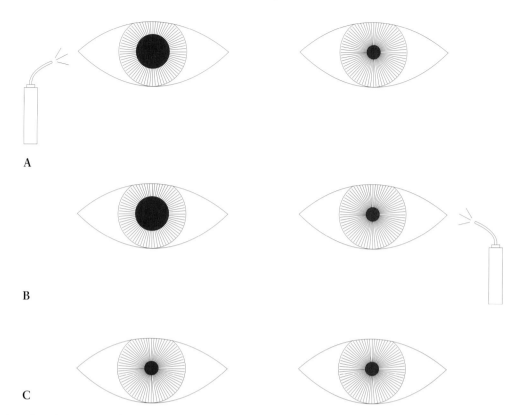

FIGURE 13-13. Argyll-Robertson pupil OD. (A) Poor direct response OD and normal consensual response OS. (B) Normal direct response OS and poor consensual response OD. (C) Normal near response in both eyes.

tion. Decreased corneal sensitivity often occurs, as some afferent sensory fibers from the cornea pass through the short ciliary nerves and the ganglion.[41] The affected muscles exhibit cholinergic supersensitivity; this denervation hypersensitivity is a physiologic phenomenon that occurs when the fibers directly innervating muscles are injured.[42] The near response is retained but is slow and long-lasting. One theory postulates that because the density of the innervation to the ciliary muscle is much greater than the density of innervation to the sphincter, some ciliary muscle nerve fibers remain intact and, with near stimulation, these fibers release acetylcholine, which diffuses into the aqueous humor and causes the supersensitive sphincter to constrict.[43] In late stages of this condition, the miotic near reaction might be difficult to demonstrate because the pupil becomes tonic, but the accommodative facility appears to recover, perhaps due to regeneration of the fibers.[15]

✍ CLINICAL COMMENT: ADIE'S TONIC PUPIL
If the cause of the tonic pupil is not apparent, the syndrome is called **Adie's tonic pupil**. The typical patient with Adie's pupil is a woman aged 20–40 years; 90% of these patients also have diminished tendon reflexes. Because of this systemic manifes-

tation, it is believed that similar degenerative processes are occurring in the ciliary ganglion and in the dorsal column of the spinal cord[44]; however, the etiology is unknown.[45] Sometimes, if pupillary constriction in early Adie's pupil is examined with the biomicroscope, segmental constriction affecting just a section of the iris is evident.[46]

In the differential diagnosis of Adie's pupil, a very mild, direct-acting cholinergic agonist can be used, as the sphincter muscle is supersensitive.[15, 47] A dilute concentration of pilocarpine (0.125%) has minimal effect on a normal sphincter but will cause significant clinical miosis in a supersensitive sphincter. With one drop instilled in each eye, the Adie's pupil should show a much greater constriction than the normal pupil (Figure 13-14).

✍ CLINICAL COMMENT: FIXED, DILATED PUPIL
Recent onset of a fixed, dilated pupil could be due to an accidental drug-induced mydriasis. Investigation of the individual's profession might indicate the handling of drugs (pharmacists, nurses) or chemicals that could exert such an effect (farmers, crop dusters, exterminators). Such a pupil will not respond to 0.125% pilocarpine.

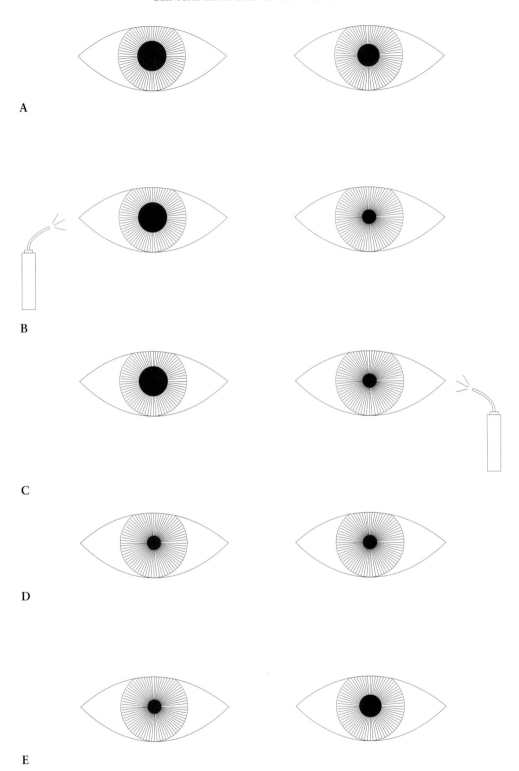

Figure 13-14. Adie's pupil OD. (A) Presenting anisocoria; right pupil is larger than the left. (B) Poor direct response OD and normal consensual response OS. (C) Normal direct response OS and poor consensual response OD. (D) Slow and long-lasting near response. (E) Pilocarpine 0.125% instilled in both eyes. Miosis OD, no response OS.

DISRUPTION IN THE SYMPATHETIC PATHWAY

An interruption in the sympathetic pathway will cause miosis. The usual tone that the dilator muscle normally exerts is not present, and there is no counteracting pull against the sphincter muscle, making the pupil smaller than normal. **Anisocoria** (a difference in pupil size) will be present under normal room-light conditions but will be more pronounced in dim light, with the normal eye having the larger pupil.

✍ CLINICAL COMMENT: HORNER'S SYNDROME

Features of the Syndrome

Damage to the sympathetic pathway to the head can cause **Horner's syndrome**, which consists of ptosis, miosis, and facial anhidrosis (absence of sweat secretion). Loss of innervation to the smooth muscle of the upper eyelid causes ptosis, whereas loss of innervation to the lower eyelid causes it to rise slightly such that the palpebral fissure appears narrow, simulating enophthalmos.

The damage can occur anywhere along the sympathetic pathway in the brain, spinal cord, preganglionic path, or postganglionic path. Involvement of the central neuron, which sends its fiber from the hypothalamus through the spinal cord to a synapse with the preganglionic neuron in the cervical dorsal column, can cause other problems (e.g., vertigo) to occur.

The preganglionic fibers leave the dorsal column of the spinal cord, pass into the chest, course over the apex of the lung, and loop around the subclavian artery en route to the superior cervical ganglion (Figure 13-15). These fibers can be damaged in thoracic injury or surgery or in metastatic disease involving the chest.[6]

The postganglionic fibers that enter the skull via the carotid plexus could be damaged by a fracture of the skull base or an injury to the internal carotid artery. Damage along the rest of the postganglionic neuron would involve the nasociliary or long ciliary nerves.

Differential Diagnosis

The location of the disruption of the sympathetic pathway is useful in determining appropriate care. In the differential diagnosis of Horner's syndrome, diagnostic drugs used to determine the site of interruption include cocaine and hydroxyamphetamine, the effects of which are shown in Figures 13-16 and 13-17. If the sympathetic pathway is intact, instillation of one drop of a 5% or 10% ophthalmic cocaine solution, an indirect-acting adrenergic agonist, causes dilation.[48, 49] In contrast, with a disruption anywhere in the pathway, norepinephrine

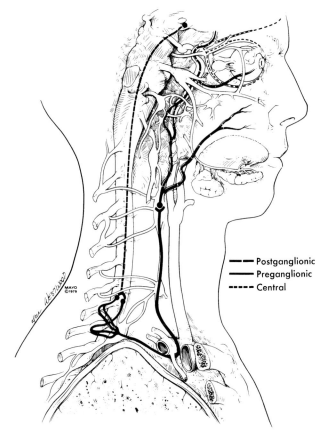

FIGURE 13-15. Sympathetic innervation of the eye. (Reprinted from WF Maloney, BR Younge, NJ Moyer. Evaluation of the causes and accuracy of pharmacologic localization in Horner's syndrome. Am J Ophthalmol 1980;90:394. With permission from the Mayo Foundation.)

--- Postganglionic
— Preganglionic
····· Central

is lacking in the neuromuscular junction, and therefore cocaine has little or no effect, and the pupil dilates poorly.

Hydroxyamphetamine 1.0% can be administered to determine whether the damage is in the preganglionic or postganglionic pathway.[50–52] A topical administration of this indirect-acting adrenergic agonist acts on the postganglionic fiber, causing release of norepinephrine. If the lesion is in the preganglionic pathway, the postganglionic fiber still is viable and will contain stores of norepinephrine. Instillation of hydroxyamphetamine will cause release of the neurotransmitter, and dilation will occur. If the disruption is in the postganglionic pathway, norepinephrine will not be stored in the nerve endings, and therefore no dilation will occur with instillation of hydroxyamphetamine.

In the presence of preganglionic and central lesions, the pupil on the affected side usually dilates more than the normal eye with hydroxyampheta-

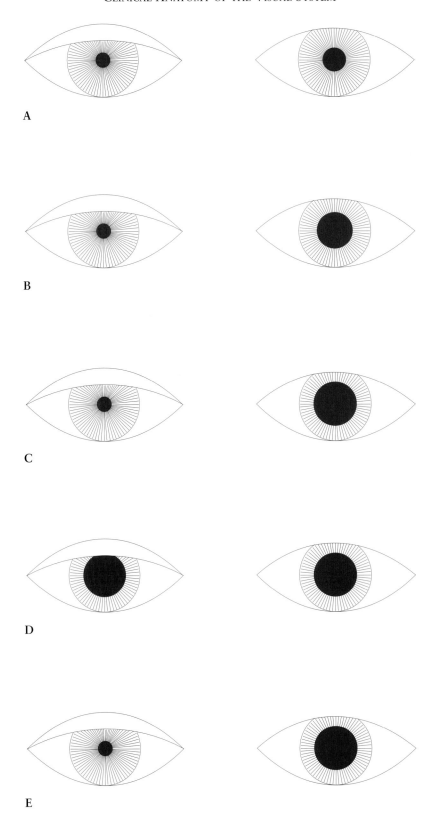

FIGURE 13-16. Horner's syndrome. (A) Presenting anisocoria; left pupil is larger than the right. Ptosis OD. (B) Anisocoria greater in dim illumination. (C) Cocaine 5% instilled OU. No response OD, mydriasis OS, interruption in sympathetic pathway OD. (D) Hydroxyamphetamine 1% instilled OU. Mydriasis OU, interruption in preganglionic pathway OD. (E) Hydroxyamphetamine 1% instilled OU. No response OD, mydriasis OS, interruption in postganglionic pathway OD.

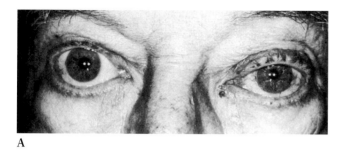

A

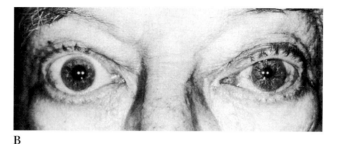

B

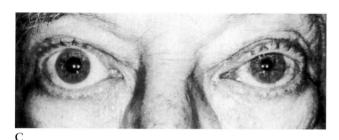

C

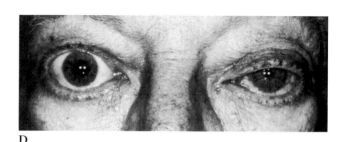

D

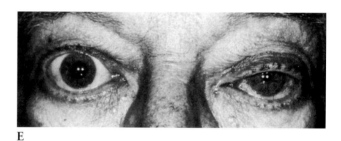

E

FIGURE 13-17. Dilation lag in 72-year-old man with left Horner's syndrome. (A) Obvious anisocoria in bright illumination. Note greater anisocoria at 4–5 seconds in darkness (B) as compared to the anisocoria at 10–12 seconds in darkness (C). (D) Cocaine test for Horner's syndrome. Following instillation of 10% cocaine into each eye, there is dilation of the normal right pupil but absence of dilation in left Horner's pupil. (E) Hydroxyamphetamine test in Horner's syndrome. Following instillation of 1% hydroxyamphetamine into each eye, there is dilation of the normal right pupil but absence of dilation of the left Horner's pupil, indicating a postganglionic lesion. (Reprinted with permission from JD Bartlett, SD Jaanus. Clinical Ocular Pharmacology [2nd ed]. Boston: Butterworth–Heinemann, 1989;437, 439, 441.)

mine instillation, either because of enhanced receptor sensitivity or because adrenergic nerve endings have accumulated more norepinephrine.[53]

REFERENCES

1. Olmsted JMD, Morgan MW. The influence of the cervical sympathetic nerve on the lens of the eye. Am J Physiol 1941;133:720.

2. Olmsted JMD. The role of the autonomic nervous system in accommodation for near and far vision. J Nerv Ment Dis 1944;99:794.

3. Morgan MW. The nervous control of accommodation. Am J Optom 1944;21:87.

4. Gilmartin B. A review of the role of sympathetic innervation of the ciliary muscle in ocular accommodation. Ophthalmic Physiol Opt 1986;6(1):23.

5. Rosenfield M, Gilmartin B. Oculomotor consequences of beta-adrenoceptor antagonism during sustained near vision. Ophthalmic Physiol Opt 1987;7(2):127.

6. Maloney WF, Younge BR, Moyer NJ. Evaluation of the causes and accuracy of pharmacologic localization in Horner's syndrome. Am J Ophthalmol 1980;90:394.

7. Doxanas MT, Anderson RL. Clinical Orbital Anatomy. Baltimore: Williams & Wilkins, 1984;93, 131.

8. Pick TP, Howden R (eds). Gray's Anatomy (15th ed). New York: Crown, 1977;799.

9. Warwick R. Eugene Wolff's Anatomy of the Eye and Orbit (7th ed). Philadelphia: Saunders, 1976;306.

10. Mohney JB, Morgan MW, Olmsted JMD, et al. The pathway of sympathetic nerves to the ciliary muscles in the eye. Am J Physiol 1942;135:759.

11. Ruskell GL. Sympathetic innervation of the ciliary muscle in monkeys. Exp Eye Res 1973;16:183.

12. Gilmartin B, Hogan RE. The relationship between tonic accommodation and ciliary muscle innervation. Invest Ophthalmol Vis Sci 1985;26:1024.

13. Gilmartin B, Bullimore MA, Rosenfield M, et al. Pharmacological effects on accommodative adaptation. Optom Vis Sci 1992;69(4):276.

14. Warwick R. The ocular parasympathetic nerve supply and its mesencephalic sources. J Anat 1954;88:71.

15. Ruskell GL. Accommodation and the nerve pathway to the ciliary muscle: a review. Ophthalmic Physiol Opt 1990;10(3):239.

16. Burde RM. Direct parasympathetic pathway to the eye: revisited. Brain Res 1988;463:158.

17. Reiner A, Erichsen JT, Cabot JB, et al. Neurotransmitter organization of the nucleus of Edinger-Westphal and its projection to the avian ciliary ganglion. Vis Neurosci 1991;6(5):451.

18. Duke-Elder W. The Anatomy of the Visual System (Vol 2). System of Ophthalmology. St. Louis: Mosby, 1961;497.

19. Stephens KG. Effect of the sympathetic nervous system on accommodation. Am J Optom Physiol Optics 1985;62(6):402.

20. Miller RJ, Takahama M. Arousal-related changes in dark focus accommodation and dark vergence. Invest Ophthalmol Vis Sci 1988;29(7):1168.

21. Tornqvist G. The relative importance of the parasympathetic and sympathetic nervous systems for accommodation in monkeys. Invest Ophthalmol Vis Sci 1967;6:612.

22. Hurwitz BS, Dacidowitz J, Chin NB, et al. The effects of the sympathetic nervous system on accommodation: I. Beta sympathetic nervous system. Arch Ophthalmol 1972;87:668.

23. Tornqvist G. Effect of cervical sympathetic stimulation on accommodation in monkeys. Acta Physiol Scand 1967;67:363.

24. VanAlphen GWHM. The adrenergic receptors of the intraocular muscles of the human eye. Invest Ophthalmol Vis Sci 1976;15:502.

25. Wax MB, Molinoff PB. Distribution and properties of beta-adrenergic receptors in human iris/ciliary body [ARVO abstract]. Invest Ophthalmol Vis Sci 1984;25(Suppl):305.

26. Monkhouse WS. The anatomy of the facial nerve. Ear Nose Throat J 1990;69:677.

27. Ruskell GL. An ocular parasympathetic nerve pathway of facial nerve origin and its influence on intraocular pressure. Exp Eye Res 1970;106:323.

28. Rodriguez-Vazquez JF, Merida-Velasco JR, Jimenez-Collado J. Orbital muscle of Müller: observations on human fetuses measuring 35–150 mm. Acta Anat (Basel) 1990;139(4):300.

29. Ruskell GL. Facial nerve distribution to the eye. Am J Optom Physiol Optics 1985;62(11):793.

30. Stjernschantz J, Bill A. Vasomotor effects of facial nerve stimulation: non-cholinergic vasodilation in the eye. Acta Physiol Scand 1980;109:45.

31. Wobig JL. The Lacrimal Apparatus. In MJ Reeh, JL Wobig, JD Wirtschafter (eds), Ophthalmic Anatomy. San Francisco: American Academy of Ophthalmology, 1981;55.

32. Jaanus SD, Pagano VT, Bartlett JD. Drugs Affecting the Autonomic Nervous System. In JD Bartlett, SD Jaanus (eds), Clinical Ocular Pharmacology (3rd ed). Boston, MA: Butterworth–Heinemann, 1995;168.

33. Thompson HS. The Pupil. In WM Hart Jr (ed), Adler's Physiology of the Eye (9th ed). St. Louis: Mosby, 1992;412.

34. Newman SA, Miller NR. The optic tract syndrome neuro-ophthalmologic considerations. Arch Ophthalmol 1983;101:1241.

35. Johnson LN. The effect of light intensity on measurement of the relative afferent pupillary defect. Am J Ophthalmol 1990;109(4):481.

36. Lam BL, Thompson HS. Brightness sense and the relative afferent pupillary defect. Am J Ophthalmol 1989;108(4):462.

37. Sadun AA, Bassi CJ, Lessell S. Why cataracts do not produce afferent pupillary defects. Am J Ophthalmol 1990;110(6):712.

38. Lam BL, Thompson HS. A unilateral cataract produces a relative afferent pupillary defect in the contralateral eye. Ophthalmology 1990;97(3):334.

39. Loewenfeld IE. The Argyll Robertson pupil, 1869–1969: a critical survey of the literature. Surv Ophthalmol 1969;14:199.

40. Thompson HS. Light-near dissociation of the pupil. Ophthalmologica 1984;189:21.

41. Purcell JJ, Krachmer JH, Thompson HS. Corneal sensation in Adie's syndrome. Am J Ophthalmol 1977;84:496.

42. Scheie HG. Site of disturbance in Adie's syndrome. Arch Ophthalmol 1940;24:225.

43. Wirtschafter JD, Volk CR, Sawchuk RJ. Transaqueous diffusion of acetylcholine to denervated iris sphincter muscle: a mechanism for the tonic pupil syndrome. Ann Neurol 1978;4:1.

44. Selhorst JB, Madge G, Ghatak N. The neuropathology of the Holmes-Adie syndrome. Ann Neurol 1984;16:138.

45. Harriman DGF, Garland H. The pathology of Adie's syndrome. Brain 1968;91:401.

46. Thompson HS. Segmental palsy of the iris sphincter in Adie's syndrome. Arch Ophthalmol 1978;96:1615.

47. Bourgon P, Pilley SFJ, Thompson HS. Cholinergic supersensitivity of the iris sphincter in Adie's tonic pupil. Am J Ophthalmol 1978;85:373.

48. Kardon RH, Denison CE, Brown CK, et al. Critical evaluation of the cocaine test in the diagnosis of Horner's syndrome. Arch Ophthalmol 1990;108(3):384.

49. Thompson HS, Mensher JH. Horner's syndrome. Am J Ophthalmol 1974;72:472.

50. Cremer SA, Thompson HS, Digre KB, Kardon RH. Hydroxyamphetamine mydriasis in normal subjects. Am J Ophthalmol 1990;110(1):66.

51. Thompson HS, Mensher JH. Adrenergic mydriasis in Horner's syndrome. Hydroxyamphetamine test for diagnosis of postganglionic defects. Am J Ophthalmol 1971;72:472.

52. Selvesen R, di-Souza CD, Sjaastad O. Horner's syndrome. Sweat gland and pupillary responsiveness in two cases with a probable 3rd neurone dysfunction. Cephalalgia 1989;9(1):63.

53. Cremer SA, Thompson HS, Digre KB, et al. Hydroxyamphetamine mydriasis in Horner's syndrome. Am J Ophthalmol 1990;110(1):71.

SUGGESTED READING

Warwick R (ed). Eugene Wolff's Anatomy of the Eye and Orbit (7th ed). Philadelphia: Saunders, 1976;396.

Wirtschafter JD. The Anatomy of the Brain. In MJ Reeh, JL Wobig, JD Wirtschafter (eds), Ophthalmic Anatomy. San Francisco: American Academy of Ophthalmology, 1981;187.

Wobig JL. The Orbital Nerves. In MJ Reeh, JL Wobig, JD Wirtschafter (eds), Ophthalmic Anatomy. San Francisco: American Academy of Ophthalmology, 1981;73.

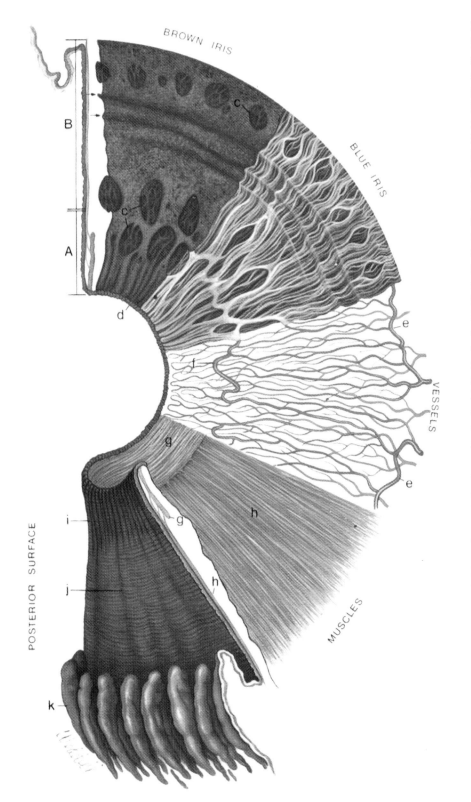

PLATE 3-1. Surfaces and layers of the iris. Beginning at the upper left and proceeding clockwise, the iris cross-section shows the pupillary (*A*) and ciliary portions (*B*), and the surface view shows a brown iris with its dense, matted anterior border layer. Circular contraction furrows are shown (arrows) in the ciliary portion of the iris. Fuch's crypts (*c*) are seen at either side of the collarette in the pupillary and ciliary portion and peripherally near the iris root. The pigment ruff is seen at the pupillary edge (*d*). The blue iris surface shows a less dense anterior border layer and more prominent trabeculae. The iris vessels are shown beginning at the major arterial circle in the ciliary body (*e*). Radial branches of the arteries and veins extend toward the pupillary region. The arteries form the incomplete minor arterial circle (*f*), from which branches extend toward the pupil, forming capillary arcades. The sector below it demonstrates the circular arrangement of the sphincter muscle (*g*) and the radial processes of the dilator muscle (*h*). The posterior surface of the iris shows the radial contraction furrows (*i*) and the structural folds of Schwalbe (*j*). Circular contraction folds also are present in the ciliary portion. The pars plicata of the ciliary body is at (*k*). (Reprinted with permission from MJ Hogan, JA Alvarado, JE Weddell. Histology of the Human Eye. Philadelphia: Saunders, 1971;207.)

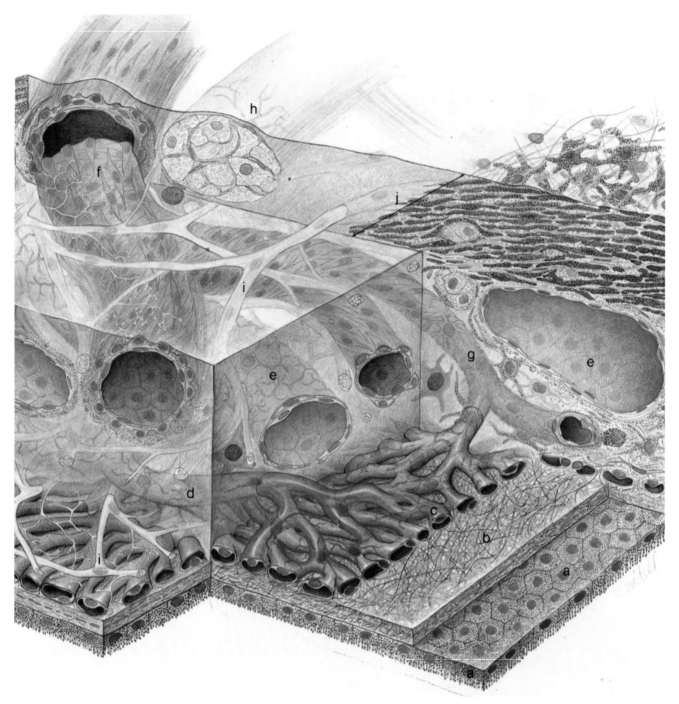

PLATE 3-2. Drawing of the choroidal blood supply and innervation and Bruch's membrane. The pigment epithelium of the retina (*a*) is in close contact with Bruch's membrane (*b*). The elastica of Bruch's membrane is blue, and the meshes contain collagen fibrils. The choriocapillaris (*c*) forms an intricate network along the inner choroid. Venules (*d*) leave the choriocapillaris to join the vortex system (*e*). The short ciliary artery is shown at (*f*), before its branching (*g*) to form the choriocapillaris. A short ciliary nerve enters the choroid at (*h*) and sends ramifying branches into the choroidal stroma (*i*). The suprachoroidea, with its star-shaped melanocytes, is at (*j*). (Reprinted with permission from MJ Hogan, JA Alvarado, JE Weddell. Histology of the Human Eye. Philadelphia: Saunders, 1971;375.)

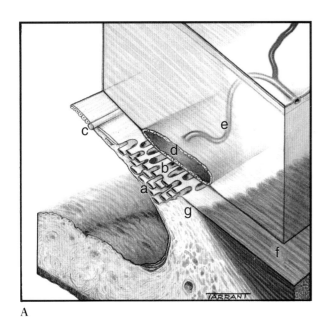

A

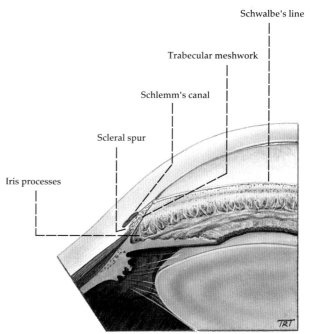

Schwalbe's line

Trabecular meshwork

Schlemm's canal

Scleral spur

Iris processes

B

PLATE 6-1. (A) Anatomy of outflow channels: (*a*) uveal mesh-work; (*b*) corneoscleral meshwork; (*c*) Schwalbe's line; (*d*) Schlemm's canal; (*e*) collector channels; (*f*) longitudinal muscle of ciliary body; and (*g*) scleral spur. (B) Anatomy of anterior chamber angle structures. (Reprinted with permission from JJ Kanski. Clinical Ophthalmology [3rd ed]. Oxford: Butterworth–Heinemann, 1995;234, 240.)

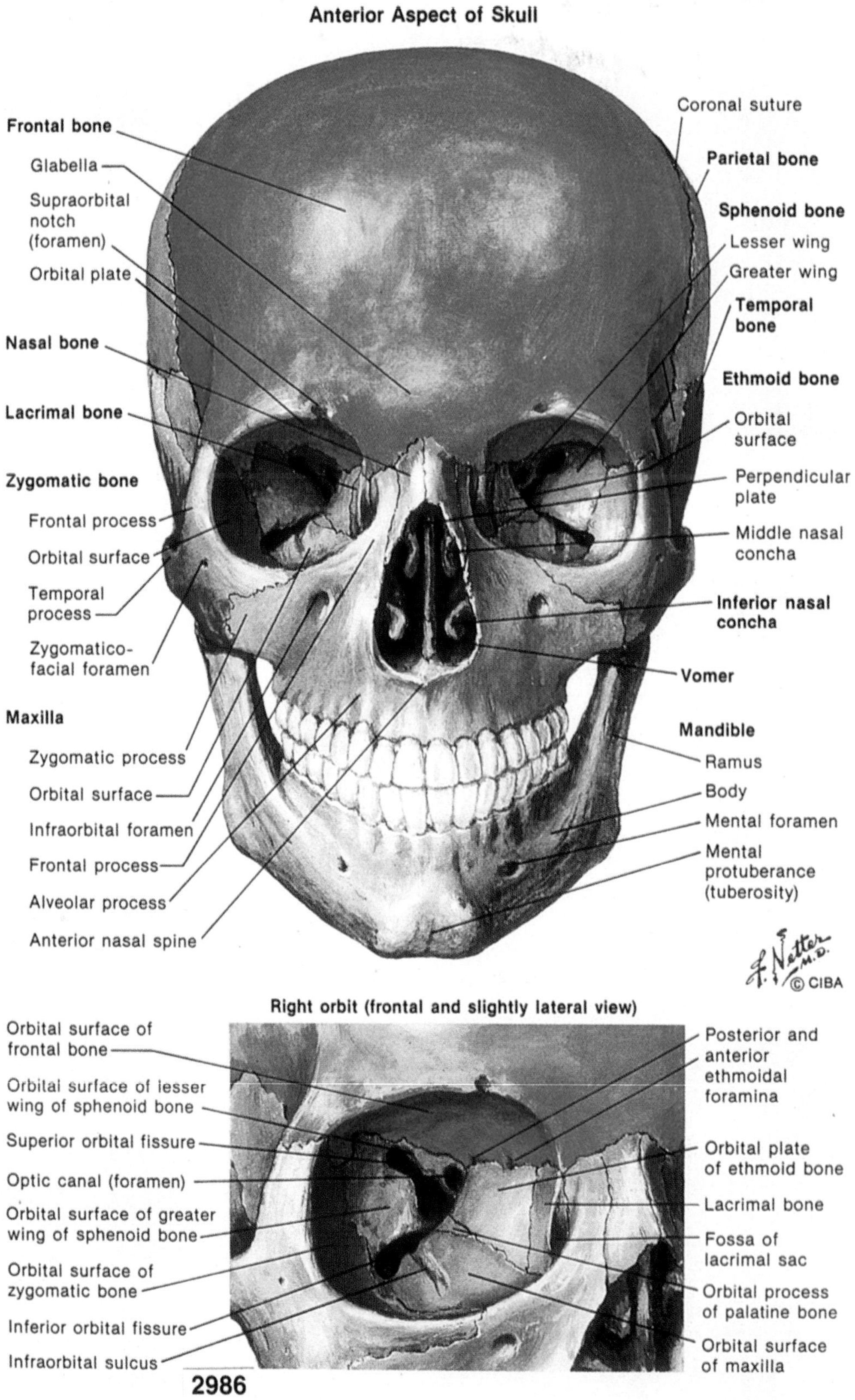

Anterior Aspect of Skull

Frontal bone

Glabella

Supraorbital notch (foramen)

Orbital plate

Nasal bone

Lacrimal bone

Zygomatic bone

Frontal process

Orbital surface

Temporal process

Zygomatico-facial foramen

Maxilla

Zygomatic process

Orbital surface

Infraorbital foramen

Frontal process

Alveolar process

Anterior nasal spine

Coronal suture

Parietal bone

Sphenoid bone

Lesser wing

Greater wing

Temporal bone

Ethmoid bone

Orbital surface

Perpendicular plate

Middle nasal concha

Inferior nasal concha

Vomer

Mandible

Ramus

Body

Mental foramen

Mental protuberance (tuberosity)

Right orbit (frontal and slightly lateral view)

Orbital surface of frontal bone

Orbital surface of lesser wing of sphenoid bone

Superior orbital fissure

Optic canal (foramen)

Orbital surface of greater wing of sphenoid bone

Orbital surface of zygomatic bone

Inferior orbital fissure

Infraorbital sulcus

Posterior and anterior ethmoidal foramina

Orbital plate of ethmoid bone

Lacrimal bone

Fossa of lacrimal sac

Orbital process of palatine bone

Orbital surface of maxilla

2986

PLATE 8-1. (Top) Anterior aspect of skull. (Bottom) Right orbit (front and slightly lateral view). (Reprinted with permission from F Netter. Nervous Systems: I. The Ciba Collection of Medical Illustrations. West Caldwell, NJ: Ciba, 1986;3. Copyright 1986 Ciba-Geigy Corporation.)

Autonomic Nerves in Head

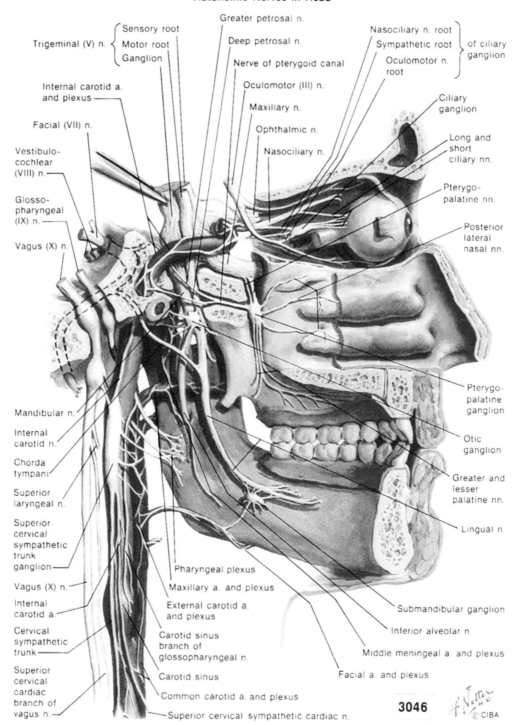

Trigeminal (V) n. { Sensory root / Motor root / Ganglion

Greater petrosal n.

Deep petrosal n.

Nerve of pterygoid canal

Oculomotor (III) n.

Maxillary n.

Ophthalmic n.

Nasociliary n.

Nasociliary n. root / Sympathetic root / Oculomotor n. root } of ciliary ganglion

Internal carotid a. and plexus

Facial (VII) n.

Vestibulo-cochlear (VIII) n.

Glosso-pharyngeal (IX) n.

Vagus (X) n.

Ciliary ganglion

Long and short ciliary nn.

Pterygo-palatine nn.

Posterior lateral nasal nn.

Pterygo-palatine ganglion

Otic ganglion

Greater and lesser palatine nn.

Lingual n.

Mandibular n.

Internal carotid n.

Chorda tympani

Superior laryngeal n.

Superior cervical sympathetic trunk ganglion

Vagus (X) n.

Internal carotid a.

Cervical sympathetic trunk

Superior cervical cardiac branch of vagus n.

Pharyngeal plexus

Maxillary a. and plexus

External carotid a. and plexus

Carotid sinus branch of glossopharyngeal n.

Carotid sinus

Common carotid a. and plexus

Superior cervical sympathetic cardiac n.

Submandibular ganglion

Inferior alveolar n.

Middle meningeal a. and plexus

Facial a. and plexus

3046

PLATE 11-1. Autonomic nerves in the head. (Reprinted with permission from F Netter. Nervous Systems: I. The Ciba Collection of Medical Illustrations. West Caldwell, NJ: Ciba, 1986;73. Copyright 1986 Ciba-Geigy Corporation.)

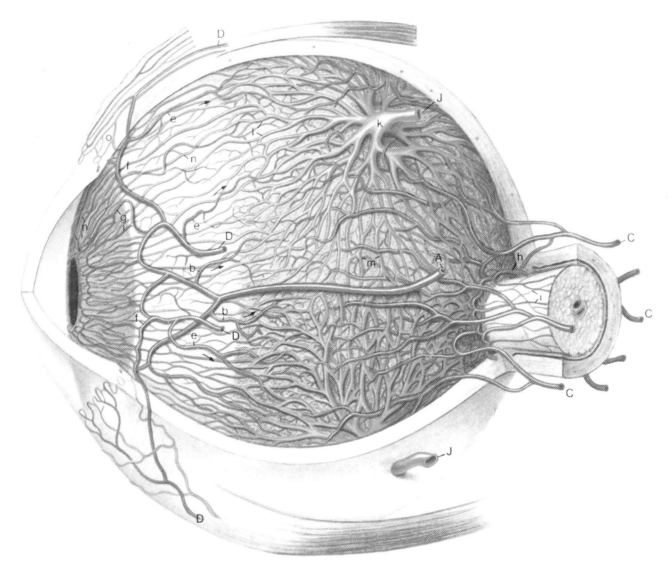

PLATE 11-2. The uveal blood vessels. The blood supply of the eye is derived from the ophthalmic artery. Except for the central retinal artery that supplies the inner retina, almost the entire blood supply of the eye comes from the uveal vessels. There are two long posterior ciliary arteries, one entering the uvea nasally and one temporally along the horizontal meridian of the eye near the optic nerve (A). These two arteries give off three to five branches (b) at the ora serrata, which pass directly back to form the anterior choriocapillaris. These capillaries nourish the retina from the equator forward. The short posterior ciliary arteries enter the choroid around the optic nerve (C). They divide rather rapidly to form the posterior choriocapillaris that nourishes the retina as far anteriorly as the equator (the choriocapillaris is not shown in this drawing). This system of capillaries is continuous with those derived from the long posterior ciliary arteries. The anterior ciliary arteries (D) pass forward with the rectus muscles, then pierce the sclera to enter the ciliary body. Before joining the major circle of the iris, they give off 8–12 branches (e) that pass back through the ciliary muscle to join the anterior choriocapillaris. The major circle of the iris (f) lies in the pars plicata and sends branches posteriorly into the ciliary body as well as forward into the iris (g). The circle of Zinn (h) is formed by pial branches (i) as well as branches from the short posterior ciliary arteries. The circle lies in the sclera and furnishes part of the blood supply to the optic nerve and disc. The vortex veins exit from the eye through the posterior sclera (J) after forming an ampulla (k) near the internal sclera. Venous branches that join the anterior and posterior part of the vortex system are meridionally oriented and are fairly straight (l), whereas those joining the vortices on their medial and lateral sides are oriented circularly about the eye (m). The venous return from the iris and ciliary body (n) is mainly posterior into the vortex system, but some veins cross the anterior sclera and limbus (o) to enter the episcleral system of veins. (Reprinted with permission from MJ Hogan, JA Alvarado, JE Weddell. Histology of the Human Eye. Philadelphia: Saunders, 1971;326.)

PLATE 12-1. Nerves of orbit, ciliary ganglion, and cavernous sinus. (Reprinted with permission from F Netter. Nervous Systems: I. The Ciba Collection of Medical Illustrations. West Caldwell, NJ: Ciba, 1986;97. Copyright 1986 Ciba-Geigy Corporation.)

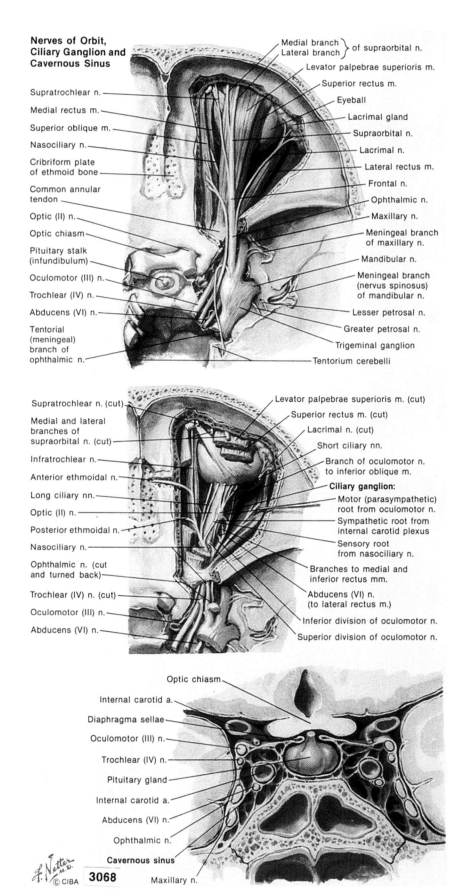

Nerves of Orbit, Ciliary Ganglion and Cavernous Sinus

Medial branch / Lateral branch } of supraorbital n.
Levator palpebrae superioris m.
Superior rectus m.
Eyeball
Lacrimal gland
Supraorbital n.
Lacrimal n.
Lateral rectus m.
Frontal n.
Ophthalmic n.
Maxillary n.
Meningeal branch of maxillary n.
Mandibular n.
Meningeal branch (nervus spinosus) of mandibular n.
Lesser petrosal n.
Greater petrosal n.
Trigeminal ganglion
Tentorium cerebelli

Supratrochlear n.
Medial rectus m.
Superior oblique m.
Nasociliary n.
Cribriform plate of ethmoid bone
Common annular tendon
Optic (II) n.
Optic chiasm
Pituitary stalk (infundibulum)
Oculomotor (III) n.
Trochlear (IV) n.
Abducens (VI) n.
Tentorial (meningeal) branch of ophthalmic n.

Supratrochlear n. (cut)
Medial and lateral branches of supraorbital n. (cut)
Infratrochlear n.
Anterior ethmoidal n.
Long ciliary nn.
Optic (II) n.
Posterior ethmoidal n.
Nasociliary n.
Ophthalmic n. (cut and turned back)
Trochlear (IV) n. (cut)
Oculomotor (III) n.
Abducens (VI) n.

Levator palpebrae superioris m. (cut)
Superior rectus m. (cut)
Lacrimal n. (cut)
Short ciliary nn.
Branch of oculomotor n. to inferior oblique m.
Ciliary ganglion:
Motor (parasympathetic) root from oculomotor n.
Sympathetic root from internal carotid plexus
Sensory root from nasociliary n.
Branches to medial and inferior rectus mm.
Abducens (VI) n. (to lateral rectus m.)
Inferior division of oculomotor n.
Superior division of oculomotor n.

Optic chiasm
Internal carotid a.
Diaphragma sellae
Oculomotor (III) n.
Trochlear (IV) n.
Pituitary gland
Internal carotid a.
Abducens (VI) n.
Ophthalmic n.
Cavernous sinus
Maxillary n.

3068

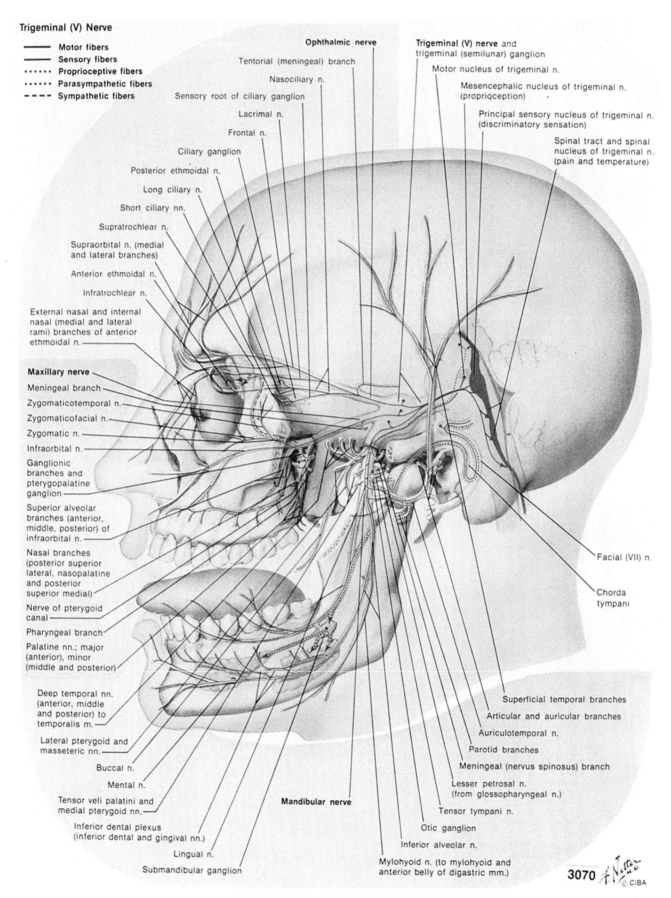

Trigeminal (V) Nerve

——— Motor fibers
——— Sensory fibers
······ Proprioceptive fibers
•••••• Parasympathetic fibers
– – – Sympathetic fibers

Ophthalmic nerve
Tentorial (meningeal) branch
Nasociliary n.
Sensory root of ciliary ganglion
Lacrimal n.
Frontal n.
Ciliary ganglion
Posterior ethmoidal n.
Long ciliary n.
Short ciliary nn.
Supratrochlear n.
Supraorbital n. (medial and lateral branches)
Anterior ethmoidal n.
Infratrochlear n.
External nasal and internal nasal (medial and lateral rami) branches of anterior ethmoidal n.

Trigeminal (V) nerve and trigeminal (semilunar) ganglion
Motor nucleus of trigeminal n.
Mesencephalic nucleus of trigeminal n. (proprioception)
Principal sensory nucleus of trigeminal n. (discriminatory sensation)
Spinal tract and spinal nucleus of trigeminal n. (pain and temperature)

Maxillary nerve
Meningeal branch
Zygomaticotemporal n.
Zygomaticofacial n.
Zygomatic n.
Infraorbital n.
Ganglionic branches and pterygopalatine ganglion
Superior alveolar branches (anterior, middle, posterior) of infraorbital n.
Nasal branches (posterior superior lateral, nasopalatine and posterior superior medial)
Nerve of pterygoid canal
Pharyngeal branch
Palatine nn.; major (anterior), minor (middle and posterior)

Deep temporal nn. (anterior, middle and posterior) to temporalis m.
Lateral pterygoid and masseteric nn.
Buccal n.
Mental n.
Tensor veli palatini and medial pterygoid nn.
Inferior dental plexus (inferior dental and gingival nn.)
Lingual n.
Submandibular ganglion

Facial (VII) n.
Chorda tympani

Superficial temporal branches
Articular and auricular branches
Auriculotemporal n.
Parotid branches
Meningeal (nervus spinosus) branch
Lesser petrosal n. (from glossopharyngeal n.)
Tensor tympani n.
Otic ganglion
Inferior alveolar n.
Mylohyoid n. (to mylohyoid and anterior belly of digastric mm.)

Mandibular nerve

3070

PLATE 12-2. Trigeminal nerve (cranial nerve V). (Reprinted with permission from F Netter. Nervous Systems: I. The Ciba Collection of Medical Illustrations. West Caldwell, NJ: Ciba, 1986;101. Copyright 1986 Ciba-Geigy Corporation.)

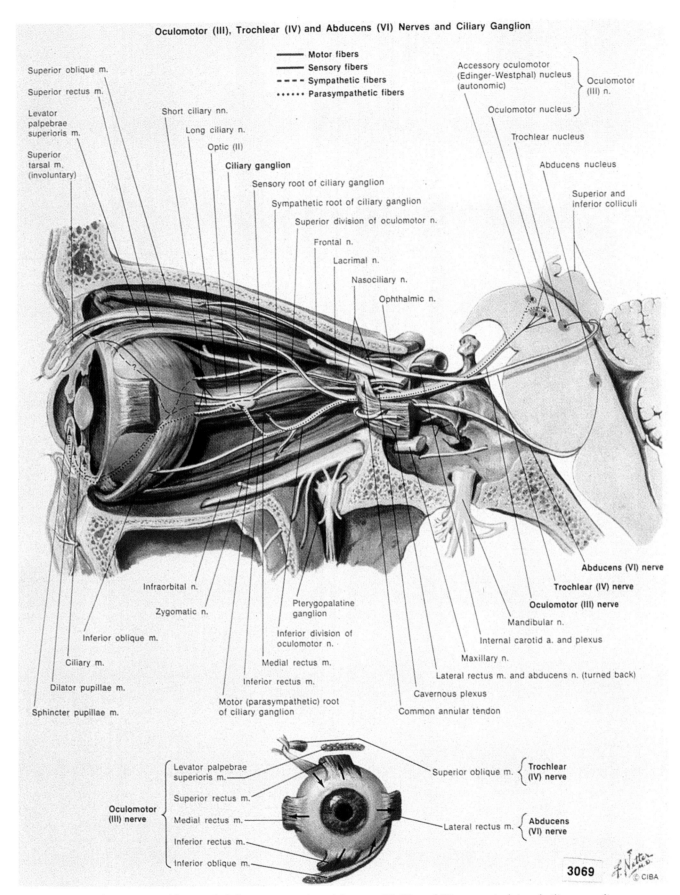

Oculomotor (III), Trochlear (IV) and Abducens (VI) Nerves and Ciliary Ganglion

Motor fibers
Sensory fibers
Sympathetic fibers
Parasympathetic fibers

Superior oblique m.
Superior rectus m.
Levator palpebrae superioris m.
Superior tarsal m. (involuntary)

Short ciliary nn.
Long ciliary n.
Optic (II)
Ciliary ganglion
Sensory root of ciliary ganglion
Sympathetic root of ciliary ganglion
Superior division of oculomotor n.
Frontal n.
Lacrimal n.
Nasociliary n.
Ophthalmic n.

Accessory oculomotor (Edinger-Westphal) nucleus (autonomic)
Oculomotor (III) n.
Oculomotor nucleus
Trochlear nucleus
Abducens nucleus
Superior and inferior colliculi

Infraorbital n.
Zygomatic n.
Inferior oblique m.
Ciliary m.
Dilator pupillae m.
Sphincter pupillae m.

Pterygopalatine ganglion
Inferior division of oculomotor n.
Medial rectus m.
Inferior rectus m.
Motor (parasympathetic) root of ciliary ganglion

Abducens (VI) nerve
Trochlear (IV) nerve
Oculomotor (III) nerve
Mandibular n.
Internal carotid a. and plexus
Maxillary n.
Lateral rectus m. and abducens n. (turned back)
Cavernous plexus
Common annular tendon

Oculomotor (III) nerve
Levator palpebrae superioris m.
Superior rectus m.
Medial rectus m.
Inferior rectus m.
Inferior oblique m.

Superior oblique m. — Trochlear (IV) nerve
Lateral rectus m. — Abducens (VI) nerve

3069

PLATE 12-3. Oculomotor, trochlear, and abducens nerves (cranial nerves III, VI, and VI, respectively) and ciliary ganglion. (Reprinted with permission from F Netter. Nervous Systems: I. The Ciba Collection of Medical Illustrations. West Caldwell, NJ: Ciba, 1986;99. Copyright 1986 Ciba-Geigy Corporation.)

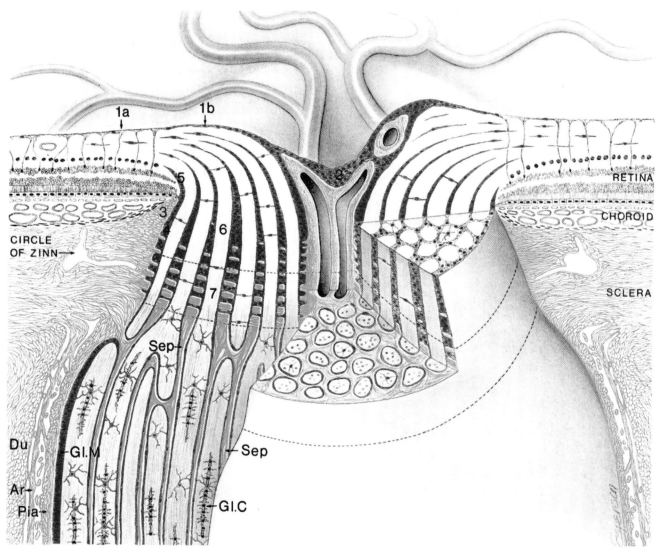

PLATE 14-1. The intraocular and part of the orbital optic nerve. Where the retina terminates at the optic disc edge, the Müller cells (*1a*) are in continuity with the astrocytes, forming the internal limiting membrane of Elschnig (*1b*). In some specimens, Elschnigís membrane is thickened in the central portion of the disc to form the central meniscus of Kuhnt (*2*). At the posterior termination of the choroid on the temporal side, the border tissue of Elschnig (*3*) lies between the astrocytes surrounding the optic nerve canal (*4*) and the stroma of the choroid. On the nasal side, the choroidal stroma is directly adjacent to the astrocytes surrounding the nerve. This collection of astrocytes (*4*) surrounding the canal is known as the **border tissue of Jacoby**. It is continuous with a similar glial lining called the **intermediary tissue of Kuhnt** (*5*) at the termination of the retina. The nerve fibers of the retina are segregated into approximately 1,000 bundles or fascicles by astrocytes (*6*). On reaching the lamina cribrosa (upper dotted line), the nerve fascicles (*7*) and their surrounding astrocytes are separated from one another by connective tissue (drawn in blue). This connective tissue is the cribriform plate, which is an extension of scleral collagen and elastic fibers through the nerve. The external choroid also sends some connective tissue to the anterior part of the lamina. At the external part of the lamina cribrosa (lower dotted line), the nerve fibers become myelinated, and columns of oligodendrocytes (*Gl.C*) (black and white cells) and a few astrocytes (red-colored cells) are present within the nerve fascicles. The astrocytes surrounding the fascicles form a thinner layer here than in the laminar and prelaminar portion. The bundles continue to be separated by connective tissue all the way to the chiasm (*Sep*). This connective tissue is derived from the pia mater and is known as the **septal tissue**. A mantle of astrocytes (*Gl.M*), continuous anteriorly with the border tissue of Jacoby, surrounds the nerve along its orbital course. The dura (*Du*), arachnoid (*Ar*), and pia mater (*Pia*) are shown. The central retinal vessels are surrounded by a perivascular connective tissue throughout its course in the nerve; this connective tissue blends with the connective tissue of the cribriform plate in the lamina cribrosa; it is called the **central supporting connective-tissue strand**. (Reprinted with permission from D Anderson, W Hoyt. Ultrastructure of interorbital portion of human and monkey optic nerve. Arch Ophthalmol 1969;82:506.)

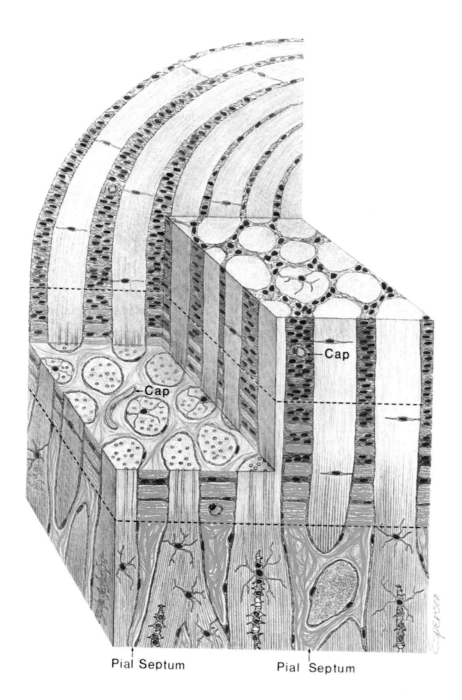

Pial Septum   Pial Septum

PLATE 14-2. Detailed view of the prelaminar, laminar, and postlaminar optic nerve. The nerve bundles are drawn in black and white, the astrocytes in red, oligodendrocytes in black and white, and the connective tissue in blue. In the prelaminar region, the nerves coming from the retina become segregated into bundles that are invested with a tubelike layer of astrocytes. The astrocytes and their processes are oriented perpendicular to the nerve bundles. Capillaries (*Cap*) course within the astrocytic tubes in the prelaminar region. As the lamina cribrosa is reached (upper dotted line), the nerve fascicles are separated from one another by a layer of astrocytes, which in turn is covered by a mantle of connective tissue containing collagen, elastic fibers, fibroblasts, and capillaries. In the posterior lamina cribrosa (lower dotted line), the nerves become myelinated, and columns of oligodendrocytes and a few astrocytes are found within the fascicles. The astrocytes separating the nerve fascicles in the laminar and postlaminar regions form a thinner layer than in the prelaminar portion. The connective tissue of the lamina cribrosa is continuous posteriorly with the pial septa. (Reprinted with permission from D Anderson. Ultrastructure of human and monkey lamina cribrosa and optic nerve head. Arch Ophthalmol 1969;82:800.)

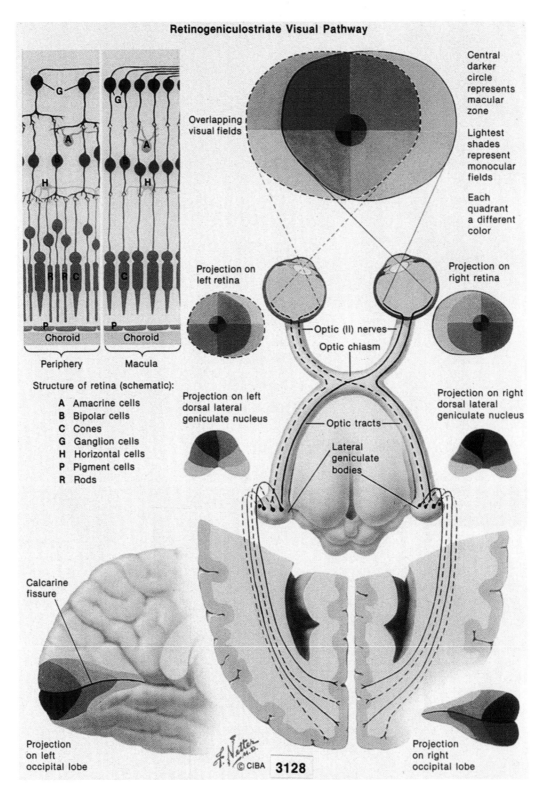

Retinogeniculostriate Visual Pathway

Central darker circle represents macular zone

Lightest shades represent monocular fields

Each quadrant a different color

Overlapping visual fields

Projection on left retina

Projection on right retina

Optic (II) nerves

Optic chiasm

Structure of retina (schematic):

A Amacrine cells
B Bipolar cells
C Cones
G Ganglion cells
H Horizontal cells
P Pigment cells
R Rods

Choroid

Periphery   Macula

Projection on left dorsal lateral geniculate nucleus

Projection on right dorsal lateral geniculate nucleus

Optic tracts

Lateral geniculate bodies

Calcarine fissure

Projection on left occipital lobe

Projection on right occipital lobe

Plate 14-3. Retinogeniculostriate visual pathway. (Reprinted with permission from F Netter. Nervous Systems: I. The Ciba Collection of Medical Illustrations. West Caldwell, NJ: Ciba, 1986;172. Copyright 1986 Ciba-Geigy Corporation.)

The Visual Pathway

The visual pathway consists of the series of cells and synapses that carry visual information from the environment to the brain for processing. It includes the retina, the optic nerve, the optic chiasm, the optic tract, the lateral geniculate body, the optic radiations, and the striate cortex (Figure 14-1). The first cell in the pathway—a special sensory cell, the photoreceptor—converts light energy into a neuronal signal passed to the bipolar cell and then to the ganglion cell; all these cells and synapses lie within the retina. The axons of the ganglion cells exit the retina via the optic nerve, with the nasal fibers from each eye crossing in the optic chiasm and terminating in the opposite side of the brain. The optic tract carries these fibers from the chiasm to the lateral geniculate body, where the next synapse occurs. The fibers leave the lateral geniculate body as the optic radiations that terminate in the visual cortex of the occipital lobe. From various points in this pathway, information about the visual environment is transferred to visual association areas and to related neurologic centers.

The structures of the visual pathway, the orientation of the fibers within each structure, and a brief overview of characteristic field defects associated with specific locations within the visual pathway are discussed here. Most of the current knowledge of the visual pathway is based on degeneration studies using laboratory animals, particularly monkeys and cats.[1-3] This type of investigation uses the fact that damage to a neuron causes the cell and its processes to degenerate. After a small area of nerve tissue is damaged, researchers make serial sections of the tissue through which the neuronal processes are believed to pass. By examining these sections under the microscope, they identify the pathway by determining the location of the degenerating processes. In some such studies, small lesions were made in the retina, and the degeneration was followed through the optic nerve, chiasm, and tract into the lateral geniculate body.[1, 3] In others, lesions were made in the striate cortex, and the degeneration was followed through the optic radiations toward the lateral geniculate body.[2] Whenever possible, reference to studies on the human pathway are cited.

ANATOMY OF THE VISUAL PATHWAY STRUCTURES

The anatomy of the retina and optic disc are discussed in Chapter 4.

Optic Nerve

The retinal nerve fibers make a 90-degree turn at the optic disc and exit as the **optic nerve**. This nerve consists of visual fibers that will terminate in the lateral geniculate body, pupillomotor fibers that terminate in the midbrain, and fibers to the superior colliculus. Various counts of the optic nerve fibers range from 1 to 2.22 million, with size ranging from small-diameter macular fibers to larger-caliber extramacular fibers.[1, 2, 4, 5]

The nerve is 5–6 cm long and can be divided into four segments on the basis of location: intraocular (0.7–1.0 mm), intraorbital (3 cm), intracanalicular (6–10 mm), and intracranial (10–16 mm).[5-7]

The intraocular section of the optic nerve can be divided into prelaminar and laminar sections on the basis of association with the lamina cribrosa. In the prelaminar optic nerve, a glial tissue network provides structural support for the delicate nerve fibers; sheaths of astrocytes bundle the nerve fibers into fascicles, con-

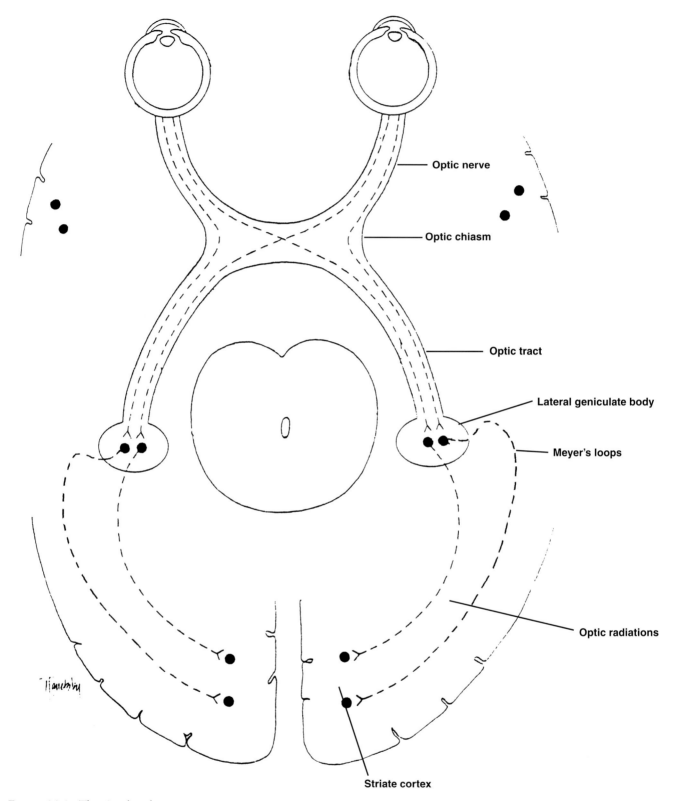

FIGURE 14-1. The visual pathway.

taining approximately 1,000 fibers each.[6] The optic nerve fibers are separated from the retinal layers by a ring of glial tissue, the intermediary tissue (of Kuhnt). The continuation of this glial tissue, the border tissue (of Jacoby), separates the choroid from the optic nerve fibers, and a ring of collagenous tissue of scleral derivation—the marginal (or border) tissue (of Elschnig)—lies outer to the glial sheaths.[6] These layers are shown in Plate 14-1.

The intraorbital (postlaminar) length exceeds the distance from the globe to the apex of the orbit, giving the nerve a slight sine wave–shaped curve, allowing for full eye excursions without stretching the nerve.[5, 8] Within the orbit, the nerve is surrounded by the rectus muscles; the sheaths of the superior and medial recti are adherent to the sheath of the optic nerve (hence the pain associated with eye movements in optic neuritis).[6]

The nerve is surrounded by three meningeal sheaths continuous with the meningeal coverings of the cranial contents. The outermost, the dura mater, is tough, dense connective tissue containing numerous elastic fibers.[6] Next to it, the thin collagenous membrane of the arachnoid sends a fine network of trabeculae through the subarachnoid space and connects to the innermost layer, the pia mater. The subarachnoid space around the optic nerve is continuous with the intracranial subarachnoid space and contains cerebrospinal fluid. The loose, vascular connective tissue of the pia mater branches, sending blood vessels and connective-tissue septa into the nerve (see Plate 14-1). All three of these layers fuse and become continuous with the sclera.[6]

As the unmyelinated retinal fibers pass through the scleral perforations of the lamina cribrosa, they become myelinated by oligodendrocytes, as no Schwann cells exist in the central nervous system. A sheath of connective tissue branching from and continuous with the pia mater meningeal covering is added to the glial sheath of each fascicle posterior to the lamina (Plate 14-2). These additional tissues double the diameter of the nerve as it leaves the eye, being approximately 1.5 mm in diameter at the level of the retina and approximately 3 mm in diameter after its exit from the globe. The septa that separate the fiber fascicles end near the chiasm.[6]

The anterior perforated substance, the root of the olfactory tract, and the anterior cerebral artery lie superior to the optic nerve in its intracranial path. The sphenoid sinus is medial, with only a thin plate of bone separating it from the nerve.[6] The internal carotid artery is below and then lateral to the nerve, and the ophthalmic artery enters the optic canal within the dural sheath of the nerve.

Optic Chiasm

The **optic chiasm** is roughly rectangular, approximately 15 mm in its horizontal diameter, 8 mm anterior to pos-

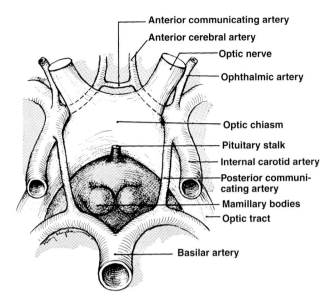

FIGURE 14-2. Relationship of chiasm to the vessels of the circle of Willis. (Reprinted with permission from DO Harrington. The Visual Fields [5th ed]. St. Louis: Mosby, 1981;90.)

terior, and 4 mm high.[5, 7, 9] It, too, is surrounded by the meningeal sheaths and cerebrospinal fluid.

The chiasm lies within the circle of Willis (Figure 14-2), a circle of blood vessels that is a common location of aneurysms.[5] The anterior cerebral and anterior communicating arteries are anterior to the chiasm, and an internal carotid artery lies on each lateral side. Above the chiasm is the floor of the third ventricle, and below is the pituitary gland (Figure 14-3). The position of the optic chiasm above the sella turcica (the fossa in which the pituitary gland sits) can vary from being directly above it to a position that is referred to as **prefixed** (if the optic nerves are short) or **postfixed** (if the optic nerves are long).[9]

Posterior to the chiasm, the visual pathway continues into both the right and left sides of the brain. However, the structures on only one side are described.

Optic Tract

The **optic tract** is a cylindric, slightly flattened band of fibers that is approximately 3.5 mm high and 5.1 mm long and runs from the posterior lateral corner of the chiasm to the lateral geniculate body.[7] Most of the fibers (which are still the axons of the retinal ganglion cells) terminate in the lateral geniculate body. Other fibers (the afferent fibers of the pupillomotor reflex) leave the tract before reaching the lateral geniculate body and pass by way of the superior brachium to the pretectal nucleus in the midbrain. Still others terminate in the superior colliculus.[6]

The tract lies along the upper anterior and then the lateral surface of the cerebral peduncle and is parallel to the posterior cerebral artery. The globus pallidus is

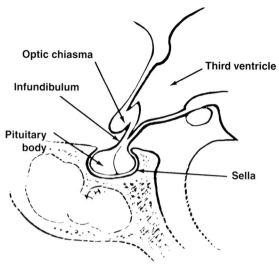

FIGURE 14-3. Sagittal section through chiasm, showing its relationship to third ventricle, pituitary body, pituitary stalk, sella turcica, and sphenoid sinus. (Reprinted with permission from DO Harrington. The Visual Fields [5th ed]. St. Louis: Mosby, 1981;76.)

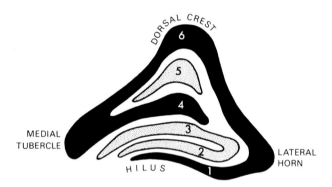

FIGURE 14-4. Laminae in right lateral geniculate body. Crossed retinal projections terminate in laminae 1, 4, and 6. Uncrossed projections terminate in laminae 2, 3, and 5. Selective partial involvement of one or more of these laminae will produce asymmetric homonymous visual field defects, depending on the extent of laminar damage. (Reprinted with permission from DO Harrington. The Visual Fields [5th ed]. St. Louis: Mosby, 1981;77.)

above, the internal capsule is medial, and the hippocampus is below the tract.[6]

Lateral Geniculate Body

Information from all the sensory systems except the olfactory pass through the thalamus before being transferred to the cerebral cortex; visual information is processed in the lateral geniculate body and then is

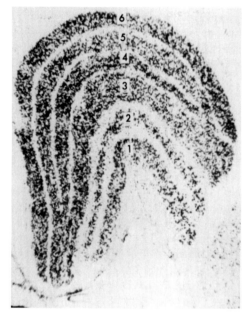

FIGURE 14-5. Coronal section of rhesus monkey lateral geniculate body, stained to show neuronal cell bodies. Layers are numbered from ventral to dorsal, and medial aspect is on right. (Reprinted with permission from WM Hart Jr [ed], Adler's Physiology of the Eye [9th ed]. St. Louis: Mosby, 1992;435.)

relayed to higher cortical centers.[10] The **lateral geniculate body (lateral geniculate nucleus)** is located on the dorsal lateral aspect of the thalamus and resembles an asymmetric cone, the rounded apex of which is oriented laterally (Figures 14-4 and 14-5). It contains six layers, which become fragmented and irregular at the sides of the structure. The retinal axons terminate here, synapsing within each layer. The fibers that leave the lateral geniculate body project to the visual cortex.

The layers of the lateral geniculate body are numbered from 1 to 6, beginning inferiorly. They contain two types of cells: Layers 1 and 2 contain larger cells and are called the **magnocellular layers**, and layers 3–6 contain smaller cells and are called the **parvocellular layers**. The retinal ganglion cells that project to the magnocellular layers are morphologically different from those that project to the parvocellular layers (see Chapter 4). The magnocellular layers project to a specific area of the visual cortex, whereas the parvocellular layers project to other areas, including a region in the parastriate cortex.[5] The magnocellular axons have a faster speed of conductance than do the parvocellular axons.[10]

The lateral geniculate body is not a simple relay station but is a center for processing; it also receives input from cortical and subcortical centers and reciprocal innervation from the visual cortex.[5, 11] The precise nature of the processing that occurs is not understood fully.[12]

FIGURE 14-6. The visual pathway from retina to calcarine fissure of occipital lobe. Cutaway view from gross dissections shows distribution of visual fibers in optic radiation. (Reprinted with permission from DO Harrington. The Visual Fields [5th ed]. St. Louis: Mosby, 1981;79.)

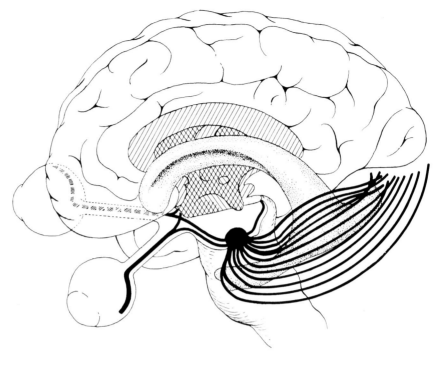

FIGURE 14-7. Medial surface of cerebral cortex showing striate cortex of occipital lobe.

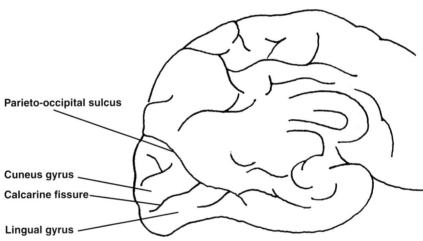

Parieto-occipital sulcus

Cuneus gyrus

Calcarine fissure

Lingual gyrus

The optic tract enters the lateral geniculate body anteriorly; the internal capsule is lateral, the medial geniculate nucleus is medial, and the inferior horn of the lateral ventricle is posterolateral to the lateral geniculate body.[6] The axons leave the lateral geniculate body neurons as the optic radiations.

Optic Radiations (Geniculocalcarine Tract)

The **optic radiations** spread out fanwise as they leave the lateral geniculate body, deep in the white matter of the cerebral hemispheres, sweeping laterally and inferiorly around the anterior tip of the temporal horn of the lateral ventricle (Figure 14-6). Some fibers loop into the temporal lobe before passing back to the parietal lobe en route to the occipital lobe. Within the parietal lobe, the fibers pass lateral to the occipital horn of the lateral ventricle before terminating in the striate cortex.[6]

Primary Visual Cortex (Striate Cortex)

The **primary visual cortex (Brodmann area 17** or, according to more recent nomenclature, **V1**), is located almost entirely on the medial surface of the occipital lobe; just a small portion (perhaps 1 cm long) extends around the posterior pole onto the lateral surface. The visual cortex is called also the **striate cortex** because a white myelinated fiber layer—the white stria of Gennari—is characteristic of this area.[5] The **calcarine fissure** extends from the parieto-occipital sulcus to the posterior pole, dividing the visual cortex into an upper portion (the **cuneus gyrus**) and a lower part (the **lingual gyrus**) (Figure 14-7);

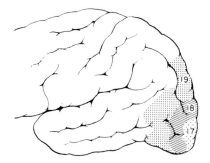
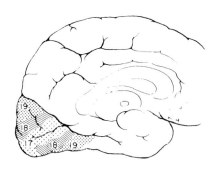

FIGURE 14-8. Visual area or striate cortex in occipital lobe. Lateral and medial views show Brodmann's area 17 (striate area), 18 (parastriate area), and 19 (peristriate area). Area 17 is sharply delineated cortical termination of visual pathway. (Reprinted with permission from DO Harrington. The Visual Fields [5th ed]. St. Louis: Mosby, 1981;79.)

most of the primary visual cortex is buried in the tissue within the calcarine fissure.

The cells of the striate cortex are organized into horizontal layers, some of which contain multiple sublayers, and vertical columns. The magnocellular and parvocellular layers of the lateral geniculate body project to specific areas and specific layers of the striate cortex.[13, 14] Certain cortical regions are active during motion stimulation, whereas others are active during color vision.[15] The magnocellular areas probably mediate moving targets and low-spatial-frequency contrast sensitivity, and the parvocellular areas likely mediate color and high-spatial-frequency contrast sensitivity.[16–19]

Projections from the lateral geniculate body also distribute in a vertical organization, according to the eye of origin, forming alternating parallel ocular dominance columns.[14, 20, 21] These columns are lacking in the area of the cortex representing the physiologic blind spot that receives information exclusively from one eye.[10] A second system of columns, specific for stimulus orientation, respond on the basis of the direction of a light slit or edge.[14] Contour analysis and binocular vision are two functions of the visual cortex, and such processing is a function of both its horizontal and vertical organization.

The striate cortex performs basic analysis of the visual information relayed from the lateral geniculate body and transmits this information to the higher visual association areas that provide further interpretation.[10] These areas surround the striate cortex, lying on the lateral aspects of the occipital cortex. Historically, they were called **Brodmann areas 18 and 19** (Figure 14-8) and now are known to contain several distinct cortical areas (designated **V2, V3, V4,** and **V5**), in which visual processing occurs; a study involving the macaque monkey has identified 32 such areas associated with visual processing.[10] The visual and visual-association areas in one hemisphere are connected to the corresponding areas in the other hemisphere via the posterior portion of the corpus callosum.[5]

Noninvasive magnetic imaging techniques have been developed that are sensitive to changes in blood flow and oxygenation occurring with neuronal activity, and these techniques are currently used to study the human visual system in vivo. Innovative work is being done to identify the areas of visual cortex and associated visual areas activated during visual stimulation and visual processing, to detect the storage areas for learned visual patterns, and to establish the pathway of activation in the cortex on recall and recognition of a visual pattern.[22–28]

Extrastriate Visual Systems

The striate cortex is connected to other areas of the brain including the superior colliculus and the frontal eye fields. The superior colliculus, which has a complete retinotopic map of the contralateral field of vision, receives communication from fibers exiting the posterior optic tract and from the striate cortex. The superior colliculus does not analyze sensory information for perception but is important for visual orientation, foveation, and the control of saccadic eye movements.[10]

The frontal eye fields, in the frontal lobe, receive fibers from the striate cortex that contribute to the control of conjugate eye movements. Both voluntary and reflex ocular movements are mediated in this area, as are pupillary responses to near objects (see Chapter 13).[6]

BLOOD SUPPLY TO THE VISUAL PATHWAY

The structures of the visual pathway have an extensive blood supply. Figure 14-9 shows many of the involved vessels. The outer retinal layers receive nutrition from the choroid, whereas the inner retina is supplied by the central retinal artery. The circle of Zinn-Haller, the anastomotic ring of branches of the short ciliary arteries, and the peripapillary choroidal vessels supply the optic disc.[5] The intraorbital portion of the optic nerve is supplied by branches from the ophthalmic artery, and the intracranial optic nerve is nourished by branches of the ophthalmic, anterior cerebral, anterior communicating, and internal carotid arteries.[5, 6]

The blood supply to the chiasm is rich and anastomotic, arterioles from the circle of Willis forming capillary beds at two levels.[29, 30] The superior network is supplied by the anterior cerebral and anterior communi-

FIGURE 14-9. Vascular supply of visual pathway from retina to occipital cortex. (Reprinted with permission from DO Harrington. The Visual Fields [5th ed]. St. Louis: Mosby, 1981;87.)

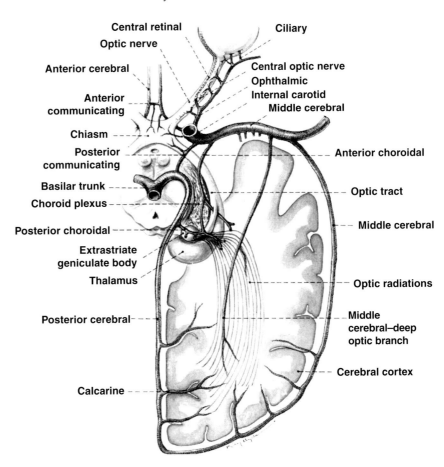

Central retinal
Optic nerve
Ciliary
Anterior cerebral
Central optic nerve
Ophthalmic
Internal carotid
Middle cerebral
Anterior communicating
Chiasm
Posterior communicating
Anterior choroidal
Basilar trunk
Optic tract
Choroid plexus
Middle cerebral
Posterior choroidal
Extrastriate geniculate body
Optic radiations
Thalamus
Middle cerebral–deep optic branch
Posterior cerebral
Cerebral cortex
Calcarine

cating arteries, whereas the inferior network is supplied by the internal carotid, posterior cerebral, and posterior communicating arteries.[5, 6, 9] The anterior choroidal artery, a branch of the internal carotid, is a primary supplier of the optic tract, though small branches from the middle cerebral artery also contribute.[5, 6, 9, 31, 32] The blood supply to the lateral geniculate body is derived from the anterior choroidal artery and the lateral choroidal and posterior choroidal branches of the posterior cerebral artery.[6, 31, 33]

The optic radiations can be divided into three sections: The anterior radiations, which pass laterally over the inferior horn of the ventricle, are supplied by the anterior choroidal artery and the middle cerebral artery; the group of fibers passing lateral to the ventricle is supplied by the deep optic branch of the middle cerebral artery; and branches of the posterior cerebral artery, including the calcarine branch, supply the posterior radiations as they spread out in the occipital lobe. Branches from the middle cerebral artery also make a contribution.[5, 6, 9] The calcarine branch of the posterior cerebral artery is the major blood supply for the striate cortex, often supplemented by the posterior temporal or parieto-occipital branch of the posterior

cerebral artery or the occipital branch of the middle cerebral artery.[5, 6, 9, 34]

FIBER ORIENTATION AND VISUAL FIELDS

With the eye looking straight ahead and fixating on an object, one is able to detect other objects around the point of regard, although the details may not be discernible. This entire visible area is termed the **visual field**. Information from the visual field is taken in by the retina and processed through the afferent visual sensory pathway. The location and orderly arrangement of the fibers throughout this pathway have been extensively studied. Damage in the afferent visual pathway will cause a defect in the visual field. Knowledge of the fiber patterns in the pathway can help to identify the location of the lesion on the basis of the resultant visual field defect.

Retina

The axons of the retinal ganglion cells form characteristic patterns in the nerve fiber layer. The group of fibers that course from the macular area to the optic

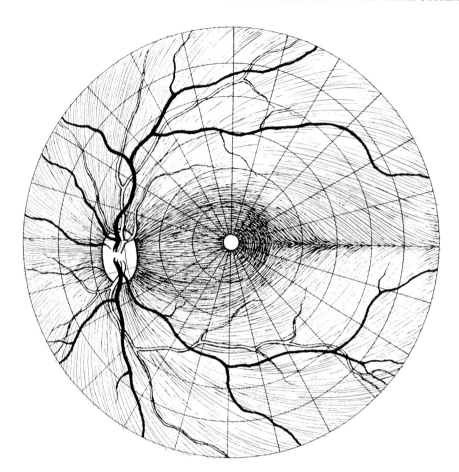

FIGURE 14-10. Nerve fiber pattern of retina in its relationship to retinal vascular tree. (Reprinted with permission from DO Harrington. The Visual Fields [5th ed]. St. Louis: Mosby, 1981;69.)

disc is called the **papillomacular bundle**. The superior and inferior temporal fibers, separated at the one hundred eightieth meridian by the horizontal raphe, must arch superiorly and inferiorly around the macular area, forming characteristic arcuate patterns in their course to the optic disc; the temporal retinal vessels usually do not cross the horizontal raphe either. The nasal fibers can travel directly to the optic disc and are described as radiating (Figure 14-10). Nasal and temporal fibers are separated by a theoretic vertical line passing through the center of the fovea. In the monkey and cat, the long nerve fibers, from peripheral retina, are more vitread in location than are the short peripapillary fibers, with extensive intermingling in the prelaminar optic nerve.[35]

Optic Disc

All of the axons in the nerve fiber layer come together at the optic disc, creating a specific pattern. The nasal fibers radiate directly to the nasal side of the disc, whereas the papillomacular bundle courses directly to the temporal side of the disc.[35-37] The fibers from the superior temporal retina arch around the papillomacular bundle to enter the superior pole of the disc; fibers from the inferior temporal retina curve below the papillomacular bun-

dle to the inferior pole.[37] The macular fibers take up approximately one-third of the disc, although the macular area encompasses only one-twentieth of the retinal area.[1, 6] The temporal fibers occupy approximately one-third of the disc, as do the nasal fibers (Figure 14-11A). The boundaries between each set of fibers are not always clear-cut in all parts of the pathway.

Optic Nerve

Near the lamina cribrosa, the fibers have the same orientation as they do in the disc but, within a short distance, the macular fibers move to the center of the nerve.[3, 6] The rest of the fibers take up their logical positions: superior temporal fibers in the superior temporal optic nerve, inferior temporal fibers in the inferior temporal nerve, the superior nasal fibers in the superior nasal nerve, and the inferior nasal fibers in the inferior nasal optic nerve (see Figure 14-11B).

Optic Chiasm

In the optic chiasm, the nasal fibers cross (decussate); the ratio of crossed to uncrossed fibers in the chiasm is approximately 53 to 47.[38] The inferior nasal retinal fibers are inferior in the anterior chiasm; they cross to the

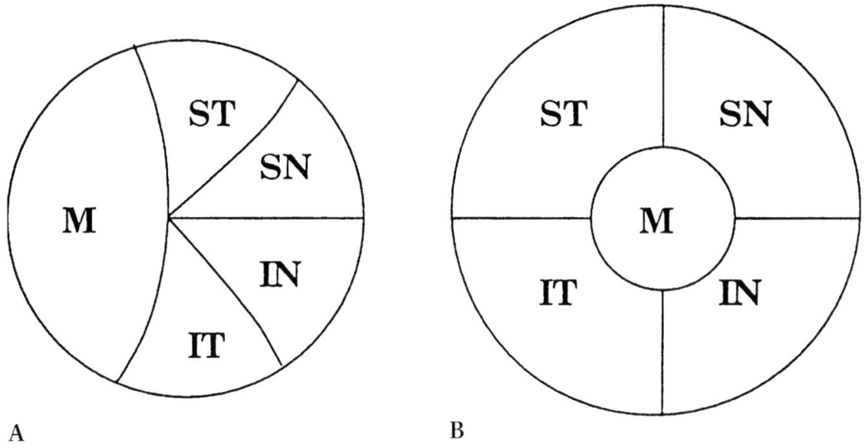

FIGURE 14-11. (A) Surface of optic disc. Shown is orientation of nerve fibers as they enter the optic disc. (B) Coronal section shows the orientation of the nerve fibers in the optic nerve proximal to chiasm. (Right disc and nerve viewed from front.) (ST = superior temporal; SN = superior nasal; IT = inferior temporal; IN = inferior nasal; M = macular.)

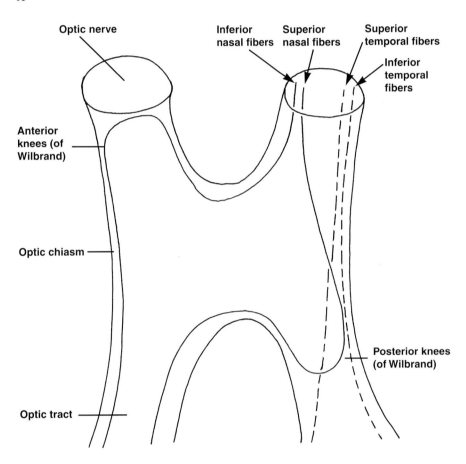

FIGURE 14-12. Fiber orientation through the chiasm. Temporal fibers (dotted lines) pass through the chiasm and exit in the ipsilateral optic tract. Nasal fibers (solid lines) cross in the chiasm to exit in the contralateral optic tract. (See text for further detail.)

other side and many loop into the terminal part of the opposite optic nerve before turning to run back through the chiasm into the contralateral optic tract (Figure 14-12).[1] These anterior loops (**Wilbrand's knees**) bring fibers from the opposite eye into the posterior optic nerve.[39] The superior nasal fibers enter the superior chiasm, where they cross and then leave the chiasm in the contralateral optic tract; some of these fibers loop posteriorly into the optic tract on the same side before crossing (see Figure 14-12).[1, 6] The fibers from the temporal retina course directly back through the chiasm into the optic tract. The nasal macular fibers cross primarily in the posterior aspect of the chiasm.[5]

A few fibers have been identified that exit the posterior of the chiasm and enter the hypothalamus. Studies suggest that these fibers represent light-dark input, affecting the circadian rhythm.[5, 40]

Optic Tract

As the fibers leave the chiasm in the optic tract, the crossed and uncrossed fibers intermingle. The superior fibers (the

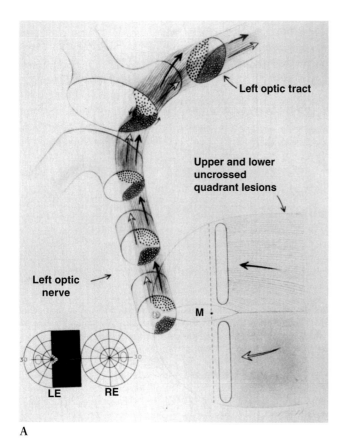

A

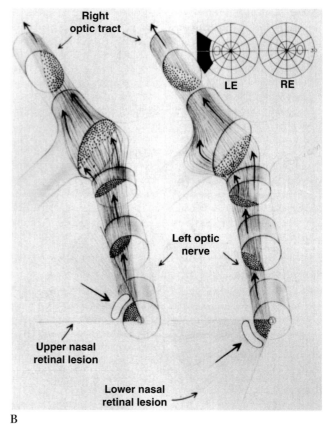

B

FIGURE 14-13. Course of uncrossed retinal ganglion cell axons through optic nerve, chiasm, and tract of monkey. Left retina is represented below on right. Vertical white bars are lesions made by photocoagulator; macula (M) has not been damaged. Hypothetical visual field defect produced by these lesions is shown in lower left. (LE = left eye; RE = right eye.) (B) Course of crossed retinal ganglion cell axons. Photocoagulator lesions in left retina are indicated by white crescents in retinal diagrams at bottom of figure; hypothetical visual field defects produced by these lesions are shown at upper right. (Reprinted with permission from WF Hoyt, O Luis. Visual fiber anatomy in the infra-geniculate pathway of the primate uncrossed and crossed retinal quadrant fiber projections studied with Nauta silver stain. Arch Ophthalmol 1962;68:428.)

fibers from both the ipsilateral superior temporal retina and the contralateral superior nasal retina) move to the medial side of the tract. The fibers from the inferior retina (ipsilateral inferior temporal retinal fibers and contralateral inferior nasal retinal fibers) occupy the lateral area of the tract.[1, 3] Figure 14-13 shows the regrouping that occurs as the fibers pass through the chiasm and into the optic tract. The macular fibers, crossed and uncrossed, are located between these two groups (Figure 14-14).[1]

Lateral Geniculate Body

Fibers from the superior retinal quadrants terminate in the medial aspect of the lateral geniculate body, whereas the inferior retinal quadrant fibers terminate in the lateral aspect.[6] A dorsal wedge, comprising two-thirds to three-fourths of the lateral geniculate body, represents the macula.[3, 41, 42] Each layer receives input from just one eye: Layers 1, 4, and 6 receive fibers from the contralateral nasal retina, whereas layers 2, 3, and 5 receive ipsilateral temporal retinal fibers (Figure 14-15).[38] Most of

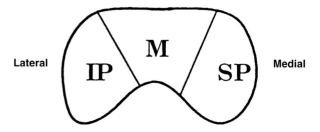

FIGURE 14-14. Coronal section showing orientation of the nerve fibers in the optic tract. (IP = inferior peripheral; M = macular; SP = superior peripheral.)

the structure, including the wedge representing macula, contains all six layers but, in the far medial and lateral aspects, some of the layers merge.[5, 41]

The anatomic structure of the human lateral geniculate body is similar to that structure in the monkey. For this reason, the detailed maps that have been made of the monkey lateral geniculate body have been applied to the human structure.[43] Each layer of the lateral geniculate

FIGURE 14-15. Retinotopic map representation in the lateral geniculate body (LGB). Fibers from ipsilateral (temporal) retina terminate in layers 2, 3, and 5 of the lateral geniculate body. Fibers from contralateral (nasal) retina terminate in layers 1, 4, and 6 of the lateral geniculate body. Fibers that originate in neighboring areas of all layers of the lateral geniculate body terminate in the same place in the striate cortex.

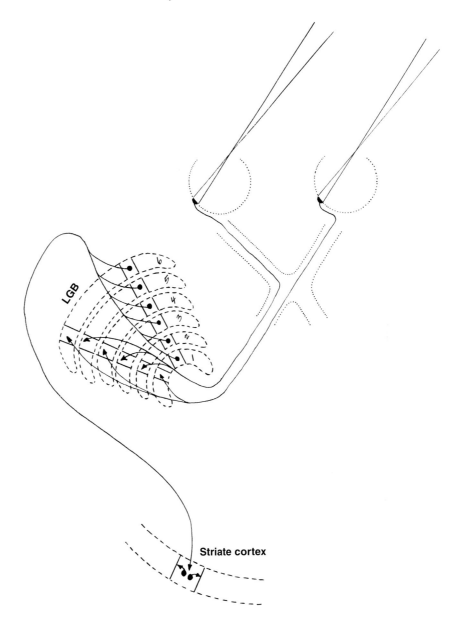

Striate cortex

body contains a retinotopic map or representation of the contralateral hemifield of vision. A retinotopic map is a "point-to-point localization" of the retina.[10] These maps are stacked on one another, such that if a line (called a **line of projection**) were passed through all six layers, perpendicular to the surface, the intercepted cells all would be carrying information about the same point in the visual field. Thus, the fibers that carry information from the same site in the visual field of each eye terminate in adjacent layers of the lateral geniculate body, right next to one another (see Figure 14-15).[6]

Optic Radiations

The fibers leaving the lateral aspect of the lateral geniculate body, representing inferior retina, follow an indirect route to the occipital lobe. They pass into the temporal

lobe and loop around the tip of the temporal horn of the lateral ventricle, forming **Meyer's loop**, before continuing into the parietal lobe; these fibers form the inferior radiations (Figure 14-16).[6] Fibers from the medial aspect of the lateral geniculate body, representing superior retina, form the superior radiations. The fibers from the macula are situated between the superior and inferior fibers.

Striate Cortex

The superior radiations terminate in the area of the striate cortex above the calcarine fissure—the cuneus gyrus—and the inferior radiations terminate in the region below the calcarine fissure— the lingual gyrus. Thus, the cuneus gyrus receives projections from superior retina and the lingual gyrus from inferior retina. Only one-third of the striate cortex is on the surface of the occipital lobe,

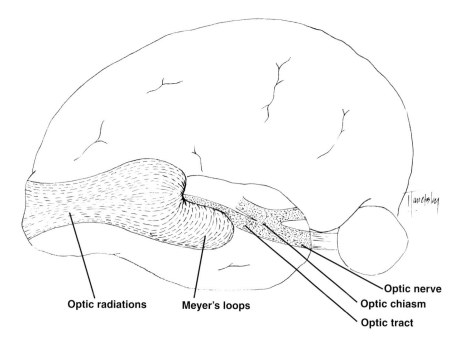

FIGURE 14-16. Location of the optic radiations in the cerebral hemisphere. Meyer's loops pass into the temporal lobe before passing into the parietal lobe.

Optic radiations   **Meyer's loops**

Optic nerve
Optic chiasm
Optic tract

the majority being buried within the calcarine fissure and only a small portion being on the posterolateral aspect of the occipital posterior pole.[44]

Fibers from the macular area terminate in the posteriormost part of the striate cortex, with the superior macular area represented in the cuneus gyrus and the inferior macula represented in the lingual gyrus. The macular projection might extend onto the posterolateral surface of the occipital cortex. The macular area representation occupies a relatively large portion of striate cortex compared to the small macular area in the retina. The macular cells are densely packed, and macular fibers are small-caliber. Because macular function involves sharp, detailed vision, the macular representation in the striate cortex is more extensive than the representation of peripheral retinal areas. The anteriormost part of the striate cortex represents the periphery of the nasal retina, corresponding to an area of visual field, the temporal crescent, that is seen by one eye only.

Retinotopic representation is present in the striate cortex. Those fibers that are adjacent to one another in the layers of the lateral geniculate body project to the same area in the visual cortex (see Figure 14-15)—that is, corresponding points from the two retinas (ipsilateral temporal and contralateral nasal) that represent the same target in the visual field will project to the same place in the primary visual cortex.

CLINICAL COMMENT: VISUAL FIELDS

The visual field is tested monocularly with the patient looking straight ahead at a fixation point and responding when a target is seen anywhere in the area surrounding that fixation point, usually described to the patient as "seen out of the corner of your eye." The

field can be divided into four quadrants by a vertical and a horizontal line that intersect at the point of fixation. The point of fixation is seen by the fovea and is eccentric because the temporal field is slightly larger than the nasal. Inversion and reversal of the field is caused by the optical system of the eye; the superior field is imaged on the inferior retina and the inferior field on the superior retina; the nasal field is imaged on the temporal retina and the temporal field on the nasal retina (Figure 14-17). This orientation is maintained in the cortex, where the superior field is projected onto the visual cortex inferior to the calcarine fissure and the inferior visual field is projected onto the cortex superior to the calcarine fissure.

The reader is cautioned to be aware of the difference between visual fibers and visual fields. Both can be described as nasal, temporal, superior, and inferior.

The visual field seen by the right eye is nearly the same as that seen by the left eye, the nasal part of the field for one eye being the same as the temporal part of the field seen by the other eye, with the exception of the far temporal periphery, which is called the **temporal crescent**. The temporal crescent is imaged on the nasal retina of one eye but not on the temporal retina of the other owing to the prominence of the nose. Within each temporal field is an absolute scotoma, the physiologic blind spot, a result of the lack of photoreceptors in the optic disc (Figure 14-18).

Because the fibers that emanate from nasal retina cross in the chiasm, the postchiasmal pathway carries information from the contralateral temporal field and the ipsilateral nasal field. These combined areas can be described as the **contralateral hemifield** (i.e., the right postchiasmal pathway carries infor-

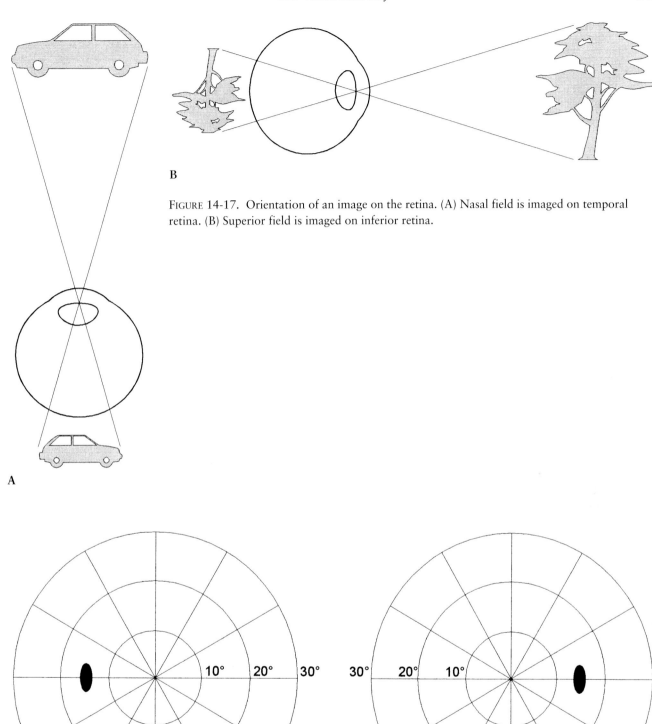

B

FIGURE 14-17. Orientation of an image on the retina. (A) Nasal field is imaged on temporal retina. (B) Superior field is imaged on inferior retina.

LEFT EYE

RIGHT EYE

FIGURE 14-18. Central visual field plots showing scotoma of physiologic blind spot in the temporal field.

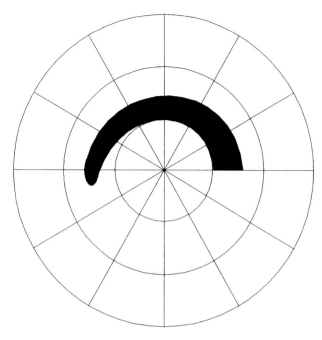

FIGURE 14-19. Visual field plot showing arcuate scotoma in field of left eye. Note nasal step.

mation from the left side of the visual field for both eyes). Hence, the left side of the field is "seen" by the right striate cortex, paralleling the involvement of the right hemisphere in the motor and sensory activities of the left side of the body. Similarly, objects in the right side of the field are "seen" by the left striate cortex (Plate 14-3). (Note that reference to the left side of the visual field is not the same thing as the visual field of the left eye.) A defect that affects the nasal field of one eye and the temporal field of the other eye is described as **homonymous**.

A defect in the field of just one eye must be caused by a disruption anterior to the chiasm. If there is a defect in the fields of both eyes, there are either two lesions—one in each prechiasmal pathway—or a single lesion in the chiasm or postchiasmal pathway where the fibers for the two eyes are brought together. The pattern of the defect as well as associated signs or symptoms might aid in determining the location of the damage.

CLINICAL COMMENT: CHARACTERISTIC DEFECTS

The regular fiber orientation in each structure of the pathway can be correlated with a specific pattern of visual field loss. A lesion of the choroid or outer retina will cause a field defect that is similar in shape to the lesion and is in the corresponding location in the field (e.g., if the lesion is in the superior nasal retina, the defect will be in the inferior temporal field).

A lesion in the nerve fiber layer will cause a field defect corresponding to the location and configura-

tion of the affected nerve fiber bundle. One of the disease processes that affects the nerve fiber layer is glaucoma. If temporal retinal fibers are affected, an arcuate defect can be produced that curves around the point of fixation from the blind spot to termination at the horizontal nasal meridian (Figure 14-19). This abrupt edge (at the horizontal meridian) is called a **nasal step** and results from the configuration of the fibers at the temporal retinal raphe. Less often, a lesion affects a nasal bundle of nerves, producing a wedge-shaped defect emanating from the physiologic blind spot into the temporal field.

Injury to the optic nerve is accompanied by a visual field defect, a relative afferent pupillary defect, and atrophy of the affected nerve fibers, which eventually is manifested at the disc. The small-diameter, tightly packed fibers of the macula have the greatest metabolic need and often are affected first in both compressive and ischemic lesions.[9]

The chiasm brings all the visual fibers together; lesions of the chiasm usually will show bitemporal or binasal defects. The most common cause of a bitemporal field defect is a pituitary gland tumor, and a visual field defect is often the first clinical sign. The crossed fibers seem to be damaged first in compressive lesions such as a tumor.[10] This susceptibility to damage might be attributable to the purported weak blood supply of the median portion of the chiasm. Consequently, the crossed fibers also are more susceptible to ischemia in a vascular event.[30] Involvement of both lateral sides of the chiasm, producing a binasal defect, might be caused by an aneurysm of the internal carotid artery that impinges on the chiasm and displaces it against the other internal carotid artery.

A single lesion at the optic chiasm and its junction with the optic nerve might be characterized by a central defect in the field of the eye on the same side as the lesion and a superior temporal defect in the field of the opposite eye, owing to the inferior nasal fibers that loop into the optic nerve from the contralateral eye.

A homonymous field defect will be produced by a single lesion in the postchiasmal pathway, as the nasal fibers of the contralateral eye join the temporal fibers of the ipsilateral eye; visual acuity usually is not affected because one-half of the fovea is sufficient for 20/20 Snellen acuity.[10] Other signs or symptoms accompanying a homonymous defect can help the diagnostician determine more exactly the site of the lesion.

A lesion involving the optic tract eventually will produce optic nerve atrophy, which usually becomes evident at the disc. Because the optic tract is relatively small in cross section, a lesion often damages all of the fibers, causing a homonymous field defect that affects the entire half of the field; if a partial hemianopsia results, the defects will be incongruent.[45] The defects in a homonymous field are congruent if the two defects are similarly shaped and are incongruent if the defect shapes are dissimilar. Because crossed fibers outnumber uncrossed fibers, a lesion of the optic tract may be accompanied be a relative afferent pupillary defect of the contralateral eye.[10]

A lesion in the lateral geniculate body would affect the contralateral field and eventually also cause optic atrophy; however, there would be no associated pupillary defect. Because of the point-to-point localization in the lateral geniculate body, lesions here produce moderately to completely congruent field defects.[31]

Damage to the optic radiations or cortex does not normally cause atrophy of the optic nerve because it does not involve the fibers of the retinal ganglion cells. A lesion of the optic radiations causes a contralateral homonymous field defect and, because the fibers are so spread out, the defect often affects only one quadrant. If a lesion of the temporal lobe involves Meyer's loop, a superior quadrant field defect will result; parietal lobe lesions more commonly cause inferior field defects.[10]

The characteristic feature of a defect in the occipital lobe is congruency. Congruency depends on how closely fibers from corresponding points of each eye and carrying the same visual field information are positioned to one another at the site of the lesion. As the fibers reach the occipital lobe and, finally, the striate cortex, the fibers emanating from corresponding points in the field come together to form a point-to-point representation of the field. Hence, a lesion here will cause a congruent defect. Figure 14-20 depicts examples of various visual field defects.

Striate Cortex Maps

Early work correlating the visual field to striate cortex was done by Holmes and Lister, who studied injured soldiers from World War I and attempted to match visual field defects with injuries from shrapnel to the occipital lobe.[46] The Holmes map was the most detailed source showing the representation of the visual field in human striate cortex. However, detailed mapping of monkey striate cortex using electrophysiologic methods revealed discrepancies between monkey and human data. These findings suggested that either monkey cortex and human cortex were not as alike as was believed or the Holmes map required some modification.

Technologies, such as magnetic resonance imaging, have been used to study the human cortex, allowing direct correlation of a lesion with a field defect. Horton and Hoyt suggested some revisions of the Holmes map to reflect more accurately the human striate cortex, as shown in Figure 14-21.[44] The primary change concerns

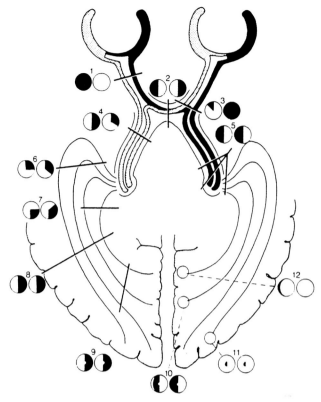

FIGURE 14-20. Visual field defects. Visual pathway is shown, as are sites of interruption of nerve fibers and resulting visual field defects. (1) Complete interruption of left optic nerve, resulting in complete loss of visual field for left eye; (2) interruption in midline of optic chiasm, resulting in bitemporal hemianopsia; (3) interruption in right optic nerve at the junction with the chiasm, resulting in complete loss of visual field for right eye and superior temporal loss in field for left eye (due to anterior knees); (4) interruption in left optic tract, resulting in an incongruent right homonymous hemianopsia; (5) complete interruption in the right optic tract, lateral geniculate body, or optic radiations, resulting in total left homonymous hemianopsia; (6) interruption in the left optic radiations involving Meyer's loop, resulting in an incongruent right homonymous hemianopsia; (7) interruption in optic radiations in left parietal lobe, resulting in an incongruent right homonymous hemianopsia; (8) interruption of all left optic radiations, resulting in total right homonymous hemianopsia; (9) interruption of fibers in left anterior striate cortex, resulting in right, homonymous hemianopsia with macular sparing; (10) interruption of fibers in right striate cortex, resulting in left homonymous hemianopsia with macular and temporal crescent sparing; (11) interruption of fibers in right posterior striate cortex, resulting in left macular homonymous hemianopsia; (12) interruption of fibers in right anterior striate cortex, resulting in left temporal crescent loss. (Reprinted with permission from WM Hart Jr [ed], Adler's Physiology of the Eye [9th ed]. St. Louis: Mosby, 1992;738.)

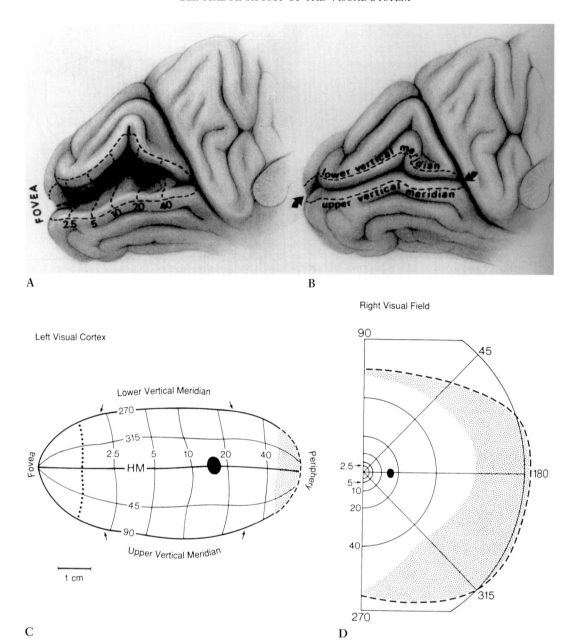

FIGURE 14-21. Revised map of the visual field in the human striate cortex. It is important to emphasize that considerable variation occurs among individuals in the exact size and location of striate cortex. This new map provides the best fit for our data. (A) View of left occipital lobe with the calcarine fissure opened, exposing the striate cortex. Dashed lines indicate the coordinates of the visual field map. The representation of the horizontal meridian runs approximately along the base of the calcarine fissure. The vertical lines mark the isoeccentricity contours from 2.5 to 40 degrees. The striate cortex wraps around the occipital pole to extend approximately 1 cm onto the lateral convexity, where the fovea is represented. (B) View of the left occipital lobe, showing the striate cortex, which is mostly hidden within the calcarine fissure (running between arrows). The boundary (dashed line) between the striate cortex (V1) and extrastriate cortex (V2) contains the representation of the vertical meridian, which usually is located along the exposed medial surface of the occipital lobe, as shown, but variation occurs in specimens. (C) Projection of the right visual hemifield (D) on the left visual cortex, depicted by transposing the map illustrated in the top left onto a flat surface. The striate cortex is an ellipse measuring approximately 80 × 40 mm, measuring roughly 2,500 mm² (40 mm × 20 mm × π = 2,500 mm²). The row of dots indicates where the striate cortex folds around the occipital pole: the small region between the dots and the foveal representation is situated on the exposed lateral convexity of the occipital lobe. The black oval marks the region of the striate cortex corresponding to the visual field coordinates of the contralateral eye's blind spot. This region of cortex receives visual input from only the ipsilateral eye. (HM = horizontal meridian.) (D) Right visual hemifield shows the V4e isopter plotted with a Goldmann perimeter. The stippled region corresponds to the monocular temporal crescent that is mapped within the most anterior 8–10% of the striate cortex (see stippled region of map in C). (Reprinted with permission from W Hoyt. Striate cortex. Arch Ophthalmol 1991;109:822.)

the extent of the area depicting macular representation. A much greater area of the visual cortex apparently is taken up by macular projection than was originally thought.[44] The macular portion extends from the posterior pole forward, with the periphery of the field represented in anterior occipital lobe and the uniocular temporal crescent in the most anterior aspect of the striate cortex adjacent to the parieto-occipital sulcus. The central 30 degrees of the visual field is apparently represented by approximately 83% of the striate cortex.[44]

Macular Sparing

Macular sparing occurs when an area of central vision remains within a homonymous field defect. Because fixational eye movements of 1 to 2 degrees do occur during the visual field examination, the area spared should involve at least 3 degrees in order for macular sparing to be confirmed clinically.[34] Because the macular area often was spared in homonymous defects caused by occipital lobe lesions, it once was supposed that the entire macula was represented in both sides of the striate cortex. We now know that this is not the case. However, even in the presence of an extensive lesion, some of the macular projection area might remain unaffected either because the posterior pole of the occipital lobe has such an extensive blood supply or because the macular projection covers a very large area.[10]

REFERENCES

1. Hoyt WF, Osman L. Visual fiber anatomy in the infrageniculate pathway of the primate. Arch Ophthalmol 1962;68:124.

2. Polyak S. The Vertebrate Visual System. Chicago: University of Chicago Press, 1957.

3. Brouwer B, Zeeman WPC. The projection of the retina in the primary optic neuron in monkeys. Brain 1926;49:1.

4. Jonas JB, Schmidt AM, Muller-Bergh JA, et al. Human optic nerve fiber count and optic disc size. Invest Ophthalmol Vis Sci 1992;33(6):2012.

5. Sadun AA, Glaser JS. Anatomy of the Visual Sensory System. In W Tasman, EA Jaeger (eds), Duane's Foundations of Clinical Ophthalmology (Vol 1). Philadelphia: Lippincott, 1994;1.

6. Warwick R. Eugene Wolff's Anatomy of the Eye and Orbit (7th ed). Philadelphia: Saunders, 1976;325.

7. Parravano JG, Toledo A, Kucharczyk W. Dimensions of the optic nerves, chiasm, and tracts. MR quantitative comparison between patients with optic atrophy and normals. J Comput Assist Tomogr 1993;17(5):688.

8. Unsold R, Hoyt WF. Band atrophy of the optic nerve. Arch Ophthalmol 1980;98:1637.

9. Harrington DO. The Visual Fields (5th ed). St. Louis: Mosby, 1981.

10. Horton JC. The Central Visual Pathways. In WM Hart Jr (ed), Adler's Physiology of the Eye (9th ed). St. Louis: Mosby, 1992;728.

11. Lachica EA, Casagrande VA. The morphology of collicular and retinal axons ending on small relay (W-like) cells of the primate lateral geniculate nucleus. Vis Neurosci 1993;10(3):403.

12. Gilbert CD, Kelly JP. The projections of cells in different layers of the cat's visual cortex. J Comp Neurol 1975;163:81.

13. Hubel DH, Wiesel TN. Laminar and columnar distribution of geniculocortical fibers in the macaque monkey. J Comp Neurol 1972;146:421.

14. Horton JC, Dagi LR, McCrane EP, et al. Arrangement of ocular dominance columns in human visual cortex. Arch Ophthalmol 1990;108(7):1025.

15. Zeki S, Watson JDG, Lueck CJ, et al. A direct demonstration of functional specialization in human visual cortex. J Neurosci 1991;11(3):641.

16. Livingstone MS, Hubel DH. Segregation of form, color, movement, and depth: anatomy, physiology, and perception. Science 1988;240:740.

17. Hockfield S, Tootell RB, Zaremba S. Molecular differences among neurons reveal an organization of human visual cortex. Proc Natl Acad Sci U S A 1990;87(8):3027.

18. Hubel DH, Livingstone MS. Color and contrast sensitivity in the lateral geniculate body and primary visual cortex in the macaque monkey. J Neurosci 1990;10(7):2223.

19. Silverman SE, Trick GL, Hart Jr WM. Motion perception is abnormal in primary open-angle glaucoma and ocular hypertension. Invest Ophthalmol Vis Sci 1990;31(4):722.

20. Hubel DH, Wiesel TN. Receptive fields and functional architecture of monkey striate cortex. J Physiol 1968;195:215.

21. Hubel DH, Wiesel TN, Stryker MP. Anatomical demonstration of orientation columns in macaque monkey. J Comp Neurol 1978;177:361.

22. Roland E, Guly'as B, Seitz RJ, et al. Functional anatomy of storage, recall, and recognition of a visual pattern in man. Neuroreport 1990;1(1):53.

23. Belliveau JW, Kennedy Jr DN, McKinstry RC, et al. Functional mapping of the human visual cortex by magnetic resonance imaging. Science 1991;254(5032):716.

24. Belliveau JW, Kwong KK, Kennedy DN, et al. Magnetic resonance imaging mapping of brain function. Human visual cortex. Invest Radiol 1992;27(Suppl 2):59.

25. Kwong KK, Belliveau JW, Chesler DA, et al. Dynamic magnetic resonance imaging of human brain activity during primary sensory stimulation. Proc Natl Acad Sci U S A 1992;89(12):5675.

26. Menon RS, Ogawa S, Kim SG, et al. Functional brain mapping using magnetic resonance imaging. Signal

changes accompanying visual stimulation. Invest Radiol 1992;27(Suppl 2):47.

27. Le Bihan D, Turner R, Zeffiro TA, et al. Activation of human primary visual cortex during visual recall: a magnetic resonance imaging study. Proc Natl Acad Sci U S A 1993;90(24):11802.

28. Ogawa S, Menon RS, Tank DW, et al. Functional brain mapping by blood oxygenation level-dependent contrast magnetic resonance imaging. A comparison of signal characteristics with a biophysical model. Biophys J 1993;64(3):803.

29. Francoisa J, Neetens A, Collette JM. Vascularization of the optic pathway. Br J Ophthalmol 1958;42:80.

30. Lao Y, Gao H, Zhong Y. Vascular architecture of the human optic chiasma and bitemporal hemianopia. Chin Med Sci J 1994;9(1):38.

31. Ferreira A, Braga FM. Microsurgical anatomy of the anterior choroidal artery [abstract]. Arq Neuropsiquiatr 1990;48(4):448.

32. Margo CE, Hamed KM, McCarty J. Congenital optic tract syndrome. Arch Ophthalmol 1991;109(8):1120.

33. Luco C, Hoppe A, Schweitzer M, et al. Visual field defects in vascular lesions of the lateral geniculate body. J Neurol Neurosurg Psychiatr 1992;55(1):12.

34. McFadzean R, Brosnahan D, Hadley D, et al. Representation of the visual field in the occipital striate cortex. Br J Ophthalmol 1994;78(3):185.

35. Ogden TE. Nerve fiber layer of the macaque retina: retinotopic organization. Invest Ophthalmol Vis Sci 1983;24:85.

36. Hoyt WF, Tudor RC. The course of parapapillary temporal retinal axons through the anterior optic nerve. Arch Ophthalmol 1963;69:503.

37. Ballantyne AJ. The nerve fiber pattern of the human retina. Trans Ophthalmol Soc U K 1946;66:179.

38. Kupfer C, Chumbley L, Downer J, et al. Quantitative histology of optic nerve, optic tract, and lateral geniculate body of man. J Anat 1967;101:393.

39. Wilbrand HL. Schema des verlaufs der sehnervenfasern durch das chiasma. Z Augenheilk 1927;59:135.

40. Moore RY. Retinohypothalmic projection in mammals: a comparative study. Brain Res 1973;49:403.

41. Kupfer C. The projection of the macula in the lateral geniculate body of man. Am J Ophthalmol 1962;54:597.

42. Hickey TL, Guillery RW. Variability of laminar patterns in the human lateral geniculate body. J Comp Neurol 1979;183:221.

43. Malpeli JG, Baker FH. The representation of the visual fields in the lateral geniculate body of *Macaca mulatta*. J Comp Neurol 1975;161:569.

44. Horton JC, Hoyt WF. The representation of the visual field in human striate cortex. Arch Ophthalmol 1991;109:816.

45. Reese BE, Cowey A. Fibre organization of the monkey's optic tract: II. Noncongruent representation of the two half-retinae. J Comp Neurol 1990;295(3):401.

46. Holmes G, Lister WT. Disturbances of vision from cerebral lesions with special reference to the cortical representation of the macula. Brain 1916;39:34.

Index

Page numbers followed by f indicate figures; page numbers followed by t indicate tables.